T0139807

Recent Results in Cancer Research

Volume 214

Series Editors

Peter-Michael Schlag, Charite Campus Mitte, Charite Comprehensive Cancer
Center, Berlin, Germany
Hans-Jörg Senn, Tumor- und Brustzentrum ZeTuP, St. Gallen, Switzerland

This book series presents comprehensive, high-quality updates on areas of current interest in basic, clinical, and translational cancer research. The scope of the series is broad, encompassing epidemiology, etiology, pathophysiology, prevention, diagnosis, and treatment. Each volume is devoted to a specific topic with the aim of providing readers with a thorough overview by acclaimed experts. While advances in understanding of the cellular, genetic, and molecular mechanisms of cancer and progress toward personalized cancer care are a particular focus, subjects such as the lifestyle, psychological, and social aspects of cancer and public policy are also covered. *Recent Results in Cancer Research* is accordingly of interest to a wide spectrum of researchers, clinicians, other health care professionals, and stakeholders. The series is listed in PubMed/Index Medicus.

More information about this series at http://www.springer.com/series/392

Matthias Theobald

Editor

Current Immunotherapeutic Strategies in Cancer

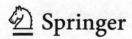 Springer

Editor
Matthias Theobald
Department of Hematology, Oncology
and Pneumology, University Cancer
Center (UCT) Mainz
Johannes Gutenberg University
Medical Center
Mainz, Germany

ISSN 0080-0015   ISSN 2197-6767   (electronic)
Recent Results in Cancer Research
ISBN 978-3-030-23767-7   ISBN 978-3-030-23765-3   (eBook)
https://doi.org/10.1007/978-3-030-23765-3

This Springer imprint is published by the registered company Springer Nature Switzerland AG
The registered company address is: Gewerbestrasse 11, 6330 Cham, Switzerland

Contents

Current Development of Monoclonal Antibodies in Cancer Therapy

Sagun Parakh, Dylan King, Hui K. Gan and Andrew M. Scott

1 Antibody Structure

Antibodies are the epitome of specificity with an estimated ten billion different antibodies produced by human B cells; there is an extraordinarily diverse range of antibodies capable of being produced by the immune system (Fanning et al. 1996). Antibodies are made up of four polypeptide chains, two identical light chains and two identical heavy chains, which are joined by disulphide bridges forming a structure that is similar to the shape of a Y (Fig. 1) (Merino 2011). Both the light and heavy chains are comprised of variable and constant domains, each with differing functions (Merino 2011). The variable domains determine antigen specificity, and the constant domains determine immunoglobulin (Ig) class. For the light chains, the constant domain differs depending on whether they are encoded by κ or λ genes (Merino 2011). Similarly, the constant domain of the heavy chain varies with 5 genes (γ, μ, α, δ and ε), and this determines the overall antibody class (IgG, IgM, IgA, IgD and IgE, respectively) (Merino 2011). Furthermore, IgA has two

S. Parakh · D. King · H. K. Gan · A. M. Scott (✉)
Tumour Targeting Laboratory, Olivia Newton-John Cancer Research Institute,
145 Studley Road, Heidelberg, Melbourne, VIC 3084, Australia
e-mail: andrew.scott@onjcri.org.au

S. Parakh · H. K. Gan
Department of Medical Oncology, Olivia Newton-John Cancer and Wellness Centre,
Austin Health, Heidelberg, Melbourne, Australia

S. Parakh · D. King · H. K. Gan · A. M. Scott
School of Cancer Medicine, La Trobe University, Melbourne, Australia

Department of Molecular Imaging and Therapy, Austin Health, Melbourne, Australia

Department of Medicine, University of Melbourne, Melbourne, Australia

© Springer Nature Switzerland AG 2020
M. Theobald (ed.), *Current Immunotherapeutic Strategies in Cancer*,
Recent Results in Cancer Research 214,
https://doi.org/10.1007/978-3-030-23765-3_1

1

Antibody structure

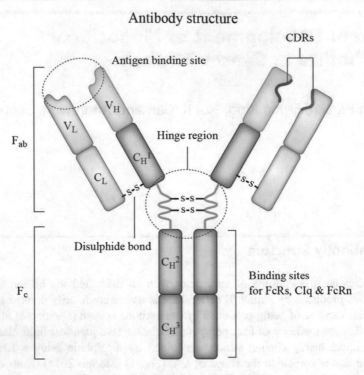

Fig. 1 Antibody structure: Antibodies are made up of four polypeptide chains, two identical light chains and two identical heavy chains, joined by disulphide bridges. Heavy chains comprise one variable (V_H) domain followed by a constant domain (C_H1), a hinge region and two more constant (C_H2 and C_H3) domains. The light chain has one variable (V_L) and one constant (C_L) domain. The two arms in the Y-shaped structure contain the antigen-binding sites, the fragment antigen-binding (Fab) region, along with the base of the Y-shaped structure called the fragment crystallizable (Fc) region. Antigen specificity in the Fab region is determined by complementarity-determining regions (CDRs) within the variable domains

subclasses, IgA1 and IgA2, and IgG, four: IgG1, IgG2, IgG3 and IgG4 (Merino 2011). In healthy people, IgG antibodies represent approximately 75% of serum antibodies, 15% are IgA, 10% are IgM, along with very small amounts of circulating IgD and IgE antibodies. IgG antibodies are the primary isotype used in cancer therapy and as such will be the major focus in the following sections.

Functionally, antibodies are divided into two parts; the two arms in the Y-shaped structure contain the antigen-binding sites and are named as the fragment antigen-binding (Fab) region, along with the base of the Y-shaped structure which mediates immunological signalling by antibodies and is called the fragment crystallizable (Fc) region. The Fab arm of an IgG antibody contains the full light chains and part of the heavy chain, each with their own constant and variable domains. Antigen specificity in the Fab region is determined by complementarity-determining regions (CDRs) within the variable domains. These CDRs have the greatest sequence variation within antibodies, and this feature gives rise to the diverse range of antigen specificities. There are three CDRs for each variable region, which means six CDRs (heavy and light) for each Fab arm and twelve in total for a single antibody molecule. The six CDRs on each Fab arm fold together to form the antigen-binding pocket, and this allows an antibody to be able to simultaneously bind two epitopes. When antibodies recognize a soluble antigen, this simultaneous binding can produce large multimeric structures called immune complexes.

Within the immune system, a principle function of antibodies is to neutralize pathogens such as bacteria and viruses. The CDRs within the variable regions of an antibody recognize a specific molecular structure of an antigen, called the epitope, present on the pathogen. Because of the random nature of antibody generation in the development of each individual B cell, there are millions of B cells circulating at any given time that each recognize a different antigen. Once a B cell encounters an invading pathogen with its unique epitope, it undergoes maturation with the help of specific T cells and produces large amounts of soluble antibody. Multiple B cells will recognize different epitopes present on the pathogen, and so many different antibodies will be produced. Once produced, these antibodies bind their antigen on the surface of the bacteria or virus to neutralize the pathogen and mark it for destruction by innate immune effector cells.

1.1 Target Antigens

Following the discovery of antibodies and their functions, it was realized that they would be potentially efficacious for the treatment and diagnosis of cancers (Rettig and Old 1989; Scott et al. 2012). Because antibodies are uniquely specific for their target antigen, they could be used to directly target tumours expressing the antigen. For ideal targeting of tumour-associated antigens (TAA), what is required is a cell surface antigen on the tumour that is mutated, overexpressed or selectively expressed when compared to normal tissue (Scott et al. 2012). Ideally, the target antigen would be homogenously expressed within the tumour and antigen secretion would be minimal, in order to reduce antibody trapping in the circulation (Scott et al. 2012). In addition to expression, antigen function and effect on downstream signalling are also taken into consideration when selecting a target.

TAAs that are targeted by therapeutic antibodies can be initially grouped on what type of cancer they target (Tables 1 and 2). Haematological cancers are usually targeted through cluster of differentiation (CD) antigens that include CD20, CD30, CD33 and CD52 (Scott et al. 2012), whereas solid tumours can be targeted through a variety of antigens that fall into different categories based on their function. The epidermal growth factor receptor (EGFR) is one such example of a TAA that has been successfully targeted in cancer therapy (Scott et al. 2012). Antibodies that target EGFR abrogate the native function of the receptor, thereby inhibiting tumour growth, and can also recruit innate immune cells through Fc-signalling to mediate killing of the tumour.

Table 1 Approved monoclonal antibodies in solid tumours

Target	Drug	Indication	Tx line	Year	Trial	Treatment arms	Endpoints		
HER2	Trastuzumab	Metastatic breast cancer	1st	1997	Slamon et al. (2001)	Chemotherapy + trastuzumab versus chemotherapy	**ORR** 50% versus 32%; $p <$ 0.001	**PFS** 7.4 versus 4.6 months; $p <$ 0.001	**OS** 25.1 versus 20.3 months p = 0.046
		Node-positive breast cancer	Adjuvant	2006	NSABP B31 + N9831 (Perez et al. 2011, 2014)	TAC ± trastuzumab	**DFS** 62% versus 74%; $p <$ 0.001		**OS** 75% versus 84%; $p <$ 0.001
		Metastatic gastric or GEJ adenocarcinoma	1st	2010	TOGA (Bang et al. 2010)	Chemotherapy ± trastuzumab	**ORR** 47% versus 35%	**PFS** 6.7 versus 5.5 months; p = 0.002	**OS** 13.8 versus 11.1 months; p = 0.046
	Pertuzumab	Metastatic breast cancer	1st	2012	CLEOPATRA (Swain et al. 2015)	Trastuzumab + docetaxel ± pertuzumab		**PFS** 18.7 versus 12.4 months; $p <$ 0.0001	**OS** 56.5 versus 40.8 months; p = 0.0002
		Breast cancer	Neo-adjuvant	2012	NEOSPHERE (Gianni et al. 2012)	T + D	**pCR** 29%	**DFS** 81%	
						P + T + D	46%	86%	
						P + T	17%	73%	
						P + D	24%	73%	
	Trastuzumab emtansine (T-DM1)	Metastatic breast cancer	2nd	2013	EMILIA (Verma et al. 2012)	T-DM1 versus capecitabine + lapatinib	**ORR** 44% versus 31%; $P <$ 0.001	**PFS** 9.6 versus 6.4 months; $P <$ 0.001	**OS** 30.9 versus 25.1 months; $p <$ 0.001

(continued)

Table 1 (continued)

Target	Drug	Indication	Tx line	Year	Trial	Treatment arms	Endpoints		
EGFR	Cetuximab	Metastatic colorectal carcinoma		2004	Van Cutsem et al. (2009, 2011)	Cetuximab + FOLFIRI versus FOLFIRI	**ORR** 57% versus 40%; $p <$ 0.001	**PFS** 9.9 versus 8.4 months; $P =$ 0.0012	**OS** 23.5 versus 20 months; $P =$ 0.0093
		Locally advanced SCCHN	1st	2006	Bonner et al. (2006, 2010)	Radiotherapy ± cetuximab		**PFS** 17.1 versus 12.4 months; $p =$ 0.005	**OS** 49 versus 29.3 months; $p =$ 0.018
		Metastatic SCCHN	2nd	2011	EXTREME (Vermorken et al. 2008)	Platinum agent + fluorouracil ± cetuximab	**ORR** 36% versus 20%; $p <$ 0.001	**PFS** 5.6 versus 3.3 months; $P <$ 0.001	**OS** 10.1 versus 7.4 months; $P =$ 0.04
	Panitumumab	Metastatic KRAS WT colorectal cancer	2nd	2006	Van Cutsem et al. (2007a)	Panitumumab versus BSC		**PFS** 13.8 versus 8.5 wks; $P <$ 0.0001	**OS** No difference
		Metastatic colorectal cancer	1st	2006	PRIME (Douillard et al. 2010)	FOLFOX4 ± panitumumab	**ORR** 54% versus 47%	**PFS** 9.6 versus 8.0 months; $p =$ 0.02	**OS** 23.9 versus 19.7 months; $P =$ 0.17
	Necitumumab	Metastatic SCC NSCLC	1st	2015	SQUIRE (Paz-Ares et al. 2016)	Gemcitabine + cisplatin ± necitumumab	**ORR** 31.2% versus 28.8%; $p =$ 0.4	**PFS** 5.7 versus 5.5 months; $P =$ 0.006	**OS** 11.5 versus 9.9 months; $p =$ 0.012

(continued)

Table 1 (continued)

Target	Drug	Indication	Tx line	Year	Trial	Treatment arms	Endpoints		
							ORR	**PFS**	**OS**
VEGF	Bevacizumab	Metastatic colorectal cancer	1st	2004	AVF2107 (Hurwitz et al. 2004)	FOLFIRI ± bevacizumab	**ORR** 45% versus 35%	**PFS** 10.6 versus 6.2 months; $p < 0.001$	**OS** 20.3 versus 15.6 months; $p < 0.001$
		Metastatic colorectal cancer	2nd	2006	ECOG E3200 (Giantonio et al. 2007)	FOLFOX versus	**ORR** 8.6%	**PFS** 4.7 months	**OS** 10.9 months
						FOLFOX + bevacizumab versus	22.7%	7.3 months	12.8 months
						Bevacizumab	3.3% ($p < 0.001$)	2.7 ($p < 0.001$)	10.2 ($P = 0.0011$)
		Metastatic NSCLC	1st	2006	ECOG E4599 (Sandler et al. 2006)	Paclitaxel + carboplatin ± bevacizumab	**ORR** 35% versus 15%; $p < 0.001$	**PFS** 6.2 versus 4.5 months; $p < 0.001$	**OS** 12.3 versus 10.3 months; $p = 0.003$
		Metastatic clear cell RCC	1st	2009	AVOREN (Escudier et al. 2010)	Interferon ± bevacizumab		**PFS** 10.2 versus 5.4 months; $p < 0.0001$	**OS** 23.3 versus 21.3 months; $p = .3360$
			1st		CALGB 90206 (Rini et al. 2008, 2010)	Interferon ± bevacizumab	**ORR** 25.5% versus 13.1%	**PFS** 8.5 versus 5.2 months; $p < 0.0001$	**OS** 18.3 versus 17.4 months; $p = 0.097$
		Glioblastoma multiforme	1st	2009	AVAGLIO (Chinot et al. 2014)	Temozolomide + RT ± bevacizumab		**PFS** 10.6 versus 6.2 months; $p < 0.001$	**OS** 16.8 versus 16.7 months; $p = 0.10$
			2nd		BELOB (Taal et al. 2014)	Lomustine			**OS**
									43%
						Bevacizumab			38%
						Combination			63%

(continued)

Table 1 (continued)

Target	Drug	Indication	Tx line	Year	Trial	Treatment arms	Endpoints		
		Metastatic EOC, fallopian tube, or peritoneal Ca	2nd Platinum resistant	2014	AURELIA (Pujade-Lauraine et al. 2014)	ICC ± chemotherapy	**ORR** 48% versus 36%; $p = 0.008$	**PFS** 8.2 versus 5.9 months; $p = 0.002$	**OS** 17 versus 13.3 months; $p = 0.004$
		Metastatic EOC, fallopian tube, or peritoneal Ca	2nd Platinum sensitive	2014	OCEANS (Aghajanian et al. 2012, 2015	Gemcitabine + carboplatin ± bevacizumab	**ORR** 79% versus 57%; $p < 0.0001$	**PFS** 12.4 versus 8.4 months; $p < 0.0001$	**OS** 33.6 versus 32.9 months; $p = 0.65$
	Ramucirumab	Metastatic gastric or GEJ adenocarcinoma	2nd line	2014	REGARD (Tsal et al. 2014)	Ramucirumab versus BSC		**PFS** 2.1 versus 1.3 months; $p < 0.001$	**OS** 5.2 versus 3.8 months; $p = 0.047$
		Metastatic gastric or GEJ adenocarcinoma	2nd line	2014	RAINBOW (Aghajanian et al. 2012)	Ramucirumab + paclitaxel versus paclitaxel	**ORR** 28% versus 16%; $p < 0.001$	**PFS** 4.4 versus 2.9 months; $p < 0.001$	**OS** 9.6 versus 7.4 months; $p = 0.017$
		Metastatic NSCLC	2nd	2014	REVEL study (Garon et al. 2014)	Ramucirumab + docetaxel versus docetaxel		**PFS** 4.5 versus 3.0 months; $p < 0.001$	**OS** 10.5 versus 9.1 months; $p = 0.024$
		Metastatic colorectal cancer	2nd	2015	RAISE (Homing et al. 2005)	FOLFIRI + ramucirumab versus FOLFIRI		**PFS** 5.7 versus 4.5 months; $p < 0.001$	**OS** 13.3 versus 11.7 months $p = 0.023$

(continued)

Table 1 (continued)

Target	Drug	Indication	Tx line	Year	Trial	Treatment arms	Endpoints		
PD1	Nivolumab	Metastatic melanoma	2nd	2014	CheckMate 037 (Larkin et al. 2016; Fuchs et al. 2014)	Nivolumab versus ICC	**ORR** 27% versus 10%	**PFS** 3.1 versus 3.7 months	**OS** 16 versus 14 months
		Metastatic NSCLC	2nd	2015	CheckMate 017 (Garon et al. 2014)	Nivolumab versus docetaxel	**ORR** 20% versus 9%	**PFS** 3.5 versus 2.8 months; $p = 0.31$	**OS** 9.2 versus 6.0 months; $p = 0.0015$
		Metastatic RCC	2nd	2015	CheckMate 025	Nivolumab versus everolimus	**ORR** 25% versus 5%; $p < 0.001$	**PFS** 4.6 versus 4.4 months; $p = 0.11$	**OS** 25.0 versus 19.6 months; $p = 0.002$
		Metastatic melanoma	1st	2015 2016	CheckMate 067 (Larkin et al. 2015; Wolchok et al. 2016)	Nivolumab + ipilimumab versus	**ORR** 58.9%	**PFS** 11.7 months	**OS** NR
						Ipilimumab versus	44.6%	2.9 months	20 months
						Nivolumab	19%	6.9 months	NR
		Metastatic head and neck cancer	2nd	2016	CheckMate 141 (Ferris et al. 2016)	Nivolumab versus ICC		**PFS** 2.0 versus 2.3 months; $p = 0.32$	**OS** 7.5 versus 5.1 months; $p = 0.01$
		Metastatic urothelial cancer	2nd	2017	CheckMate 275 (Sugimoto et al. 2003)	Nivolumab	**ORR** 19.6%	**PFS**	**OS** 7 months
	Pembrolizumab	Metastatic melanoma	1st	2014	KEYNOTE-006 (Robert et al. 2015b; Long et al. 2016)	Pembrolizumab 10 mg/kg 2wkly	**ORR** 34%	**PFS** 5.5 months	**OS** NR
						Pembrolizumab 10 mg/kg wkly	33%	4.1 months	NR
						Ipilimumab x4 3 mg/kg q3wkly	12%	2.8 months	NR

(continued)

Table 1 (continued)

Target	Drug	Indication	Tx line	Year	Trial	Treatment arms	Endpoints		
							ORR	PFS	OS
		Metastatic NSCLC	2nd	2015	KEYNOTE-010 (Ferrara 2010)	Pembrolizumab 2 mg/kg versus		3.9 months	10.4 months
						Pembrolizumab 10 mg/kg versus		4.0 months	12.7 months
						Docetaxel		4.0 months	8.5 months
		Metastatic NSCLC	1st	2016	KEYNOTE-024 (Reck et al. 2016)	Pembrolizumab versus ICC	44.8% versus 27.8%	10.3 versus 6.0 months; $p < 0.001$	80.2% versus 72.4%; $p = 0.005$
		Metastatic head and neck cancer	2nd	2016	KEYNOTE-012 (Teicher and Ellis 2008; Hillen and Griffioen 2007)	Pembrolizumab	18% (82% were durable responses ≥ 6 months)		
PDL1	Avelumab	Metastatic Merkel cell cancer	2nd	2017	JAVELIN Merkel 20C (Telang et al. 2011)	Avelumab	32% (86% were durable responses ≥ 6 months)		
	Atezolizumab	Metastatic urothelial Ca	2nd	2016	Rosenberg (Gerena-Lewis et al. 2009)	Atezolizumab	14.8% (84% were durable responses ≥ 6 months)		
		Metastatic NSCLC	2nd	2016	OAK (Rittmeyer et al. 2017; Barlesi et al. 2016)	Atezolizumab versus docetaxel			13.8 versus 9.6 months (OS)
CTLA-4	Ipilimumab	Metastatic melanoma	2nd	2011	MDX010-20 (Hodi et al. 2010b)	Ipilimumab + gp100 versus	10.9%		10 months
						Ipilimumab versus	5.7%		10 months
						gp100 alone	1.5%		6 months

BSC—Best supportive care; D—docetaxel; DFS—disease-free survival; FOLFOX—fluorouracil plus leucovorin and oxaliplatin; P—pertuzumab; TAC—paclitaxel, doxorubicin, cyclophosphamide; T—trastuzumab; TTP—time to progression; ORR—overall response rates; OS—overall survival; CLEOPATRA—clinical evaluation of pertuzumab and trastuzumab; ToGA—trastuzumab for gastric cancer; pCR—pathological complete response; RT—radiotherapy; SCC—squamous cell carcinoma

Table 2 Approved monoclonal antibodies in haematological tumours

Target	Drug	Year	Indication	Study	Key endpoints		
CD20	Rituximab	2006	First-line treatment of DLBCL in combination with CHOP or other anthracycline-based chemotherapy regimens				
		2006	First-line treatment of FL combined with CVP and following CVP	CVP + rituximab versus CVP (Marcus et al. 2005)	ORR 81% versus 57% ($p < 0.0001$)	TTP 32 versus 15 months ($p < 0.0001$)	TTnT 27 versus 7 months ($p < 0.0001$)
		2010	In combination with FC for the treatment of CLL in untreated and previously treated patients	Rituximab ± FC (Hallek et al. 2010; Fischer et al. 2012)	ORR 86% versus 73%	PFS 42.5 versus 33.1 months ($p = 0.02$)	OS NR versus 86.0 months ($p = 0.001$)
				Rituximab ± FC (Robak et al. 2010)	ORR 61% versus 49%	PFS 27 versus 21.9 months ($p < 0.02$)	OS NR versus 52 months ($p = 0.2874$)
		2011	Maintenance therapy in untreated FL	Rituximab maintenance versus observation (Salles et al. 2011)	PFS 74.9% versus 57.6% ($p < 0.0001$)		No difference in OS
	[90]Y Ibritumomab tiuxetan	2002	Relapsed or refractory, low-grade follicular B cell NHL or rituximab-refractory follicular NHL	Single-arm phase II (Wiseman et al. 2002)	ORR 83%	TTP 9.4 months	DoR 11.7 months
		2009	Treatment of previously untreated follicular NHL, who achieve an objective response to first-line chemotherapy	[90]Y Ibritumomab tiuxetan versus no treatment (Hagenbeek et al. 2007; Morschhauser et al. 2013)	PFS 4.1 versus 1.1 years ($p < 0.001$)	TTnT 8.1 versus 3 years ($p < 0.001$)	
	[131]I Tositumomab[a]	2003	FL refractory to rituximab and relapsed following chemotherapy	Single-arm phase II (Horning et al. 2005)	ORR 63%	TTP 10.4 months	DoR 16 months
	Ofatumumab	2014[b]	In combination with chlorambucil, for previously untreated CLL where fludarabine-based therapy is considered inappropriate	Chlorambucil + ofatumumab versus ofatumumab (Hillmen et al. 2015)	PFS 22.4 versus 13.1 months ($p < 0.001$)		

(continued)

Table 2 (continued)

Target	Drug	Year	Indication	Study	Key endpoints		
		2016	In combination with FC in relapsed CLL	FC + ofatumumab versus FC (Robak et al. 2017)	ORR 84% versus 68%	DoR 29.6 versus 24.9 months ($p = 0.0878$)	PFS 28.9 versus 18.8 months ($p = 0.0032$)
	Obinutuzumab	2013	In combination with chlorambucil for previously untreated CLL	Obinutuzumab + chlorambucil versus chlorambucil (Goede et al. 2014, 2015)	ORR 75.9% versus 32.1%	DoR 15.2 versus 3.5 months	PFS 23 versus 11.1 months ($p < 0.001$)
		2016	In combination with bendamustine followed by obinutuzumab monotherapy for patients with FL refractory to a rituximab (Sehn et al. 2016)	Obinutuzumab + bendamustine -> obinutuzumab monotherapy versus bendamustine	ORR 78.7% versus 74.7%	DoR NR versus 11.6 months	PFS NR versus 13.8 months ($p < 0.0001$)
CD30	Brentuximab vedotin	2011	Hodgkin lymphoma after ASCT or ≥2 prior chemotherapy regimens in patients not candidates for ASCT	Single-arm phase II studies (Younes et al. 2012; Gopal et al. 2014)	ORR 75%	PFS 40.5 months	OS 9.3 months
		2011	Systemic ALCL after prior multi-agent chemotherapy regimen	Single-arm study (de Claro et al. 2012)	ORR 86%	DoR 12.6 months	
		2015	Patients with HL at high risk of relapse/progression post-ASCT consolidation	Brentuximab vedotin versus placebo	PFS 42.9 versus 24.1 months ($p = 0.0013$)		
CD38	Daratumumab	2016	For treatment of relapsed MM in combination with lenalidomide or bortezomib and dexamethasone	Daratumumab ± lenalidomide + dexamethasone (Dimopoulos et al. 2016)	ORR 93% versus 76% ($p < 0.0001$)	DoR NR versus 17.4 months	PFS NR versus 18.4 months ($p < 0.0001$)
				Daratumumab ± bortezomib + dexamethasone (Palumbo et al. 2016)	ORR 83% versus 63% ($p < 0.0001$)	TPP NR versus 7.3 months ($p < 0.0001$)	PFS NR versus 7.2 months ($p < 0.0001$)

(continued)

Table 2 (continued)

Target	Drug	Year	Indication	Study	Key endpoints		
PD-1	Nivolumab	2016	HL relapsed or progressed after auto-HSCT and post-transplantation brentuximab vedotin	Single-arm studies (Timmerman et al. 2016; Ansell et al. 2015)	ORR 65%	DoR 8.7 months	
	Pembrolizumab	2017	Refractory classical Hodgkin lymphoma	Single-arm study (Chen et al. 2016b; Moskowitz et al. 2016)	ORR 69%	DoR NR	PFS (6 months) 72.4%
SLAMF7	Elotuzumab	2015	In combination with lenalidomide and dexamethasone for multiple myeloma who received ≥ 1 therapies	Elotuzumab ± lenalidomide and dexamethasone	ORR 75.8% versus 65.5%	PFS 19.4 versus 14.9 months	

ASCT—Autologous stem cell transplantation; ALCL—anaplastic large cell lymphoma; CR—complete response; CVP—cyclophosphamide, vincristine and prednisone; CHOP—cyclophosphamide, doxorubicin, vincristine and prednisone; CLL—chronic lymphocytic leukaemia; DoR—duration of response; HL—Hodgkin's lymphoma; HSCT—haematopoietic stem cell transplantation; FC—fludarabine and cyclophosphamide; FL—follicular lymphoma; NHL—non-Hodgkin's lymphoma; NR—not reached; ORR—overall response rate; PFS—progression-free survival; TTP—time to progression; TTnT—time to next treatment

[a]Discontinued due to projected decline in sales and the availability of alternative treatments
[b]Initial approval in 2009 as part of the FDA's accelerated approval process

Target antigens are not restricted to the tumour itself, as tumour support structures like the vasculature, stroma and extracellular matrix also provide potential targets (Scott et al. 2012; Ferris et al. 2010). Vascular endothelial growth factor (VEGF) is one of the ligands for the VEGF receptor 2 (VEGFR2) where it plays a role in promoting angiogenesis in developing tumours, and both have been targeted by antibodies in cancer therapy (Holmes et al. 2007). Trapping of the ligand or blocking of the receptor is able to limit the tumours' ability to develop vascular networks, thereby reducing its capacity to grow and spread (Holmes et al. 2007). Additional to tumour support structures, the immune system itself can be targeted in cancer therapy to enhance the natural response against the tumour. For example, cytotoxic T-lymphocyte-associated antigen 4 (CTLA-4) is a cell surface receptor expressed on T cells that when activated by its ligand it functions to downregulate their responses (Leach et al. 1996; Hodi et al. 2010a). Ipilimumab is an antibody that has been developed to block CTLA-4 cytotoxic T cells, and this blocking of CTLA-4 keeps the T cells in an active state with anti-tumour capacity (Hodi et al. 2010a).

1.2 Monoclonal Antibody Formats

Monoclonal antibodies (mAbs) are produced by a single B cell clone and target one specific epitope of an antigen. The first method for the production of mAbs was the hybridoma technology introduced by Kohler and Milstein in 1975 (Kohler and Milstein 1975). This method involves immunizing mice with the antigen of interest and then isolating B cells from the spleen. These isolated B cells are then fused with myeloma cells with each fusion resulting in an immortal cell that produces unlimited quantities of identical antibody, called hybridomas. The first mAb approved for cancer therapy, rituximab, is used for the treatment of non-Hodgkin's lymphoma through targeting of the CD20 receptor on B cells (Maloney et al. 1997).

Even though the technology existed to produce large quantities of antibodies to any target antigen required, there were still several obstacles to overcome in order to achieve maximal efficacy. Because hybridoma-derived antibodies were of murine origin, their therapeutic potential is hampered by two main problems. Firstly, the murine Fc region of the antibodies has reduced binding to human Fc receptors which impair cellular effector function of immune cells and diminishes serum half-life. Secondly and most importantly, the infusion of murine antibodies into patients leads to the development of a host immune response to the foreign protein and the production of human anti-mouse antibodies (HAMA).

To overcome HAMA responses and improve the interaction with human Fc receptors, methods to produce antibodies with higher human homology were established. The first methods developed took advantage of recombinant DNA technology by isolating the mRNA sequence coding for the antibody from the hybridoma. With the murine DNA, it was then possible to substitute in human constant region DNA to reduce immunogenicity without impacting on antigen binding. This combination produced chimeric antibodies with murine variable regions and human constant regions (Morrison 1985; Neuberger et al. 1985; Norderhaug et al. 1997). Following the success of chimeric antibodies, further efforts to produce mAbs with higher human homology were researched. These chimeric antibodies could be refined further by selective alteration of the amino acids in the framework region of the variable domain portion while still keeping the original murine CDRs (Riechmann et al. 1988; Queen et al. 1989). This process of refinement is referred to as humanization and produces mAbs where the only murine sequence is limited to the CDRs.

With the technology established to produce chimeric and humanized mAbs, research continued to design methods to create "fully" human mAbs (Laffleur et al. 2012). Following the creation of transgenic mice with human germline genes for the heavy and kappa light chains, it was possible to immunize these mice to produce human antibodies that were antigen-specific (Lonberg and Huszar 1995). Platforms to produce mAbs without the use of mice were also developed that use phage display to randomly generate CDRs in Fab fragments (Winter and Milstein 1991; Smith 1985; Bazan et al. 2012). This is achieved through the use of viruses that infect bacteria (bacteriophages) that express proteins on the viral particle surface, and DNA for these random CDRs is inserted into genes for surface proteins (Bazan et al. 2012). In doing this, a large library of phage surfaces can be generated and screened against the antigen of interest, thereby creating a high-throughput method for generating novel antibodies (Bazan et al. 2012). Once identified, any positive clones can also be further refined to enhance binding through small amino acid changes in the CDRs through iterations of the phage display system (Bazan et al. 2012).

Additional to the use of full-sized antibodies, it is possible to produce smaller antibody fragments that retain antigen-binding activity. Due to their smaller size, these antibody fragments have altered pharmacokinetic properties that make them useful for the diagnosis and treatment of cancers (Chames et al. 2009; Holliger and Hudson 2005). These include monovalent Fab fragments, approximately 55 kDa, which lack an Fc and are not able to engage effector functions through FcRs. Without FcR engagement, Fab fragments have a short half-life, 12–20 h, compared to intact IgG molecules which have a half-life in serum of more than 10 days (Holliger and Hudson 2005; Flanagan and Jones 2004). This short half-life of Fab fragments makes them great tools for imaging tumours because of the rapid blood clearance. Arcitumomab is a Fab fragment of a murine monoclonal antibody that targets carcinoembryonic antigen expressed on colorectal cancers and has been used as a radioimmunoconjugate with the radioisotope technetium-99 m for tumour imaging (Hansen et al. 1990). As a result of the rapid blood clearance of arcitumomab the background observed when imaging tumours is reduced when compared to the intact IgG (Behr et al. 1995). Fab fragments are not the only antibody formats available, and single-chain variable fragments (scFv) are created by linking both the heavy and light variable domains of an antibody with flexible polypeptide linker (Holliger and Hudson 2005). This creates an even smaller molecule, approximately 28 kDa, that still retains antigen-binding capacity, and multiple scFvs can be linked together to create multivalent complexes (Holliger and Hudson 2005).

1.3 Mechanism of Action

Antibodies used in cancer therapy have various methods of mediating tumour cell death, which are intimately linked with the native function of the target antigen (Fig. 2). They can directly act on tumour cells by the blocking of growth factor receptors that are required for tumour growth (Scott et al. 2012) such as members of the ErbB family. Cetuximab is one such example, and it was the first monoclonal antibody to target EGFR and has been approved for the treatment of colorectal cancer patients (Van Cutsem et al. 2009). By binding to EGFR on the cell surface, cetuximab blocks the ligand binding site which in turn inhibits intracellular receptor signalling resulting in cell-cycle arrest, induction of apoptosis and downregulation of cell surface expression of EGFR. Trastuzumab is another example of a mAb that has been successfully used to target the human epidermal growth factor receptor type 2 (HER2).

Antibodies can also act upon stromal cells and vasculature in the tumour microenvironment to limit growth or induce tumour cell death (Scott et al. 2012). Malignant tumours are made up of rapidly dividing and growing cancer cells, and in order to support this growth, they need their own dedicated blood supply. This is achieved by the tumour releasing factors that tilt the balance within the microenvironment towards pro-angiogenesis to drive vascular growth and establish its own blood network. Bevacizumab is an antibody that targets the pro-angiogenic factor, vascular endothelial growth factor A (VEGF-A) (Yang et al. 2003). Bevacizumab works by binding to and trapping the soluble form of VEGF-A, which stops VEGF-A from working as a ligand to stimulate the vascular endothelial growth factor receptor (VEGF) expressed on endothelial cells (Willett et al. 2004).

Antibody-coated tumour cells are recognized by immune cells via interactions with specific receptors on their cell surface and trigger cellular effector functions. This interaction is mediated by the Fc domain of the antibody which contains specific binding sites for receptors on the immune cell surface (Hogarth and Pietersz 2012; Nimmerjahn and Ravetch 2008). These are known as the Fc receptors (FcRs), which are expressed on a variety of immune effector cells. Natural killer (NK) cells have the greatest reputation among anti-tumour effector cells as they have been shown to be the primary mediators of antigen-dependent cell-mediated cytotoxicity (ADCC) (Hogarth and Pietersz 2012; Nimmerjahn and Ravetch 2008). ADCC is triggered when the Fc domain of the bound therapeutic antibody is recognized by Fc gamma receptor IIIa (FcγRIIIa) on the surface of NK cells and involves the release of cytotoxic factors, such as perforin, that cause lysis of the tumour cell (Hogarth and Pietersz 2012; Nimmerjahn and Ravetch 2008). ADCC can be enhanced in therapeutic antibodies through engineering that improves the interaction of the antibody Fc domain with FcγRIIIa (Desjarlais and Lazar 2011; Desjarlais et al. 2007). This can be achieved through amino acid engineering, whereby a more favourable amino acid can be introduced to the enhance interaction with Fc (Desjarlais and Lazar 2011; Desjarlais et al. 2007). Additionally, the alteration of the glycosylation pattern of IgG Fc to reduce fucose content can provide a selective binding enhancement to FcγRIIIa and improved ADCC (50–100-fold increase).

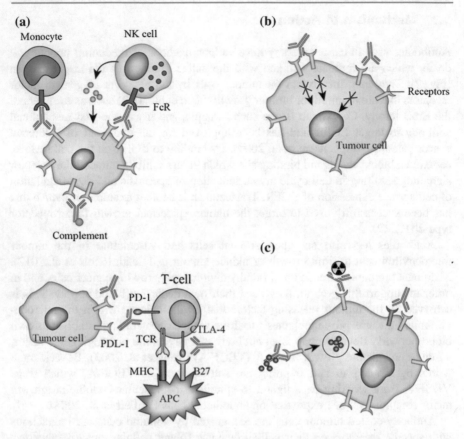

Fig. 2 Mechanisms of action of monoclonal antibodies: **a** Immune-mediated tumour cell killing through complement activation, antibody-dependent cellular cytotoxicity (ADCC), inhibition of T cell inhibitory receptors such as cytotoxic T lymphocyte-associated antigen 4 (CTLA4) and induction of phagocytosis; **b** tumour cell killing through inhibition of dimerization, kinase activation and downstream signalling leading to reduced proliferation and apoptosis; **c** conjugated antibodies to deliver toxic payloads such as a drug, toxin, small interfering RNA or radioisotope into tumour-cell-inducing cell death

Opsonized tumour cells can be phagocytosed through engagement of FcγRs, and in addition to the killing of the target cell, antigen presentation can occur to activate T cells (Nimmerjahn and Ravetch 2008; Richards et al. 2008). The process of engulfing an antibody-coated tumour cell is called antigen-dependent cellular phagocytosis (ADCP) and involves the engagement of activatory FcγRs (Nimmerjahn and Ravetch 2008; Richards et al. 2008). This could potentially provide patients with long-term immunity against tumours through the induction of the adaptive immune system in the form of anti-tumour memory T cells (Richards et al. 2008). This linking of the innate and adaptive immune system through the passive administration of anti-tumour antibodies is referred to as the vaccinal effect and has long been thought as the holy grail of antibody therapy (Richards et al. 2008;

DiLillo and Ravetch 2015). An additional Fc-mediated function of antibodies is to engage the complement system through a number of small proteins found in the blood (Duncan and Winter 1988; Ricklin et al. 2010). This involves the recruitment of these proteins to form a complex on the surface of the pathogen (Duncan and Winter 1988; Ricklin et al. 2010). This complex serves three main functions: to enhance phagocytosis, recruit immune cells, and form a membrane attack complex (MAC) that lyses the target (Ricklin et al. 2010).

Antibodies can also be used to deliver a payload directly to the tumour site due to the unique specificity for their TAA. These antibody conjugates can be used to deliver a drug, toxin, small interfering RNA (siRNA) or even a radioactive isotope in a targeted approach that often leads to improved efficacy and reduced toxicity. Trastuzumab is used as an antibody–drug conjugate (ADC) to deliver the chemotherapeutic agent DM1 directly to the tumour through receptor internalization (Barok et al. 2014; Hudis 2007). The use of trastuzumab as an ADC allows for a broad anti-tumour mechanism of action with its ability to abrogate HER2 signalling, recruit immune cells and directly kill the tumour through payload delivery.

2 Approved Monoclonal Antibodies

A summary of approved monoclonal antibodies in cancer treatment is detailed in Tables 1 and 2 with an approval history timeline shown in Fig. 3.

2.1 Anti-CD20 Monoclonal Antibodies

CD20 is a transmembrane calcium channel highly expressed on the surface of human B cells, making it an ideal target for directed therapy. It is involved in B cell activation, proliferation, differentiation (Gopal and Press 1999) and calcium flux (Bubien et al. 1993). Cross-linking of CD20 with monoclonal antibodies has shown to trigger antibody-dependent cellular cytotoxicity (ADCC) and complement-dependent cytotoxicity (CDC) in cells (Kosmas et al. 2002).

2.1.1 Rituximab
Rituximab is a chimeric anti-CD20 monoclonal antibody, which has revolutionized the management of B cell lymphoproliferative malignancies. Rituximab is one of the most widely prescribed biological agents today. It was first approved in 1997 for the treatment of relapsed indolent NHL. Today, it is used in a number of settings as induction therapy, for maintenance of disease remission and at disease relapses in NHL as well as in chronic lymphocytic leukaemia (CLL).

In 2006, rituximab was approved for use as first-line treatment in patients with diffuse large B cell (DLBCL) in combination with cyclophosphamide, doxorubicin, vincristine and prednisone (CHOP) or other anthracycline-based chemotherapy regimens based on the results of three randomized trials involving nearly 2000 treatment-naive patients (Pfreundschuh et al. 2010; Coiffier et al. 2010; Habermann

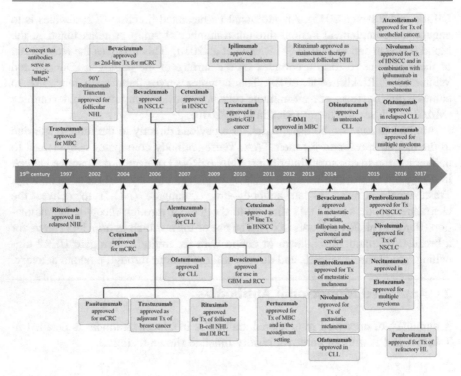

Fig. 3 Timeline of antibody approval in cancer treatment

et al. 2006). Two trials evaluated patients aged ≥ 60 years with stage 3–4 disease (E4494 (Habermann et al. 2006) and LNH 98-5/GELA (Coiffier et al. 2010)), while the M39045/MiNT (Pfreundschuh et al. 2010)-enrolled patients aged between 18 and 60 years with majority having early-stage disease. In each study, hazard ratios for the main outcome measured as well as overall survival favoured the rituximab-containing arms, with results consistent across all subgroup analysis. The benefit of rituximab was seen at long-term follow-up (Feugier et al. 2005). The benefit of rituximab in this setting however has shown to be limited to patients whose tumours do not express the bcl-6 protein (Winter et al. 2006). Also in 2006, rituximab was approved for use as first-line treatment for patients with low-grade or follicular B cell, CD20-positive NHL, in combination with cyclophosphamide, vincristine and prednisone (CVP) as well as following CVP chemotherapy (Marcus et al. 2005). Treatment with single-agent rituximab after CVP chemotherapy in patients that have responded resulted in a statistically significant reduction in PFS.

In 2010, rituximab in combination with fludarabine and cyclophosphamide (FC) was approved for the treatment of CLL in treatment-naive patients with excellent performance status as well as in patients with relapsed or refractory disease based on the positive findings of two randomized trials, ML17102 and BO17072, respectively (Hallek et al. 2010; Robak et al. 2010; Fischer et al. 2012).

The benefit of FCR however was not seen in a subgroup of patients with del(17p) by fluorescence in situ hybridization (FISH)1, TP53 mutations (Rossi et al. 2014) and unmutated immunoglobulin heavy chain variable (IGHV) gene (Thompson et al. 2016).

Rituximab in 2011 was approved for maintenance therapy in patients with previously untreated follicular CD20-positive B cell NHL after first-line treatment with rituximab in combination with chemotherapy. The approval was based on phase III PRIMA trial (Salles et al. 2011). Despite the benefit in PFS, this did not translate into an improvement in overall survival or reduce the rate of histological transformation. With no clear benefit in overall survival, reported in a number of other randomized trials, there remains a lot of debate with regard to the optimum duration of maintenance treatment.

2.1.2 Ofatumumab

Ofatumumab is a humanized type I anti-CD20 monoclonal antibody approved for the treatment of CLL in treatment-naive patients as well as patients with relapsed, treatment-refractory disease. A single-arm study evaluated ofatumumab in patients with CLL refractory to fludarabine and alemtuzumab and in patients with fludarabine-refractory CLL with bulky (>5 cm) lymphadenopathy who were not suitable for alemtuzumab. Treatment with ofatumumab resulted in improved responses rates and complete resolution of constitutional symptoms and improved performance status in almost half of all patients (Wierda et al. 2010).

In a phase III trial (COMPLEMENT 1) (Hillmen et al. 2015), the addition of ofatumumab to chemotherapy in treatment-naive patients with CLL resulted in a significant improvement in median PFS and prolonged median duration of response. After a median follow-up of 28.9 months, OS was not reached in both groups. Despite enrolling elderly patients (half of enrolled patients >70 years) and those with multiple comorbidities, the addition of ofatumumab resulted in clinically meaningful improvements.

In the COMPLEMENT 2 trial (Robak et al. 2017), patients with relapsed CLL were randomized to fludarabine and cyclophosphamide with or without ofatumumab. The addition of ofatumumab resulted in significantly longer PFS, with manageable toxicities.

2.1.3 Obinutuzumab

Obinutuzumab is the first Fc-engineered, humanized anti-CD20 monoclonal antibody to be approved in combination with chlorambucil in the management of treatment-naive patients with CLL. In the randomized phase III trial, CLL11, the median age of patients was 73 years, 68% had impaired renal function, and 76% had multiple coexisting medical conditions. Chemo-immunotherapy with either rituximab or obinutuzumab was shown to be superior to chemotherapy alone. After a follow-up of 39 months, compared with rituximab, treatment with obinutuzumab resulted in clinically meaningful PFS and TTNT with a trend towards improved OS

(Goede et al. 2014, 2015). In a subgroup analysis defined by gene mutations, obinutuzumab–chlorambucil had better outcomes and was able to overcome NOTCH1mut-associated rituximab resistance (Estenfelder et al. 2016).

In 2016, obinutuzumab was approved in combination with bendamustine followed by obinutuzumab monotherapy as maintenance therapy for the treatment rituximab-refractory follicular lymphoma based on the findings of the GADOLIN study, in which the median PFS was significantly higher in patients treated with obinutuzumab plus bendamustine (Sehn et al. 2016).

Toxicities Associated with Anti-CD20 Antibodies

Infusion reactions are the most commonly reported adverse event associated with anti-CD20 antibodies (Coiffier et al. 2008; Ghielmini et al. 2005; Kasi et al. 2012). Infusion reactions typically occur after the first infusion and within 24 h of the infusion and are dose-dependent (Ghielmini et al. 2005; Coiffier et al. 1998). Most infusion reactions are mild with severe (grade 3/4) reactions rare (Kasi et al. 2012). Grade 3/4 cytopenias have been reported in almost half of all patients treated with anti-CD20 antibodies with lymphopenia and neutropenia being the most commonly reported (Coiffier et al. 2008; Kasi et al. 2012). This incidence increases when rituximab is used in combination with chemotherapy regimens (Buske et al. 2009; Eve et al. 2009). There is an associated increase in frequency of infectious complications, with bacterial infections most commonly seen (Kasi et al. 2012; Cohen et al. 2006). A dose-dependent increase in the frequency of infections is seen in patients treated with rituximab (Avilés et al. 2007). Severe and sometimes fatal mucocutaneous reactions can occur. Also reported is JC virus reactivation, leading to progressive multifocal leukoencephalopathy (Carson et al. 2009). Pulmonary complications have been reported in 5% of patients treated with rituximab monotherapy. Hypoalbuminemia has been identified as an independent risk factor (Kang et al. 2012). The most common toxicities are infectious; however, other toxicities reported include interstitial lung disease, bronchiolitis obliterans, hypersensitivity pneumonitis and diffuse alveolar haemorrhage (Biehn et al. 2006; Tonelli et al. 2009; Heresi et al. 2008).

Resistance Mechanisms to Anti-CD20 Antibodies

The exact mechanisms of rituximab resistance remain poorly understood. Resistance mechanisms can be broadly divided into host factors such as Fc receptor polymorphisms affecting the affinity of effector cells for rituximab Fc and tumour-related factors, e.g. CD20 expression and structure, acquired CD20 mutations and tumour burden. Other general mechanisms include alterations in rituximab pharmacokinetics. Rituximab-resistant cell lines have shown to express high levels of membrane complement regulatory proteins, CD20, CD55 and CD59, which inhibit the complement cascade, thereby affecting the ability of rituximab to induce complement-dependent cytotoxicity (Takei et al. 2006). Patients with rituximab resistance transfused with fresh frozen plasma and treated with rituximab showed excellent clinical response (Klepfish et al. 2009; Xu et al. 2011).

The efficacy of ofatumumab is limited by drug resistance, which is not well characterized (Baig et al. 2010). In vitro studies using CLL cells pre- and post-treatment with ofatumumab showed a single dose of ofatumumab resulted in a marked decrease in serum complement levels, and the surviving CLL cells showed depletion in CD20 expression. These cells were resistant to in vitro ofatumumab-mediated CDC, but most retain full sensitivity to alemtuzumab-mediated CDC.

2.2 Anti-CD30 Monoclonal Antibodies

CD30, a member of the tumour necrosis factor receptor (TNFR) family, is a transmembrane glycoprotein with expression in normal tissues limited to some activated B and T cells (Younes and Kadin 2003). CD30 is highly expressed in Hodgkin lymphoma (HL) and systemic anaplastic large cell lymphoma (sALCL) cells irrespective of disease stage, line of therapy or transplant status (Francisco et al. 2003). In contrast, CD30 expression in solid tumours occurs at a lower frequency compared to haematopoietic-derived tumours; however, high expression of CD30 has shown to occur in testicular embryonal carcinoma and germ cell tumours (Dürkop et al. 2000).

2.2.1 Brentuximab Vedotin

Brentuximab vedotin (BV) is an antibody–drug conjugate (ADC) composed of a monoclonal antibody directed against CD30 that is covalently bound by a protease-cleavable linker to the anti-microtubule agent monomethyl auristatin E (MMAE) (Francisco et al. 2003). Binding of BV to CD30 results in internalization of the MMAE-CD30 complex and release of MMAE by proteolytic cleavage.

In 2011, BV received accelerated approval for the treatment of patients with CD30-positive HL that relapsed after autologous stem cell transplantation (ASCT), and relapsed sALCL, based on results of two single-arm trials (de Claro et al. 2012; Chen et al. 2016a). In 2015, brentuximab vedotin also received FDA approval for the treatment of patients with HL at high risk of relapse/progression post-ASCT consolidation. This approval was based on the AETHERA trial which showed an improvement in the median PFS in the BV group compared to 24.1 months in the placebo group (Moskowitz et al. 2015). This benefit was seen in all subgroups analysed.

Toxicities

The most frequent adverse events related to BV seen across all trails were peripheral sensory neuropathy, neutropenia, fatigue and nausea. Other toxicities reported were diarrhoea, pyrexia, upper respiratory tract infection and vomiting. In all trials, neuropathy was the leading cause of treatment discontinuation. Toxicity usually developed between 3 and 4 months after commencing treatment (Scott 2017; Garnock-Jones 2013). At the five-year follow-up of patients with relapsed/refractory HL who developed treatment-related peripheral neuropathy, majority experienced either resolution or improvement in symptoms (Chen et al. 2016a).

Mechanisms of Resistance

Currently, mechanisms of resistance to BV are unknown (Chen et al. 2015). Using two different treatment models, Chen et al. (2015) developed BV-resistant HL (L428) and ALCL (Karpas-299) cell lines to elucidate potential resistance mechanisms. Although loss of target expression was not shown in the BV-resistant HL cell line or in tissue samples of patients with HL who had relapsed or progressed after BV treatment, the alteration in signalling level may be a potential mechanism. A reduction in the dynamics of receptor cellular or receptor internalization could also reduce the efficiency of antigen targeting (Parakh et al. 2016a). In contrast, the HL cell line, but not the ALCL cell line, exhibited MMAE resistance and overexpression of MDR1 mRNA compared to the parental line. Both HL and ALCL treatment-resistant patient samples persistently expressed CD30 by immunohistochemistry (Chen et al. 2015).

2.3 Anti-CD38 Monoclonal Antibodies

CD38 is a transmembrane glycoprotein expressed by a variety of lymphoid and myeloid lineages; in particular, plasma cells express particularly high levels of CD38 (Deaglio et al. 2001). CD38 functions as an adhesion molecule, involved in the activation and proliferation of human leucocytes as well as signal transduction and intracellular calcium mobilization (Lin et al. 2004; Malavasi et al. 1994). CD38 is highly expressed in a number of haematological malignancies, in particular MM (Lin et al. 2004) and CLL (Damle et al. 1999). CD38 expression by CLL cells has shown to be associated with a more aggressive clinical course and poorer patient outcomes (Damle et al. 1999).

2.3.1 Daratumumab

Daratumumab is a humanized anti-CD38-specific antibody. In 2016, daratumumab was approved for the treatment of multiple myeloma (MM) in combination with lenalidomide and dexamethasone, or bortezomib and dexamethasone, in patients who have received prior therapy. The approval is based on two randomized trials in which daratumumab in combination with standard therapies resulted in improved response rates and PFS (Plesner et al. 2014; Palumbo et al. 2016; Dimopoulos et al. 2016).

Toxicities

The most frequently reported haematological AEs of any grade were anaemia, thrombocytopenia and neutropenia. Nearly half of all patients experienced infusion-related reactions post-cycle 1, majority of which were of low grade. Common non-haematological AEs were fatigue, nausea and diarrhoea (Sanchez et al. 2016). Another effect unique to anti-CD38 monoclonal antibodies is the high false positive results with the indirect anti-globulin test (Coombs test) (Oostendorp et al. 2015) as daratumumab binds to CD38 expressed on RBC, masking antigens in the patient's serum (Oostendorp et al. 2015).

Mechanisms of Resistance
Majority of patients treated with daratumumab eventually develop resistance (Nijhof et al. 2016). Examining patient samples pre- and post-treatment with daratumumab showed CD38 expression levels correlated with response, while expression of complement-inhibitory proteins (CIPs), membrane cofactor protein (CD46), decay-accelerating factor (CD55) and protectin (CD59) levels increased at time of progression and correlated with development of antibody resistance. Treating MM cells from patients who developed daratumumab resistance with ATRA led to increased CD38 levels and decreased CD55 and CD59 expression to almost pretreatment values (Nijhof et al. 2015, 2016). Furthermore, in the light of the immune-effector-mediated mechanism of daratumumab, T cell exhaustion could affect its effectiveness.

2.4 Anti-CD52 Monoclonal Antibodies

CD52 is a glycosylphosphatidylinositol-anchored antigen highly expressed on normal and neoplastic lymphoid cells. Erythrocytes, platelets and bone marrow stem cells lack CD52 surface expression (Xia et al. 1991). The CD52 antigen is also expressed on subsets of tumour cells, including T cell prolymphocytic leukaemia, CLL, hairy cell leukaemia, NHL and acute lymphoblastic leukaemia (Ginaldi et al. 1998). The exact biological function of CD52 is yet to be elucidated; however, some evidence suggests that it may be involved in T cell migration and costimulation (Watanabe et al. 2006).

2.4.1 Alemtuzumab
Alemtuzumab is an anti-CD52 humanized monoclonal antibody approved in 2007 for use as a single agent in the treatment of patients with B cell CLL (B-CLL) refractory to alkylating agents and failed fludarabine therapy. Alemtuzumab initially received accelerated approval in 2001 based on the findings of three single-arm phase II studies (Osterborg et al. 1997; Rai et al. 2002; Keating et al. 2002). Full approval was given following results of the larger randomized phase III trial, CAM 307 (Hillmen et al. 2007).

Toxicities
The most common adverse events associated with alemtuzumab are infusion-related side effects, myelosuppression and infections (Fraser et al. 2007). Grade 3/4 reactions however were noted in up to 20% of patients. The incidence of infusion-related side effects was similar regardless of the treatment setting and was most severe on first exposure to the drug (Osterborg et al. 1997; Rai et al. 2002; Keating et al. 2002; Liggett et al. 2005; Ferrajoli et al. 2003). The subcutaneous

administration of alemtuzumab had a significantly lower incidence of grade 3/4 infusion-related toxicity (Lundin et al. 2002). Majority of patients treated with alemtuzumab will experience transient cytopenias; patients with relapsed/refractory disease or those who have received prior treatment are at higher risk (Fraser et al. 2007). Thrombocytopenia commonly occurs first and develops in the first 2 weeks of therapy, while neutropenia occurs by week 6 (Keating et al. 2002). The route of administration of alemtuzumab does not influence the development of haematological toxicity. Significant infections were reported in 42–55% of patients with pretreated CLL during alemtuzumab therapy (Rai et al. 2002; Keating et al. 2002). The most frequently observed opportunistic infection during alemtuzumab therapy is CMV reactivation, reported in 15–25% of patients (Nguyen et al. 2002).

Mechanisms of Resistance
Mechanisms of resistance to alemtuzumab have not yet been fully elucidated; in vitro analysis of CLL cells from patients with progressive untreated CLL has shown a subpopulation of CLL cells intrinsically resistant to alemtuzumab CDC and spontaneous apoptosis, despite effective complement activation. Possible explanations include insufficient complement activation, increased activity of complement resistance factors or low target antigen expression (Baig et al. 2010, 2012; Zent et al. 2005). Future studies are needed to examine these resistance mechanisms.

2.5 Anti-signalling Lymphocytic Activation Molecule (SLAM) Monoclonal Antibodies

Signalling lymphocytic activation molecule (SLAM) F7 (aka CS1, CD subset 2, CD319 or CRACC) is a cell surface receptor that belongs to the SLAM family. It has no normal tissue expression; however, it is widely expressed in haematopoietic cells, in particular, on normal and malignant plasma cells as well as on all NK cells, most CD8+ T cells, activated B cells, mature dendritic cells (Hsi et al. 2008). While the exact role of SLAM7 in MM cells is not entirely clear (Tai et al. 2008), it has been shown to play an important role in the interaction between MM cells and bone marrow stromal cells (Tai et al. 2008) and regulates NK cell cytolytic activity by coupling with the SLAM-associated protein family adapter Ewing's sarcoma-associated transcript 2 (EAT-2) (Kumaresan et al. 2002). Importantly, SLAM7 expression is not affected by stage of disease or prior treatment (van Rhee et al. 2009).

2.5.1 Elotuzumab

Elotuzumab is a humanized monoclonal antibody that targets the extracellular domain of SLAM7 expressed both on MM and NK cells. In 2015, elotuzumab was approved for the treatment of MM in combination with lenalidomide and dexamethasone in treatment-refractory patients based on the findings of phase III study,

ELOQUENT-2 (Lonial et al. 2015). The benefit of elotuzumab was consistent across all subgroups including patients with resistance to the most recent line of therapy and patients ≥ 65 years or had a high-risk cytogenetic profile, i.e. had 17p deletion (Lonial et al. 2016). Furthermore, the addition of elotuzumab also resulted in improved health-related quality of life (Lonial et al. 2015).

Toxicities
Elotuzumab has been well tolerated in trials (Lonial et al. 2012, 2015; Zonder et al. 2012; Usmani et al. 2015; Richardson et al. 2015). The most common grade 3/4 haematological toxicities reported include lymphocytopenia, neutropenia and neutropenia. Of the non-haematological toxicities, commonly reported were fatigue, diarrhoea and pneumonia. Infusion reactions were seen in most patients; however, majority were of lower grade (grade 1/2) in severity.

2.6 Anti-epidermal Growth Factor Receptor (EGFR) Monoclonal Antibodies

Epidermal growth factor receptor (also known as EGFR or ErbB1) is a member of ErbB family of receptor tyrosine kinases (RTK), which also include ErbB2 (HER2), ErbB3 (HER3) and ErbB4 (HER4) (Olayioye et al. 2000). In many different cancer cell types, signalling through EGFR becomes dysregulated by several mechanisms, including overproduction of ligands, overexpression of receptors, mutational activation of receptors or downstream signalling components or structural alterations, such as the truncated EGFRvIII variant, resulting in constitutive kinase activation of EGFR signalling (Kruser and Wheeler 2010; Dhomen et al. 2012).

2.6.1 Cetuximab
Cetuximab is a chimeric monoclonal antibody approved in 2004 for use as a single agent for the treatment EGFR-expressing mCRC after failure of both irinotecan- and oxaliplatin-based chemotherapy regimens (Jonker et al. 2007). Patients with KRAS WT tumours had significantly higher PFS and OS rates and significantly higher rates of surgery for metastases (Van Cutsem et al. 2009, 2011). Approval of cetuximab and its efficacy in the wild-type subgroup was based on outcomes of this study and two supporting trials, CA225025 and OPUS.

Cetuximab has also been approved for use in combination with radiation therapy for the treatment of locally or regionally advanced SCCHN as well as for use as a single agent for the treatment of patients with advanced SCCHN who have progressed on prior platinum-based therapy (Bonner et al. 2006, 2010). In 2011, cetuximab was approved for use in combination with platinum-based therapy plus 5-fluorouracil (5-FU) for the first-line treatment of patients with advanced SCCHN (Vermorken et al. 2008). Addition of cetuximab to chemotherapy significantly prolonged OS, PFS and ORR with no difference in response rates seen in HPV-negative or positive tumours (Vermorken et al. 2014).

2.6.2 Panitumumab

Panitumumab is a fully humanized monoclonal antibody against the extracellular domain of EGFR (Yang et al. 2001). Panitumumab is the first fully human monoclonal antibody approved for the treatment of colorectal cancer. Panitumumab first received accelerated approval in 2006 as monotherapy for the treatment of patients with EGFR-expressing mCRC with disease progression on or following fluoropyrimidine-, oxaliplatin- and irinotecan-containing chemotherapy regimens (Van Cutsem et al. 2007a). Benefit of panitumumab was limited to patients whose tumours were WT for KRAS exon 2 (Van Cutsem et al. 2007b; Amado et al. 2008). The lack of survival benefit in this study was likely to due to crossover to the panitumumab arm (Amado et al. 2008). In 2014, further approval was granted for use in combination with fluorouracil plus leucovorin and oxaliplatin chemotherapy regimen in the first-line setting for patients with KRAS WT (exon 2 in codons 12 or 13) mCRC (Douillard et al. 2010). As seen in other studies, the survival benefit was seen in patient with KRAS WT tumours; furthermore, patients with other RAS mutations in KRAS exons 3 and 4 and in NRAS exons 2, 3 and 4, i.e. other than in exon 2, had also experienced inferior PFS and OS with the addition of panitumumab (Douillard et al. 2013).

2.6.3 Necitumumab

Necitumumab is a humanized anti-EGFR monoclonal antibody approved in 2015 for use as first-line treatment in combination with cisplatin and gemcitabine in patients with advanced squamous cell carcinoma (SCC) NSCLC, on the findings of phase III study, SQUIRE (Thatcher et al. 2015; Paz-Ares et al. 2016). In a subgroup analysis, patients with EGFR-expressing tumours had outcomes similar to the unselected population of the SQUIRE study and no benefit has been seen in patients with non-EGFR-expressing tumours (Paz-Ares et al. 2016).

Toxicities Associated with Anti-EGFR Antibodies

Almost all patients treated with anti-EGFR monoclonal antibodies experience dermatological toxicities in a dose-dependent manner; while majority are typically of low grade, it can significantly impact QoL and adherence to treatment grade (Thatcher et al. 2015; Paz-Ares et al. 2015; Mitchell et al. 2007). Dermatologic toxicities may to lead to dose modification or discontinuation by 36 and 72%, respectively (Boone et al. 2007). Dermatological toxicities, of which an acneiform rash is the commonest, also include papulopustular eruptions, hair changes, periungual and nail plate abnormalities, xerosis, telangiectasia and pruritus (Segaert and Van Cutsem 2005). Pruritus, of any grade, more commonly occurs in patients treated with panitumumab as compared to cetuximab (Ensslin et al. 2013). A papulopustular rash typically develops early, occurring within six weeks of commencing treatment (Mitchell et al. 2007). It is shown to be predictive of response and positively correlate with survival (Bonomi et al. 2015; Peeters et al. 2009; Fakih and Vincent 2010). Preemptive skin treatment has shown to reduce the incidence and severity of panitumumab-associated skin toxicities (Lacouture et al. 2010; Kobayashi et al. 2015). Ocular toxicities such as conjunctivitis and blepharitis have been reported with use of anti-EGFR antibodies and result from inflammation of the meibomian glands which contain EGFR-expressing cells (Van Cutsem et al. 2007b; Tonini et al. 2005). Similarly, anti-EGFR therapies result in tubular damage at the ascending loop of Henle, the site of magnesium resorption, due to high EGFR expression and result in a magnesium-wasting syndrome in almost a third of patients (Van Cutsem et al. 2007a). Diarrhoea is a commonly encountered toxicity and reported in about 20% of patients with the incidence and severity significantly increasing when these agents were used in combination with chemotherapy (Fakih and Vincent 2010). Severe infusion reactions occur more commonly in patients treated with cetuximab as compared to panitumumab or necitumumab (Fakih and Vincent 2010) and likely mediated due to preexisting IgE antibodies (Chung et al. 2008). While the incidence of pulmonary fibrosis is low, <1%, prescribing information contains warnings of pulmonary fibrosis and interstitial lung disease (ILD). Importantly, phase III INSPIRE trial (Paz-Ares et al. 2015), evaluating the benefit of necitumumab to doublet chemotherapy in treatment-naive patients with advanced non-squamous NSCLC was prematurely stopped due to more fatal thromboembolic events in the necitumumab arm, 8% versus 4% with chemotherapy alone.

Mechanisms of Resistance to Anti-EGFR Antibodies

Our current understanding of resistance mechanisms to anti-EGFR antibodies is largely from studies involving colorectal cancer (CRC) and extrapolated to head and neck cancers as little information is available for resistance mechanisms to anti-EGFR antibodies in this setting. Primary or acquired resistance to anti-EGFR treatment often results due to activation of downstream signalling pathways from mutations in KRAS and NRAS (exon 2–4), BRAF (exon 15) and PIK3CA (exon 20), as well as gene amplification of KRAS (Misale et al. 2014; Sorich et al. 2015). The most common cause of resistance to anti-EGFR antibodies is the presence of RAS mutations; no benefit was seen in patients with metastatic colorectal cancer (mCRC) whose tumours harbour KRAS mutations with the addition of cetuximab or panitumumab in the first- or second-line settings (Van Cutsem et al. 2009; Amado et al. 2008; Douillard et al. 2010; Karapetis et al. 2008; Bokemeyer et al. 2012; Peeters et al. 2010). Approximately, 40% of CRC patients have a mutation in exon 2 of the KRAS gene (Amado et al. 2008) and 5–9% of patients with mCRC have a mutation in BRAF gene (Van Cutsem et al. 2009; Tol et al. 2009). While the role BRAF V600 mutation as a predictive marker of resistance to anti-EGFR antibodies is still unclear (Douillard et al. 2010; Bokemeyer et al. 2012), it has shown to be associated with poor outcomes in mCRC (Bokemeyer et al. 2012; Tol et al. 2009). Almost 40% of patients who do not have a KRAS or BRAF mutation do not respond to anti-EGFR treatment strongly implicating pathways other than the MAPK pathway. Mutations in PI3KCA (phosphatidylinositol-4,5-bisphosphate 3-kinase, catalytic subunit alpha) or loss of PTEN, which frequently coexists with RAS mutations, has also shown to be associated with resistance to anti-EGFR treatment in some studies and correlated with poorer survival rates (Laurent-Puig et al. 2009; Perrone et al. 2009; Frattini et al. 2007; Loupakis et al. 2009). Genetic alterations have been shown to develop and increase in tumours during the course of anti-EGFR therapy, with more than one mutation often present (Arena et al. 2015). Another mechanism of resistance is through the activation of alternative signalling pathways including HER2 or MET gene amplifications (Yonesaka et al. 2011; Bertotti et al. 2011; Bardelli et al. 2013). Significant and durable responses were seen in a "proof-of-concept" trial with therapies targeting these pathways in patients with treatment-refractory KRAS wild-type (wt) and HER2-positive mCRC (Siena et al. 2015). Preclinical studies into non-genetic mechanisms of resistance suggest ongoing oncogenic dependency to EGFR signalling through increased EGFR expression and alterations in EGFR trafficking and degradation (Iida et al. 2013) as well as overexpression and ectopic production of EGFR ligands in treatment-refractory tumour cells (Hobor et al. 2014).

2.7 HER2 Targeting Monoclonal Antibodies

HER2 is a unique member of the ErbB family. Its extracellular domain is unable to bind to any known natural ligand (Klapper et al. 1999), and HER2 naturally adopts a conformation state that favour dimerization (Garrett et al. 2002). HER2 overexpression and amplification has been identified in a variety of cancer types; it has shown to be associated with poor outcomes in breast and gastric/gastroesophageal junction (GEJ) cancers (Reichelt et al. 2007; Gowryshankar et al. 2013; Nagaraja et al. 2016; Burstein 2005; Slamon et al. 1987; Tanner et al. 2005; Andrulis et al. 1998); however, its effect on other tumour types is not well defined (Berchuck et al. 1990; Tuefferd et al. 2007; Santin et al. 2005; Morrison et al. 2006; Grushko et al. 2008). Amplification or overexpression of HER2 also serves as a predictive biomarker for anti-HER2 treatment in a variety of tumour types including breast, gastric and gynaecological cancers (Slamon et al. 1987; Tanner et al. 2005; Andrulis et al. 1998; Berchuck et al. 1990; Morrison et al. 2006; Yonemura et al. 1991; Mineo et al. 2007; Liu et al. 2010a; Santin et al. 2008). Given the compelling nature of HER2 as a target for cancer therapy, a number of monoclonal antibodies targeting HER2 have been developed.

2.7.1 Trastuzumab
Trastuzumab has revolutionized the treatment of patients with HER2-positive breast cancer and provided vital insights into the biology of HER2. Trastuzumab has been approved for use in patients with breast cancer that overexpresses HER2 in all settings, either as monotherapy or in combination with chemotherapy. In 1998, almost ten years after its initial development, trastuzumab was the first HER2-targeting monoclonal antibody to receive approval for use in patients with HER2 overexpressing/amplified metastatic breast cancer (Slamon et al. 2001). In 2006, based on the joint analysis of the NSABP B31/N9831 (Perez et al. 2011, 2014) studies, trastuzumab was approved for use in combination with doxorubicin,

cyclophosphamide and paclitaxel for the adjuvant treatment of patients with early-stage HER2-positive, node-positive breast cancer. Final analysis of these studies confirmed the addition of trastuzumab resulted in superior OS. Based on the results of the BCIRG 006 study (Slamon et al. 2009), which evaluated a non-anthracycline containing adjuvant regimen, the FDA also approved trastuzumab for use in combination with docetaxel and carboplatin.

Trastuzumab is the first biological to show survival benefit in patients with advanced gastric cancer in the pivotal phase III trial, ToGA, leading to its approval in HER2-positive gastric cancer in combination with chemotherapy (Bang et al. 2010).

2.7.2 Pertuzumab

Pertuzumab, the first-in-class of agents known as HER dimerization inhibitors (Adams et al. 2006), binds to the extracellular dimerization domain II of HER2; an epitope distinct from the epitope for trastuzumab, inhibiting dimerization between HER receptors (Adams et al. 2006). In 2012, pertuzumab was approved as first-line treatment in combination with trastuzumab and docetaxel chemotherapy for the treatment of patients with HER2-positive metastatic breast cancer. The approval was granted on the findings of phase III trial, the CLEOPATRA study (Swain et al. 2015).

Pertuzumab is the first therapeutic to be approved for the neo-adjuvant treatment of breast cancer. Approval for this indication was based on the findings of phase II NEOSPHERE study (Gianni et al. 2012) and supported by the TRYPHAENA study (Schneeweiss et al. 2013). In both studies, the addition of pertuzumab improved pCR rates significantly. In phase III APHINITY trial (NCT01358877), the addition of pertuzumab to trastuzumab in patients with HER2-positive early breast cancer did not appear to significantly affect the invasive disease-free survival after a median follow-up of three years. The benefit of pertuzumab appeared slightly greater among patients with node-positive disease (Von Minckwitz et al. 2017).

2.7.3 Trastuzumab Emtansine (T-DM1)

Ado-trastuzumab emtansine (T-DM1) is the first anti-HER2 ADC to be approved in solid tumours. It is composed of trastuzumab linked to potent cytotoxic agent DM1, an inhibitor of microtubule dimerization (Junttila et al. 2011). T-DM1 has been approved for use as a single agent in the treatment of HER2-positive, metastatic breast cancer in patients who have previously received trastuzumab and a taxane (Verma et al. 2012).

Toxicities Associated with Anti-HER2 Antibodies

Cardiac toxicity is the most common and significant adverse event associated with trastuzumab therapy. Presentations may vary from an asymptomatic drop in left ventricular ejection fraction (LVEF) to symptomatic congestive cardiac failure. Proposed mechanisms include altered balance between anti- and pro-apoptotic proteins affecting mitochondrial function and inhibition of NRG-1-mediated activation of HER2 affecting sarcomere function (Kuramochi et al. 2006; Grazette et al. 2004; Lemarié et al. 2008). Rates of cardiac dysfunction from trastuzumab monotherapy ranged from 2 to 4.7% (Cobleigh et al. 1999; Vogel et al. 2002). A Cochrane Review of eight randomized clinical trials (B31, BCIRG 006, Buzdar, FinHer, HERA, N9831, NOAH and PACS-04 trials), involving over 10,000 patients, showed trastuzumab-containing regimens were associated with higher risk of congestive heart failure (RR 5.11; $p < 0.0001$) and LVEF decline (RR 1.83; $p = 0.0008$) (Moja et al. 2012). Trials focusing on neo-adjuvant therapy (Budzar, NAOH, HERA) reported low rates of symptomatic cardiotoxicity (0–1.7%), which is likely due to selection bias. Risk factors shown to be associated with trastuzumab-induced cardiotoxicity include hypertension, diabetes, previous anthracycline use and older age (Jawa et al. 2016). Importantly, the incidence of any grade cardiac toxicity did not significantly increase with the combination of trastuzumab and pertuzumab (Swain et al. 2013). The most common non-cardiac toxicity are infusion reactions, commonly occurring at first exposure, and do not recur at subsequent infusions (Slamon et al. 2001). Other commonly reported toxicities include arthralgia, myalgia, fatigue, dyspnea, nail changes, rash, headache, insomnia, thrombosis/embolism and diarrhoea (Trastuzumab FDA Label 2008). Rare but significant toxicities reported in less than 1% of patients include interstitial pneumonitis, grade 4/5 neutropenia, glomerulopathy causing nephrotic syndrome (Trastuzumab FDA Label 2008).

Mechanisms of Resistance to Anti-HER Antibodies

Primary resistance to single-agent trastuzumab is seen in approximately 70% of HER2-overexpressing breast cancers, with nearly all patients eventually developing resistance during treatment (Cobleigh et al. 1999; Spector and Blackwell 2009). While mechanism of resistance to trastuzumab has been extensively investigated, mechanisms of resistance to pertuzumab are poorly understood (Wuerkenbieke et al. 2015). Some of the proposed mechanisms of resistance to trastuzumab include:

i. Altered activation of downstream pathways such as the PI3K/AKT/mTOR pathway, by either PIK3CA mutation or loss of function of phosphatase and tensin homolog (PTEN) tumour suppressor gene (Nagata et al. 2004; Klos et al. 2003; Berns et al. 2007; Kataoka et al. 2010). Despite preclinical evidence, the relationship between PIK3CA mutations and trastuzumab benefit remains unclear, with no statistically significant association demonstrated with PTEN loss or PIK3CA mutation and benefit to trastuzumab in some studies (Loi et al. 2013; Wang et al. 2013; Pogue-Geile et al. 2015; Perez et al. 2013), while a positive correlation was seen between PI3K alterations and pCR rates (Schneeweiss et al. 2013; Untch et al. 2010).

ii. Dependence on signalling through alternative growth factor receptors including GFR, p95ErbB2, ErbB3, insulin-like growth factor receptor (IGF-1R), leading to hyperactivation of the PI3K-Akt signalling pathway (Nahta and Esteva 2006; Zhuang et al. 2010; Shattuck et al. 2008; O'Brien et al. 2010; Yakes et al. 2002; Lu et al. 2001; Garrett and Arteaga 2011; Nahta 2012).

iii. Impaired trastuzumab binding or masking of binding epitopes.

iv. Overexpression of EGFR or HER3 ligands (Ritter et al. 2007; Freudenberg et al. 2009).
v. Altered immune mechanisms affecting ADCC response due to polymorphisms within Fcγ receptors on immune cells affecting the affinity for trastuzumab Fc region binding (Hamid et al. 2013); increased expression of killer inhibitory receptors (KIRs) on NK cells, which can suppress NK activity (Kim et al. 2013) or immunosuppression through cytokines produced by tumour cells (Weber et al. 2015b).
vi. Binding of p27^{kip1} to the CDK2/cyclin E1 complex prevents cell-cycle progression and cell proliferation.

Similar to trastuzumab, patients with HER2-positive breast cancer treated with T-DM1 have either primary resistance to T-DM1 or develop resistance during treatment (Verma et al. 2012; Hurvitz et al. 2013; Wildiers et al. 2013). In preclinical models, efficacy of T-DM1 varied depending on the tumour mass in trastuzumab- and lapatinib-resistant human breast cancer xenograft models (Barok et al. 2011a), with resistance developing even after a long latency period (Barok et al. 2011b). Resistance mechanisms to T-DM1 have not been fully elucidated; potential mechanisms include reduced antigen expression (Burris et al. 2011), impaired internalization and endosomal trafficking of the HER2-T-DM1 complexes as well as development of resistance to the toxic payload or trastuzumab (Li et al. 2010).

2.8 Immune Checkpoint Inhibitors

Therapies targeting immune checkpoints and their ligands have shown impressive and durable responses in solid tumours and haematological malignancies. Immune checkpoint inhibitors approved by the FDA include ipilimumab, a monoclonal antibody that targets CTLA-4; nivolumab and pembrolizumab are highly selective humanized monoclonal antibodies against the PD-1 receptor. There are over 500 open clinical trials on ClinicalTrials.gov evaluating pembrolizumab and nivolumab in a variety of tumour types as monotherapies as well as in combination with other conventional and experimental therapies.

2.8.1 Ipilimumab
In a phase III trial (MDX010-20) (Hodi et al. 2010b), patients with treatment-refractory metastatic melanoma treated with ipilimumab had significantly improved ORR and OS at 24 months. The trial population included patients with previously treated brain metastases and those treated with prior IL-2 therapy. Efficacy data from this trial led to the approval of ipilimumab in patients with previously treated metastatic melanoma in 2011. In 2015, the approval was further expanded for use as adjuvant therapy in patients with resected stage III melanoma supported by the EORTC 18071 trial (Eggermont et al. 2015, 2016). After a median follow-up of 5.3 years, patients treated with ipilimumab had significantly better

relapse-free survival (RFS), OS and distant metastasis-free survival (DMFS). Despite the clear benefit of ipilimumab, treatment is associated with significant toxicity, with almost all patients expressing toxicity of any grade. Grade 3/4 adverse events occurred in almost 42% of patients with five treatment-related deaths. The dose of ipilimumab used in this trial was 10 mg/kg which is significantly higher than the dose used in the metastatic setting (3 mg/kg) and, thus, may be associated with increased toxicity. This is the approved dose for use in the adjuvant setting.

2.8.2 Nivolumab

In 2016, based on results from early phase studies (Timmerman et al. 2016; Ansell et al. 2015), nivolumab was approved for the treatment of classical HL in patients that relapsed or progressed after ASCT and post-transplantation brentuximab vedotin (BV). The CheckMate 205 (Timmerman et al. 2016) exclusively evaluated nivolumab in patients with classical HL (cHL) including BV-naïve patients and patients who received post-ASCT BV ($n = 240$); the CheckMate 039 (Ansell et al. 2015) was a dose escalation study that included a cohort of patients with cHL ($n = 23$).

Nivolumab has been approved for use in patients with metastatic melanoma in a number of clinical settings. Nivolumab was first approved in 2014 for use in patients with refractory unresectable metastatic melanoma that have progressed following ipilimumab and, if BRAF V600 mutation-positive, a BRAF inhibitor. Approval was based on the findings of phase III CheckMate 037 III trial (Weber et al. 2015a; Larkin et al. 2016). Despite having more patients in the nivolumab arm with brain metastases and higher pretreatment LDH levels, patients treated with nivolumab had a higher ORR and longer median duration of response. In a phase III study of treatment-naive patients with BRAF-wt advanced melanoma, nivolumab demonstrated superior ORR, prolonged PFS and improved OS rate at 1 year when compared with dacarbazine (Robert et al. 2015a).

In 2015, nivolumab was the first immunotherapy agent approved for the treatment of advanced squamous and non-squamous cell cancer (NSCLC), in patients who have progressed on platinum-based chemotherapy based on the findings of phase III CheckMate 017 study (Brahmer et al. 2015). PD-L1 expression was not prognostic or predictive (Brahmer et al. 2015). Phase III CheckMate 057 trial (Borghaei et al. 2015; Horn et al. 2015) randomized patients with advanced non-squamous NSCLC who progressed during or after first-line treatment with platinum-based chemotherapy to nivolumab or docetaxel. Nivolumab showed significantly higher ORRs and longer median OS rates. In patients with PD-L1 expressing tumours ($\geq 1\%$), nivolumab treatment was associated with longer OS, PFS and higher ORR, while OS and PFS were similar between the two arms in patients with PD-L1 negative tumours (<1%). Nivolumab in the first-line setting in patients with NSCLC with $\geq 5\%$ PD-L1 tumour expression failed to show superior PFS versus platinum-based doublet chemotherapy (Socinski et al. 2016).

Patients with advanced clear cell renal cell carcinoma (RCC) treated with nivolumab in phase I and II studies showed one-third of patients were alive at

5 years in phase I study and 3 years in phase II study (McDermott et al. 2016). Interim analysis of phase III CheckMate 025 trial showed patients treated with nivolumab had significantly higher ORR, increased OS and improved quality of life compared with everolimus. PD-L1 expression did not influence survival (Motzer et al. 2015; Cella et al. 2016). Based on these findings, nivolumab was approved for metastatic RCC in late 2015.

In 2016, based on the results of the Checkmate 141 phase III trial (Ferris et al. 2016), nivolumab was approved for the treatment recurrent or metastatic squamous cell carcinoma of the head and neck (SCCHN) in patients who have had disease progression on or after platinum-based therapy. Patients with tumours that had PD-L1 expression ≥ 1% and were HPV-positive derived greatest survival benefit.

Nivolumab has shown activity in patients with metastatic urothelial carcinoma whose disease progressed after previous platinum-based chemotherapy in early phase clinical trials (Sharma et al. 2016, 2017). In a phase I trial (CheckMate 032) (Sharma et al. 2016), an ORR of 24% was achieved with toxicities consistent with previous studies. In the larger single-arm phase II study (CheckMate 275) (Sharma et al. 2017), overall ORR of 19.6% was achieved across all levels of PD-L1 expression. Nivolumab was approved in February 2017.

2.8.3 Pembrolizumab

Pembrolizumab has been approved as first-line treatment for patients with metastatic melanoma as well as for those with ipilimumab-refractory disease. In phase I study (Ribas et al. 2016; Manders et al. 2016), high PD-L1 expression correlated with a higher response rate, longer PFS and OS; however, patients with no PD-L1 expression also showed durable responses. In phase II KEYNOTE-002 trial (Ribas et al. 2015; Hamid et al. 2016), patients treated with pembrolizumab regimens had a significantly improved ORRs and median PFS compared with the chemotherapy group. More than half of patients treated with chemotherapy crossed over and received pembrolizumab after developing progressive disease. In the KEYNOTE-006 trial (Robert et al. 2015b; Long et al. 2016), patients with advanced, refractory melanoma receiving pembrolizumab had significantly higher ORRs, compared to those receiving ipilimumab. Overall survival was significantly prolonged with both pembrolizumab schedules compared with ipilimumab.

Pembrolizumab has been approved for the treatment of patients with pretreated advanced NSCLC that expresses PD-L1 (≥ 1% membranous staining), as determined by the 22C3 pharmDx test. FDA approval was based on the findings of the large phase I study, KEYNOTE-001 (Garon et al. 2015). Response rates correlated with PD-L1 expression, but were independent of dose and schedule of pembrolizumab and tumour histology. The large KEYNOTE-010 study (Herbst et al. 2016) enrolled over 1000 previously treated patients with advanced NSCLC, with PD-L1 expression at least 1%. Patients treated with pembrolizumab had a greater survival benefit compared with docetaxel. Responses and survival rates directly correlated with PD-L1 expression. The KEYNOTE-024 trial (Reck et al. 2016) evaluated pembrolizumab as first-line therapy in treatment-naive patients with advanced NSCLC having ≥ 50% tumour cell PD-L1 staining. Patients with EGFR mutations or ALK translocations were not included. Pembrolizumab was associated with prolonged PFS and improved OS at six months compared with platinum doublet chemotherapy. Based on these results, the FDA in 2016 approved pembrolizumab as first-line therapy for patients with metastatic NSCLC whose tumours have $\geq 50\%$ PD-L1 without EGFR or ALK genomic tumour aberrations.

In 2016, pembrolizumab received accelerated approval for the treatment of patients with recurrent or metastatic SCCHN with disease progression on or after platinum-containing chemotherapy, based on data from the KEYNOTE-012 study (Seiwert et al. 2016; Chow et al. 2016). Response rates were similar in human papillomavirus (HPV)-positive and negative patients.

In phase Ib KEYNOTE-013 study (Armand et al. 2016), pembrolizumab showed high anti-tumour activity (ORR = 65%) in refractory classical Hodgkin lymphoma (cHL) patients. Based on the results of the phase II KEYNOTE-087 study in patients with refractory cHL (Chen et al. 2016b; Moskowitz et al. 2016), pembrolizumab recieved regulatory approval for the treatment of relapsed or refractory cHL in 2017.

2.8.4 Avelumab

Avelumab is an anti-PD-L1 antibody, approved in March 2017, for use in patients with metastatic Merkel cell carcinoma based on the results of the JAVELIN Merkel 200 trial (Kaufman et al. 2016). In this single-arm study, avelumab demonstrated an ORR of 32%, including 8 complete responses. Responses were durable, lasting more than six months in 86% of patients, and more than 12 months in 45% of patients (Kaufman et al. 2016). Avelumab is the first FDA-approved drug to treat this indication.

2.8.5 Atezolizumab

Atezolizumab is the first a humanized anti-PD-L1 monoclonal antibody approved for the treatment of advanced urothelial carcinoma that has progressed during or after previous platinum-based chemotherapy (Rosenberg et al. 2016). While responses correlated with PD-L1 expression, objective responses were also seen in patients with no PD-L1 expression.

Atezolizumab is the first anti-PD-L1 antibody to be approved for the treatment of previously treated patients with metastatic NSCLC based on results from the randomized phase III OAK (Rittmeyer et al. 2017; Barlesi et al. 2016) and phase II POPLAR studies (Fehrenbacher et al. 2016). In both studies, greatest benefit was seen in patients with high PD-L1 expression on tumours or tumour-infiltrating immune cells.

2.9 Combination of Immune Checkpoint Inhibitors

2.9.1 Nivolumab and Ipilimumab

In early phase clinical trials in patients with metastatic melanoma, the combination of nivolumab and ipilimumab has shown to result in improved overall responses and OS, albeit increased grade 3/4 toxicities (Wolchok et al. 2013; Postow et al. 2015;

Hodi et al. 2016). In a large phase III study, CheckMate 067, the combination resulted in a longer median PFS and higher response rates in treatment-naïve patients with metastatic melanoma, with the greatest benefit seen in those with positive PD-L1 expression. As seen with the early phase studies, grade 3/4 adverse events were significantly higher in the combination arm, leading to discontinuation of treatment in more than a third of patients (Larkin et al. 2015; Wolchok et al. 2016). In 2015, nivolumab in combination with ipilimumab was approved for use in treatment-naive patients with BRAF wild-type metastatic melanoma. This indication was further expanded to include BRAF V600 mutation-positive patients in 2016.

Early phase trials report higher response rates with the combination of nivolumab and ipilimumab in patients with mRCC than with PD-1 inhibition alone (Hammers et al. 2014; Motzer et al. 2014). A phase III trial comparing nivolumab plus ipilimumab to sunitinib in treatment-naive mRCC patients is ongoing (NCT02231749).

The CheckMate 012 study evaluated three dosing schedules of nivolumab plus ipilimumab in chemo-naive patients with NSCLC (Hellmann et al. 2017). Confirmed objective responses were seen in 38–47% with higher responses seen in those with PD-L1 expression $\geq 1\%$. Phase I/II study, CheckMate 032, evaluated the efficacy and safety of nivolumab alone and in different dosing combinations with ipilimumab in patients with platinum-refractory small cell lung cancer (SCLC) (Antonia et al. 2016). While durable responses were seen with nivolumab monotherapy, higher response rates were seen when nivolumab was combined with ipilimumab; however, this also resulted in higher grade 3/4 treatment-related adverse events.

2.9.2 Pembrolizumab and Ipilimumab

In phase I KEYNOTE-029 non-randomized expansion cohort (NCT02089685), patients with metastatic melanoma received pembrolizumab with ipilimumab followed by pembrolizumab monotherapy. After a median follow-up of 17 months, the ORR was 61%, with a CR achieved in 15%; the median PFS and OS rates were not reached (Carlino et al. 2017). In the same trial, patients with previously treated mRCC had a DCR of 50% and ORR of 20% with two PRs (Choueiri et al. 2017). In a phase I/II study, pembrolizumab in combination with pazopanib in mRCC was prematurely terminated due to significant hepatotoxicity with the combination (Chowdhury et al. 2017).

Toxicities Associated with Immune Checkpoint Inhibitors
Fatigue is among the most common side effect reported with immune checkpoint inhibitors and has been reported in almost 40% of patients treated with ipilimumab and anti-PD-1 agents and in up to 24% of patients treated with anti-PD-L1 agents (Naidoo et al. 2015). Dermatological toxicities have been reported in almost half of all patients treated, although less than 2% are considered severe (grade 3 or 4) (Naidoo et al. 2015). Dermatological irAEs typically manifest early, occurring after

the third week of treatment (Weber et al. 2012), however can occur at any time during treatment, including after treatment discontinuation (Parakh et al. 2016b). Gastrointestinal toxicities associated with ipilimumab typically occur 6–8 weeks after commencement of therapy (Weber et al. 2012), with diarrhoea of any grade reported in approximately 30%; however, severe (grade 3/4) diarrhoea is seen in <10% of patients (Hodi et al. 2010b). In comparison, gastrointestinal toxicities associated with anti-PD1 inhibitors have a lower incidence and grade 3/4 immune-mediated colitis is seen in 1–2% of cases (Topalian et al. 2014). Clinically significant endocrinopathy occurs in <10% of patients treated with ipilimumab and may present with nonspecific symptoms such as such as nausea, headache, fatigue and vision changes, often leading to delayed diagnosis (Corsello et al. 2013). Significant endocrinopathies reported include hypophysitis, hypothyroidism, hyperthyroidism and adrenal insufficiency. The incidence of endocrinopathies due to anti-PD-1/PD-L1 antibodies is not known, and the mechanism underlying it is not fully elucidated. Hepatic adverse events typically occur 8–12 weeks after commencing treatment (Bernardo et al. 2013; Wolchok et al. 2010) and are usually present as asymptomatic elevations in AST and ALT levels (Postow 2015). The incidence is <5% with anti-PD-1/PD-L1, and grade 3/4 toxicity is rare (Hamid et al. 2013). Pathologic appearances of immune-checkpoint-inhibitor-induced autoimmune hepatitis include panlobular hepatitis, perivenular infiltrates or infiltrates surrounding the primary biliary ducts (Kim et al. 2013). Pneumonitis has been rarely described with ipilimumab therapy and is more commonly reported in association with PD-1 inhibitors (Weber et al. 2015b). Pneumonitis has been reported in <10% of patients receiving anti-PD-1/PD-L1 therapy either alone or in combination and occurs more commonly in patients with lung cancer (Brahmer et al. 2015; Rizvi et al. 2015). The incidence of adverse events is typically more frequent and more severe with higher doses of ipilimumab and with combined immunotherapy regimens (Eggermont et al. 2015; Larkin et al. 2015). Rare toxicities involving other organ systems have been reported with ipilimumab and anti-PD1 therapies (Naidoo et al. 2015). Investigation and management of immune-related adverse events should be managed as per established algorithms (YERVOY™ (ipilimumab) 2011).

Mechanisms of Resistance to Immune Checkpoint Inhibitors

Comparing pretreatment and relapse tumour samples of patients with metastatic melanoma who initially responded to treatment, mutations in genes encoding JAK1 or JAK2 were identified resulting in insensitivity to the anti-proliferative effects of interferon γ on cancer cells as well as a truncating mutation in the gene for the antigen-presenting protein beta-2-microglobulin (B2M) leading to loss of expression of major histocompatibility complex (MHC) (Zaretsky et al. 2016). Other proposed mechanisms of resistance to immune checkpoint therapies include loss of PTEN inhibiting the recruitment of T cells and increasing expression of immunosuppressive cytokines (Peng et al. 2016); upregulation of genes involving regulation of mesenchymal transition, cell adhesion, extracellular matrix remodelling and angiogenesis (Hugo et al. 2016); expression of indoleamine 2,3-dioxygenase (IDO) which suppresses effector T cells and activates regulatory T cells (Holmgaard et al. 2013).

2.10 Anti-VEGF Antibodies

Vascular endothelial growth factor (VEGF) A is a member of a family of growth factors that also includes VEGFB, VEGFC, VEGFD and placental growth factor (PLGF). VEGF-A secreted by tumour cells, and surrounding stroma drives the proliferation of endothelial cells and development of abnormal vasculature (Carmeliet 2005). VEGF is typically overexpressed in tumours and correlates with invasiveness, increased vascular density, metastasis, tumour recurrence and poor prognosis (Kerbel 2008).

2.10.1 Bevacizumab
Bevacizumab is the first approved humanized monoclonal antibody targeting VEGF-A, preventing the interaction of VEGF to its receptors (Flt-1 and KDR) on the surface of endothelial cells (Ferrara et al. 2004). Bevacizumab has been approved in combination with chemotherapy for the treatment of a number of tumour types including mCRC (Hurwitz et al. 2004; Giantonio et al. 2007), metastatic ovarian cancer (Pujade-Lauraine et al. 2014), metastatic clear cell renal cell carcinomas (mRCC) (Lonser et al. 2003), recurrent GBM (Friedman et al. 2009; Cloughesy et al. 2010) and NSCLC (Sandler et al. 2006; Soria et al. 2012).

2.10.2 Ramucirumab
Ramucirumab is a fully humanized monoclonal antibody targeting the extracellular domain of VEGF receptor-2 (VEGFR-2). Ramucirumab has been approved as monotherapy and in combination with paclitaxel chemotherapy for the treatment of patients with advanced gastric or GEJ adenocarcinoma whose disease has progressed on fluoropyrimidine- or platinum-containing chemotherapy based on the findings of the placebo-controlled REGARD (Fuchs et al. 2014) and RAINBOW (Wilke et al. 2014) trials, respectively.

In late 2014, ramucirumab was approved in combination with docetaxel as second-line therapy for patients with metastatic NSCLC who have received platinum-based chemotherapy. Approval was based on the findings of the REVEL study (Garon et al. 2014).

The efficacy of ramucirumab as second-line treatment in combination with FOLFIRI in patients with mCRC who progressed after first-line therapy with bevacizumab and FOLFOX chemotherapy was addressed in phase III RAISE trial (Tabernero et al. 2015). In view of the modest but significant benefit, ramucirumab was approved for use as second-line therapy in combination with FOLFIRI in 2015.

Toxicities Associated with Anti-VEGF Therapies

Bevacizumab and ramucirumab are generally well tolerated; discontinuation rates due to bevacizumab-related toxicity across all studies are between 8.4 and 21% (Braghiroli et al. 2012). Hypertension is the most common adverse event associated with anti-VEGF therapies (Spratlin et al. 2010). A meta-analysis showed the incidence of all-grade hypertension in patients receiving bevacizumab in variety of tumour types was 23.6% with 8% being grade ≥ 3 (Ranpura et al. 2010). Due to the high incidence of fatal pulmonary haemorrhage (31%), bevacizumab is contraindicated in patients with squamous cell NSCLC (Johnson et al. 2004). The incidence of $\geq$ grade 3 proteinuria ranged from 0.7 to 7.4% across clinical trials (Liu et al. 2010b); the incidence increased when using bevacizumab in combination with chemotherapy; using higher dosages of bevacizumab and tumour type, renal cell carcinoma was associated with the highest risk (cumulative incidence 10.2%) (Wu et al. 2010). While the exact mechanism of proteinuria is unclear and is likely a maybe a class effect of VEGF inhibitors (Eremina et al. 2003; Sugimoto et al. 2003). Fatal hemorrhage is more likely to occur in patients receiving bevacizumab compared to those on chemotherapy only, with the incidence of grade ≥ 3 hemorrhagic events 0.4–6.9% (Liu et al. 2010b; Hapani et al. 2010). The risk of bleeding was more with higher doses of bevacizumab and in patients with NSCLC (11.5%). Patients with primary brain tumours are not at higher risk of haemorrhage when compared to patients with other tumour types (Hapani et al. 2010). Mechanisms of bevacizumab-induced haemorrhage include impaired platelet activation, endothelial damage affecting vascular integrity, and deregulation of nitric oxide affecting platelet–endothelium interaction (Brandes et al. 2015). Patients treated with bevacizumab are at increased risk of venous and arterial thromboembolism, with an overall incidence of approximately 7.5 and 3.8%, respectively (Semrad et al. 2007; Scappaticci et al. 2007). The risk of developing an arterial thromboembolic event during treatment was increased in patients with a prior history of thromboembolism and diabetes and in elderly patients (Scappaticci et al. 2007). While the incidence of gastrointestinal perforation due to bevacizumab treatment is less than 1%, it is associated with a high mortality rate of 21.7%. Patients receiving a higher dose of bevacizumab, prior to radiation treatment, and those with GBM, colorectal, ovarian and renal cell cancer were at higher risk (Liu et al. 2010b; Hapani et al. 2009). Consistent with bevacizumab's mechanism of action, wound breakdown rates range 0–6% and is due to impaired cicatrization and platelet activation, mechanisms vital in wound repair (Liu et al. 2010b). Other rare but serious complications include posterior reversible encephalopathy syndrome. The addition of ramucirumab to chemotherapy resulted in higher number of grade ≥ 3 toxicities when compared to chemotherapy alone; in particular, a higher incidence neutropenic events, leucopenia, hypertension and fatigue were reported (Wilke et al. 2014; Garon et al. 2014; Tabernero et al. 2015).

Mechanisms of Resistance to Anti-VEGF Antibodies

A number of mechanisms of resistance to VEGF inhibitors have been proposed and covered in detail in a number of review papers (Van Beijnum et al. 2015; Bergers and Hanahan 2008). Some of the key mechanisms are discussed below. The activation of angiogenesis pathways can occur through the upregulation of alternate pro-angiogenic growth factors including angiopoietins, fibroblast growth factors (FGFs), transforming growth factors (TGFs) and placental growth factor (PlGF). Moreover, inhibition of a specific growth factor has shown to induce the expression of other growth factors depending on the tumour type. The expression of many growth factors has shown to be induced by hypoxia in preclinical and clinical models, which occurs as a result of the anti-angiogenic therapy. Another mechanism of resistance proposed is the infiltration of bone-marrow-derived cells into the tumour microenvironment which leads to tumour growth and angiogenesis through VEGF-independent pathways. These cells include monocytes/macrophages, myeloid-derived suppressor cells (MDSC), endothelial progenitor cells (EPC) and cancer-associated fibroblasts (CAF) (Ferrara 2010). Disruption of endothelial cell progenitor function by anti-VEGFR2 monoclonal antibodies results in decreased angiogenesis in tumour xenografts and inhibits tumour growth (Shaked et al. 2005). Pericytes or periendothelial cells regulate endothelial differentiation and proliferation and stabilize newly formed vessels (Teicher and Ellis 2008). Moreover, they have shown to have a protective effect on endothelial cells from anti-angiogenic therapies and have been implicated in clinical resistance to these agents (Bergers and Hanahan 2008). Other mechanisms by which tumour cells evade effects of anti-VEGF therapy is through the development of different growth patterns (Hillen and Griffioen 2007) including intussusceptive angiogenesis, vessel co-option and vasculogenic mimicry (Van Beijnum et al. 2015).

2.11 Immunotoxins

Denileukin diftitox is the first FDA-approved immunotoxin for the treatment of recurrent cutaneous T cell lymphoma (CTCL). This fusion protein–toxin combines the truncated form of DT (DAB389) to IL-2 protein, enabling the targeting of the CD25 subunit of the IL-2 receptor (Re et al. 1996). In the pivotal phase III trial, 30% of the 71 patients with pretreated CTCL randomized to two doses of denileukin diftitox had an objective response (20% CR; 10% PR) with a 6.9-month median duration of response. No difference in efficacy was noted between the two doses. Toxicities reported included flu-like symptoms, acute infusion-related events, VLS and elevations of hepatic transaminases. Nearly all patients developed HATA by the second treatment (Olsen et al. 2001). The potency of denileukin diftitox is limited because of the lack of high affinity IL-2 receptors in a large percentage of cases, usually owing to lack of CD122 (Kreitman 2009). Denileukin diftitox has also been evaluated in combination with other treatments for haematological and solid cancers including melanoma (Telang et al. 2011), non-small cell lung cancer (NSCLC) (Gerena-Lewis et al. 2009), pancreatic (NCT00726037; this study has been terminated) and ovarian cancers (Barnett et al. 2006). In NSCLC, high levels of soluble IL-2R have been associated with early recurrence and a poorer outcome (Naumnik and Chyczewska 2000; Kawashima et al. 2000), while the inhibitory effect of denileukin diftitox on human regulatory T cells resulted in clinical improvements in patients with ovarian cancer and melanoma.

2.12   Radioimmunotherapy

2.12.1   Iodine-131 Recombinant Chimeric Tumour Necrosis Therapy

Iodine-131 recombinant chimeric tumour necrosis therapy (^{131}I-chTNT) is the first radioimmunoconjugate to be approved in 2003, for the treatment of advanced lung cancer by the China Food and Drug Administration. ^{131}I-chTNT has not been approved for this indication in the USA or European Union (EU). TNT-1 targets an intracellular histone/DNA epitope present in necrotic and degenerating areas of tumours. In the pivotal study, 62 of a total of 107 patients with treatment-refractory solid tumours received two doses of ^{131}I-chTNT, while another 45 patients received an intratumoral injection. An ORR of 34.6% was achieved (CR in 3.7% and PR 30.8%) in all patients and 33% in patients with NSCLC. Due to the study design, the impact of treatment on OS is not established.

2.12.2   Ibritumomab Tiuxetan

Ibritumomab tiuxetan comprises of the murine IgG1 anti-CD20 antibody ibritumomab bound to tiuxetan, a chelator agent, covalently linked to the radiolabeled isotope ^{90}Y (Witzig 2002). Y90 is pure emitting beta radioisotope with a penetration of only 5–10 mm at an energy of 2.3 MeV (Witzig 2002). Initial approval for ibritumomab tiuxetan was based on the findings of the pivotal phase III study (Wiseman et al. 2002), in which patients with relapsed or refractory disease were randomized to receive either Y90 ibritumomab tiuxetan or rituximab. Compared to rituximab, patients that received ibritumomab tiuxetan experienced higher ORR, time to next therapy and time to progression, with greatest benefit seen in patients with follicular histology (Gordon et al. 2004).

In a phase III trial (First-Line Indolent trial) (Hagenbeek et al. 2007; Morschhauser et al. 2013), the benefits of ibritumomab tiuxetan as consolidation therapy after induction therapies was evaluated in patients with advanced-stage follicular lymphoma in first remission. After a median follow-up of 7.3 years, PFS was significantly improved with ibritumomab tiuxetan with a prolonged median time to next treatment. The beneficial effects were superior in patients that experienced a PR after induction treatment compared with patients that had a CR (Morschhauser et al. 2008, 2013). It should be noted however only 14% of subjects received rituximab during the induction phase. The efficacy and safety of ibritumomab tiuxetan as consolidation therapy post-chemotherapy has been shown by several additional trials (Hainsworth et al. 2009; Jacobs et al. 2008; Provencio et al. 2014).

Common Toxicities

Common toxicities reported with radioimmunotherapy (RIT) are infusion reactions, cytopenias, and cutaneous and mucocutaneous reactions, with discontinuation of treatment required in cases where toxicities have prolonged and severe (Rizzieri 2016). Cytopenias are commonly seen 4–6 weeks post-treatment, with recovery 9–20 days after nadir; however, severe cytopenias persisting more than 12 weeks can occur and are influenced by the presence of bone marrow involvement and prior treatment (Witzig et al. 1999; Knox et al. 1996). There is an increased incidence of myelodysplastic syndrome (MDS) and acute myeloid leukaemia (AML) in patients treated with RIT. In the FIT trial, after a median follow-up of 7.3 years, 4.2% patients treated with RIT consolidation developed treatment-related MDS/AM, with a median time from randomization to diagnosis of MDS/AML 57 months (range 22–84) (Morschhauser et al. 2013). Previous exposure to fludarabine-containing regimens and an abnormally low baseline platelet count are associated with significantly higher rates of MDS/AML. In another study in elderly patients with NHL who underwent an autograft after high-dose radioimmunotherapy (HD-RIT) the 5-year cumulative incidence of sMDS/AML was 8.2% (Guidetti et al. 2011).

2.13 Trifunctional Antibody

Catumaxomab was the first-in-class trifunctional antibody to be approved in 2009 in the EU for the intraperitoneal\treatment of malignant ascites secondary to epithelial cancers. It is characterized by its unique ability to target epithelial cell adhesion molecules (EpCAM) on tumour cells, CD3 antigen on T cells, and type I, IIa, and III Fcγ receptors on accessory cells (Ruf et al. 2007). Catumaxomab exerts its anti-tumour effects via T-cell-mediated lysis, ADCC and phagocytosis via activation of Fcγ receptors on accessory cells (Zeidler et al. 1999, 2000). In a pivotal phase II/III study (Heiss et al. 2010), patients were randomized to receive catumaxomab plus paracentesis or paracentesis alone. The primary endpoint was puncture-free survival (defined as the time after last infusion to first need for therapeutic paracentesis or death, whichever occurred first). Treatment with catumaxomab significantly prolonged puncture-free survival (median 46 vs. 11 days; $p < 0.0001$) and median time to next paracentesis (77 vs. 13 days; $p < 0.0001$). In addition, there was a trend towards prolonged OS with catumaxomab.

Toxicities Associated with Catumaxomab

Catumaxomab was generally well tolerated, over 80% of patients received the full treatment course, and most adverse events were reported as low grade (Heiss et al. 2010). The most common drug-related adverse events were cytokine-release-related symptoms. Other toxicities included transient derangement of liver function and transient lymphopenia, lymphocytosis and anaemia. Symptomatic grade 3/4 adverse reactions were experienced by 37.5% of the catumaxomab patients in the pivotal study, and most were managed with symptomatic treatment.

3 Novel Antibodies

Despite the success of monoclonal antibodies, patients do not adequately respond to monospecific therapy, and resistance to treatment or tumour recurrence is often observed.

3.1 Bispecific Antibodies

Compared to monotherapy, using either two antibodies to target a receptor or combinatorial approaches with monoclonal antibodies and standard therapies is more effective and may abrogate resistance. Previous strategies to target dual domains of the same receptor have typically involved two different antibodies. Bispecific antibodies (bsAbs) are uniquely developed antibodies capable of binding two different epitopes, on the same or different antigens. Examples of novel bispecific antibodies in development are summarized in the table. Bispecific antibodies are produced through a variety of methods including through quadroma (hybrid hydrioma) technology, knobs-into-holes approach, CrossMAb approach, molecular cloning techniques and dual-variable-domain (DVD) immunoglobulin approach. There are two major classes of bispecific antibodies: immunoglobulin-G (IgG)-like bsAbs and small single-chain Fv (scFv)-based bsAbs. The IgG-like bispecific antibodies have a conserved constant domain and thus maintain Fc-mediated effector functions and IgG-like pharmacokinetic properties. Small scFv-based or diabody-based bsAbs are genetically engineered recombinant antibodies lacking a constant domain. They are characterized by a short half-life, high tumour specificity and tissue penetration, making them more attractive as potential therapeutics than IgG-like bsAbs. The structure of ScFvs depends on linker length, antibody sequence and external factors and is designed for use as effector cell recruiters, in particular as T cell engagers.

A promising new development is the construction of a novel bi- and tri-specific immunotoxins using anti-CD19 and anti-CD22 antibody fragments, with preclinical models showing improved therapeutic efficacy than monomeric or bivalent immunotoxins made with anti-CD19 and anti-CD22 sFv alone (Vallera et al. 2005; Flavell et al. 1997; Herrera et al. 2000). In another study, a bispecific immunotoxin comprising an anti-HER2 scFv fused to a diphtheria toxin–anti-EpCAM immunotoxin was generated for the treatment of solid tumours overexpressing HER2 and EpCAM (Stish et al. 2009). Compared with monospecific immunotoxins, increased cytotoxicity towards tumour cells expressing both antigens was observed in vitro and in xenograft tumour models. An obvious concern with this approach is the potential of enhanced toxin-related side effects with the delivery of two mAbs.

3.2 Antibody-Conjugated Therapies

By utilizing the specificity of monoclonal antibodies, potent therapeutic agents linked to antibodies can be directly delivered into tumour cells, minimizing toxicity and increasing therapeutic efficacy (Scott et al. 2012). Antibody-conjugated therapies (ACTs) comprise of three basic components: antibody, linker and payload. The effectiveness of an ACT is dependent on a number of critical factors relating to each component. These include antigen specificity and high expression of the target antigen on tumour cells, a homogeneous expression of antigen within the tumour microenvironment and increased copy number ratio of surface antigen on tumour populations (Scott et al. 2012; Teicher and Chari 2011). Stability, site of conjugation and final drug/antibody ratio (DAR) are essential parameters that impact on toxicity, efficacy and pharmacokinetic properties of the ACT, while rapid internalization of antibody conjugates and linker stability limit off-target toxicity (Bander 2013). Furthermore, this antigen should not be secreted back into the circulation limiting the potential for off-target exposure (Ritchie et al. 2013). The action of the payload once it has been released from the antibody carrier vehicle then defines the outcome of the therapeutic agent. Selection of a mAb with therapeutic efficacy of its own is also highly desirable as seen with trastuzumab within the ACT TDM-1 (Hurvitz et al. 2013; Dieras et al. 2010). The mechanisms of action of ACTs are summarized in Fig. 1, and examples of novel ADC in development are shown in Table 3. Significant strides have been made in the development of this class of therapeutics, and an overview of some promising agents in advanced clinical testing is provided here.

3.2.1 Antibody–Drug Conjugates

The monoclonal antibody, 806 (mAb806), has shown to bind to a conformationally exposed region of EGFR that is only expressed in tumour cells (Gan et al. 2012). In vitro studies demonstrated the ability of mAb806 to inhibit EGFR activation and signalling, inhibit proliferation and induce apoptosis (Gan et al. 2012). It has significant therapeutic efficacy as monotherapy and in conjunction with other therapeutics, as well as remarkable tumour specificity and uptake in tumour models (Johns et al. 2002). ABT-414 comprises the mAb806 linked to a cytotoxic payload of monomethyl auristatin F (MMAF). Preclinical data shows activity in tumour models overexpressing wild-type EGFR, EGFR amplification or EGFRvIII mutation (Luwor et al. 2001). A large phase I trial (Lassman et al. 2015) evaluated ABT-414 with radiotherapy and temozolomide (TMZ) in patients with newly diagnosed glioblastoma (GBM) (Arm A), with TMZ in patients with newly diagnosed glioblastoma who have just completed radiation and TMZ or recurrent GBM (Arm B) or as monotherapy in patients with recurrent GBM (Arm C). Almost a third of patients with recurrent GBM treated with ABT-414 as monotherapy (Arm C) were progression-free at six months (Lassman et al. 2016), when given in combination with temozolomide (Arm B) a response rate of 28% including a complete response which is ongoing at 20 months was reported. In patients with

Table 3 Examples of novel bispecific antibodies in clinical development

Antibody	Target	Indication	Development phase
Bispecific trifunctional antibody			
Catumaxomab	EpCAM CD3	Intraperitoneal treatment of malignant ascites	Approved
Ertumaxomab	HER2 CD3	HER2-overexpressing/amplified tumours	Phase I (Haense et al. 2016)
Bispecific T cell engager			
Blinatumomab[a]	CD19 CD3	Relapsed or refractory ALL	Approved (Topp et al. 2015)
Solitomab (MT110)	EpCAM CD3	Solid tumours	Phase I completed (NCT00635596)
AMG 330	CD33 CD3	Relapsed or refractory AML	Phase I recruiting (NCT02520427)
AMG-212 BAY-2010112 MT-112	PSMA CD3	Hormone-refractory prostate cancer	Phase I completed recruiting (NCT01723475)
MT111 (MEDI-565)	CEA CD3	Gastrointestinal adenocarcinoma	Phase I completed (NCT01284231)
CrossMAb			
Vanucizumab	Ang2 VEGF	Untreated metastatic colorectal cancer—in combination with FOLFOX	Phase II—completed (NCT02141295)
		Solid tumours—monotherapy and in combination with atezolizumab	Phase I—completed recruitment (NCT01688206)
		Solid tumours—in combination with a novel anti-CD40 antibody (RO7009789)	Phase I (NCT02665416)
		Solid tumours—in combination with other treatments	Phase I (NCT02715531)
Immune-mobilizing monoclonal T cell receptors against cancer (ImmTACs)			
IMCgp100	CD3 gp100	Malignant melanoma	Phase I—completed (NCT01211262; NCT01209676)
		Uveal melanoma	Phase I recruiting (NCT02570308)
		Cutaneous melanoma—in combination with durvalumab and/or tremelimumab	Phase I/II recruiting (NCT02535078)
Tetravalent bispecific tandem diabody (TandAb)			
AFM11	CD19 CD3	Relapsed or Refractory Adult B-precursor ALL	Phase I recruiting (NCT02848911)
AFM13			
Dual-affinity re-targeting (DART)			
MGD006	CD3 \CD123		
DVD-Ig			
ABT-165			

[a]In July 2017, the FDA approved blinatumomab for the treatment of relapsed or refractory B cell precursor ALL in adults and children

newly diagnosed GBM, the median PFS was 6.1 months and the median overall survival has not been reached. ABT-414 is currently in phase II/III registration trials in GBM patients (INTELANCE I (NCT02573324), INTELLANCE II (NCT02343406)).

Labetuzumab govitecan (IMMU-130) is a conjugate of a humanized antibody to carcinoembryonic antigen-related cell adhesion molecule 5 (CEACAM5), linked to the active metabolite of irinotecan, SN-38. Metastatic colon xenograft models treated with IMMU-130 showed significant anti-tumour activity and improved median survival compared to untreated mice and are superior to 5FU/leucovorin chemotherapy. Furthermore, combining IMMU-130 with bevacizumab resulted in improved efficacy (Govindan et al. 2015). After an initial phase I dose escalation study (Segal et al. 2013) in patients with treatment-refractory mCRC, four dose schedules of IMMU-130 were evaluated in phase II portion of the study (NCT01605318). Patients had a median of five prior therapies, and all patients had prior irinotecan-containing therapy. Most frequent treatment-related AEs were nausea, fatigue, vomiting and diarrhoea. Most common grade 3/4 AEs were neutropenia (15%), anaemia (6%) and diarrhoea (2%). The interim PFS and OS rates were highest in the 10 mg/kg cohort with a median PFS 4.6 months and median OS 9.3 months (Dotan et al. 2016). This dose has been taken forward for further clinical evaluation.

Sacituzumab govitecan (IMMU-132) is an antibody–drug conjugate composed of the active metabolite of irinotecan, SN-38, conjugated to an anti-Trop-2 antibody (Goldenberg et al. 2015). Sacituzumab govitecan has significant anti-tumour activity in a variety of Trop-2-positive xenograft models, including NSCLC, pancreatic, colon, gastric cancers and triple-negative breast cancer (TNBC) (Cardillo et al. 2011, 2015). Furthermore, combining IMMU-132 with a PARP inhibitor resulted in synergistic growth inhibition and anti-tumour activity in TNBC models irrespective of BRCA1/2 status when compared to monotherapy (Cardillo et al. 2017). In a phase I, heavily pretreated patients with TNBC treated with sacituzumab govitecan had an ORR 30%, including two patients with complete responses. The median response duration was 8.9, with responses occurring early, with a median onset of 1.9 months. Median PFS was 6.0 months, and median OS 16.6 months. There were three durable responses seen that lasted 13–21 months. Grade $\geq$ 3 adverse events included neutropenia (39%), leucopenia (16%), anaemia (14%) and diarrhoea (13%) (Bardia et al. 2017). In an ongoing phase I/II study (NCT01631552), sacituzumab govitecan has shown clinical activity across a variety of pretreated tumour types (Bardia et al. 2015; Tagawa et al. 2017; Camidge et al. 2016; Starodub et al. 2015). Based on the encouraging results from phase II study, sacituzumab govitecan received Breakthrough Therapy designation from FDA for the treatment of patients with triple-negative breast cancer who have failed at least 2 prior therapies for metastatic disease. A phase III study is being planned (NCT02574455).

Glembatumumab vedotin is a fully humanized monoclonal ADC that targets glycoprotein non-metastatic b (gpNMB), a transmembrane protein involved in metastasis and invasion (Maric et al. 2013). The gpNMB is shown to be overexpressed in a variety of tumour types including basal/triple-negative subtype breast cancer, melanoma, lung, pancreatic, head and neck cancer or osteosarcoma and shown to poor prognostic marker in patients with breast cancer (Rose et al. 2010; Halim et al. 2016). It is composed of the gpNMB-targeting antibody, CR011, linked to the potent cytotoxic, monomethyl auristatin E (MMAE) (Tse et al. 2006). Preclinical studies have shown glembatumumab vedotin inhibited the growth of GPNMB-positive melanoma cells in vitro and induced tumour regression in melanoma xenograft models (Tse et al. 2006; Pollack et al. 2007). A phase II, open-label study of glembatumumab vedotin in patients with advanced melanoma who had progressed on prior immune checkpoint therapy and BRAF/MEK targeted agents, if indicated, showed an objective response in 11% patients with a median duration of response 6.0 months. More than half the patients experienced disease control and tumour shrinkage. The median PFS was 4.4 months. A positive correlation between development of skin toxicity and response was noted (Ott et al. 2016). In a phase I/II study, heavily pretreated patients with advanced breast cancer, including patients with triple-negative disease, treatment with glembatumumab vedotin resulted in tumour shrinkage as well as palliation of bone pain (Peacock et al. 2009). The pivotal phase II study, METRIC (NCT01997333), is currently recruiting patients with TNBC, and results are keenly awaited. Glembatumumab vedotin is also being evaluated in uveal melanoma (NCT02363283).

PSMA ADC is fully humanized monoclonal antibody linked via a protease-cleavable linker to the cytotoxic component, MMAE. PSMA ADC showed anti-tumour activity in prostate cancer-derived xenografts which correlated with PSMA expression (DiPippo et al. 2015). A phase I study involving patients with taxane refractory metastatic prostate cancer (mCRPC) confirmed tolerability of PSMA ADC with main grade 3/4 toxicities neutropenia and peripheral neuropathy (Petrylak et al. 2011). Anti-tumour activity and reductions in circulating tumour cells and PSA were seen with PSMA ADC treatment in patients with mCRPC that had progressed following treatment with abiraterone and/or enzalutamide in a phase II study. In this study, a third of patients were chemo-naïve (Petrylak et al. 2015). PSMA ADC showed no activity in patients with progressive GBM and was associated with dose-limiting toxicity (Elinzano et al. 2016).

3.3 Immunotoxins

A promising new development is the construction of a novel bi- and tri-specific immunotoxins using anti-CD19 and anti-CD22 antibody fragments, with preclinical models showing improved therapeutic efficacy than monomeric or bivalent immunotoxins made with anti-CD19 and anti-CD22 sFv alone (Vallera et al. 2005; Flavell et al. 1997; Herrera et al. 2000). In another study, a bispecific immunotoxin comprising an anti-HER2 scFv fused to a diphtheria toxin–anti-EpCAM immunotoxin was generated for the treatment of solid tumours overexpressing HER2 and EpCAM (Stish et al. 2009). Compared with monospecific immunotoxins, increased cytotoxicity towards tumour cells expressing both antigens was observed in vitro and in xenograft tumour models. An obvious concern with this approach is the potential of enhanced toxin-related side effects with the delivery of two monoclonal antibodies.

References

Adams CW, Allison DE, Flagella K, Presta L, Clarke J, Dybdal N et al (2006) Humanization of a recombinant monoclonal antibody to produce a therapeutic HER dimerization inhibitor, pertuzumab. Cancer Immunol Immunother 55(6):717–727

Aghajanian C, Blank SV, Goff BA, Judson PL, Teneriello MG, Husain A et al (2012) OCEANS: a randomized, double-blind, placebo-controlled phase III trial of chemotherapy with or without bevacizumab in patients with platinum-sensitive recurrent epithelial ovarian, primary peritoneal, or fallopian tube cancer. J Clin Oncol 30(17):2039–2045

Aghajanian C, Goff B, Nycum LR, Wang YV, Husain A, Blank SV (2015) Final overall survival and safety analysis of OCEANS, a phase 3 trial of chemotherapy with or without bevacizumab in patients with platinum-sensitive recurrent ovarian cancer. Gynecol Oncol 139(1):10–16

Amado RG, Wolf M, Peeters M, Van Cutsem E, Siena S, Freeman DJ et al (2008) Wild-type KRAS is required for panitumumab efficacy in patients with metastatic colorectal cancer. J Clin Oncol 26(10):1626–1634

Andrulis IL, Bull SB, Blackstein ME, Sutherland D, Mak C, Sidlofsky S et al (1998) neu/erbB-2 amplification identifies a poor-prognosis group of women with node-negative breast cancer. Toronto Breast Cancer Study Group. J Clin Oncol 16(4):1340–1349

Ansell S, Armand P, Timmerman JM, Shipp MA, Garelik MBB, Zhu L et al (2015) Nivolumab in patients (pts) with relapsed or refractory classical Hodgkin lymphoma (R/R cHL): clinical outcomes from extended follow-up of a phase 1 study (CA209-039). Blood 126(23):583

Antonia SJ, López-Martin JA, Bendell J, Ott PA, Taylor M, Eder JP et al (2016) Nivolumab alone and nivolumab plus ipilimumab in recurrent small-cell lung cancer (CheckMate 032): a multicentre, open-label, phase 1/2 trial. Lancet Oncol 17(7):883–895

Arena S, Bellosillo B, Siravegna G, Martínez A, Cañadas I, Lazzari L et al (2015) Emergence of multiple EGFR extracellular mutations during cetuximab treatment in colorectal cancer. Clin Cancer Res 21(9):2157–2166

Armand P, Shipp MA, Ribrag V, Michot J-M, Zinzani PL, Kuruvilla J et al (2016) Programmed death-1 blockade with pembrolizumab in patients with classical Hodgkin lymphoma after brentuximab vedotin failure. J Clin Oncol 34(31):3733–3739

Avilés A, Nambo MJ, Neri N, Cleto S, Castañeda C, Huerta-Guzmàn J et al (2007) Dose dense (CEOP-14) vs dose dense and rituximab (CEOP-14+R) in high-risk diffuse large cell lymphoma. Med Oncol 24(1):85–89

Baig NA, Church AK, Nowakowski GS, Taylor RP, Lindorfer MA, Zent CS (2010) Complement activation and cytotoxicity in CLL cells treated with alemtuzumab and ofatumumab: evidence for multiple mechanisms of resistance to complement dependent cytotoxicity. Blood 116 (21):3575

Baig NA, Taylor RP, Lindorfer MA, Church AK, Laplant BR, Pavey ES et al (2012) Complement dependent cytotoxicity in chronic lymphocytic leukemia: ofatumumab enhances alemtuzumab complement dependent cytotoxicity and reveals cells resistant to activated complement. Leuk Lymphoma 53(11):2218–2227

Bander NH (2013) Antibody–drug conjugate target selection: critical factors. Antibody-drug conjugates. Springer, Berlin, pp 29–40

Bang Y-J, Van Cutsem E, Feyereislova A, Chung HC, Shen L, Sawaki A et al (2010) Trastuzumab in combination with chemotherapy versus chemotherapy alone for treatment of HER2-positive advanced gastric or gastro-oesophageal junction cancer (ToGA): a phase 3, open-label, randomised controlled trial. Lancet 376(9742):687–697

Bardelli A, Corso S, Bertotti A, Hobor S, Valtorta E, Siravegna G et al (2013) Amplification of the MET receptor drives resistance to anti-EGFR therapies in colorectal cancer. Cancer Discov 3 (6):658–673

Bardia A, Vahdat LT, Diamond JR, Starodub A, Moroose RL, Isakoff SJ et al (2015) Therapy of refractory/relapsed metastatic triple-negative breast cancer (TNBC) with an anti-Trop-2-SN-38 antibody-drug conjugate (ADC), sacituzumab govitecan (IMMU-132): phase I/II clinical experience. Am Soc Clin Oncol

Bardia A, Mayer IA, Diamond JR, Moroose RL, Isakoff SJ, Starodub AN et al (2017) Efficacy and safety of anti-trop-2 antibody drug conjugate sacituzumab govitecan (IMMU-132) in heavily pretreated patients with metastatic triple-negative breast cancer. J Clin Oncol JCO. 2016.70. 8297

Barlesi F, Park K, Ciardiello F, von Pawel J, Gadgeel S, Hida T et al (2016) Primary analysis from OAK, a randomized phase III study comparing atezolizumab with docetaxel in 2L/3L NSCLC. Ann Oncol 27(Suppl 6):LBA44_PR

Barnett B, Ruter J, Brumlik M, Kryczek I, Cheng P, Zou W et al (eds) (2006) A phase II trial of denileukin diftitox to treat refractory advanced-stage ovarian cancer. In: ASCO Annual meeting proceedings

Barok M, Tanner M, Köninki K, Isola J (2011a) Trastuzumab-DM1 causes tumour growth inhibition by mitotic catastrophe in trastuzumab-resistant breast cancer cells in vivo. Breast Cancer Res 13(2):R46

Barok M, Tanner M, Köninki K, Isola J (2011b) Trastuzumab-DM1 is highly effective in preclinical models of HER2-positive gastric cancer. Cancer Lett 306(2):171–179

Barok M, Joensuu H, Isola J (2014) Trastuzumab emtansine: mechanisms of action and drug resistance. Breast Cancer Res BCR 16(2):209

Bazan J, Całkosiński I, Gamian A (2012) Phage display—a powerful technique for immunotherapy: 1. Introduction and potential of therapeutic applications. Human Vaccines Immunother 8 (12):1817–1828

Behr T, Becker W, Hannappel E, Goldenberg DM, Wolf F (1995) Targeting of liver metastases of colorectal cancer with IgG, F(ab′)2, and Fab′ anti-carcinoembryonic antigen antibodies labeled with 99mTc: the role of metabolism and kinetics. Can Res 55(23 Suppl):5777s–5785s

Berchuck A, Kamel A, Whitaker R, Kerns B, Olt G, Kinney R et al (1990) Overexpression of HER-2/ncu is associated with poor survival in advanced epithelial ovarian cancer. Can Res 50 (13):4087–4091

Bergers G, Hanahan D (2008) Modes of resistance to anti-angiogenic therapy. Nat Rev Cancer 8 (8):592–603

Bernardo SG, Moskalenko M, Pan M, Shah S, Sidhu HK, Sicular S et al (2013) Elevated rates of transaminitis during ipilimumab therapy for metastatic melanoma. Melanoma Res 23(1):47–54

Berns K, Horlings HM, Hennessy BT, Madiredjo M, Hijmans EM, Beelen K et al (2007) A functional genetic approach identifies the PI3K pathway as a major determinant of trastuzumab resistance in breast cancer. Cancer Cell 12(4):395–402

Bertotti A, Migliardi G, Galimi F, Sassi F, Torti D, Isella C et al (2011) A molecularly annotated platform of patient-derived xenografts ("xenopatients") identifies HER2 as an effective therapeutic target in cetuximab-resistant colorectal cancer. Cancer Discov 1(6):508–523

Biehn SE, Kirk D, Rivera MP, Martinez AE, Khandani AH, Orlowski RZ (2006) Bronchiolitis obliterans with organizing pneumonia after rituximab therapy for non-Hodgkin's lymphoma. Hematol Oncol 24(4):234–237

Bokemeyer C, Van Cutsem E, Rougier P, Ciardiello F, Heeger S, Schlichting M et al (2012) Addition of cetuximab to chemotherapy as first-line treatment for KRAS wild-type metastatic colorectal cancer: pooled analysis of the CRYSTAL and OPUS randomised clinical trials. Eur J Cancer 48(10):1466–1475

Bonner JA, Harari PM, Giralt J, Azarnia N, Shin DM, Cohen RB et al (2006) Radiotherapy plus cetuximab for squamous-cell carcinoma of the head and neck. N Engl J Med 354(6):567–578

Bonner JA, Harari PM, Giralt J, Cohen RB, Jones CU, Sur RK et al (2010) Radiotherapy plus cetuximab for locoregionally advanced head and neck cancer: 5-year survival data from a phase 3 randomised trial, and relation between cetuximab-induced rash and survival. Lancet Oncol 11(1):21–28

Bonomi P, Peterson P, Socinski M, Reck M, Paz-Ares L, Melosky B et al (2015) Rash as a marker for the efficacy of necitumumab in the SQUIRE Study. J Thorac Oncol

Boone SL, Rademaker A, Liu D, Pfeiffer C, Mauro DJ, Lacouture ME (2007) Impact and management of skin toxicity associated with anti-epidermal growth factor receptor therapy: survey results. Oncology 72(3–4):152–159

Borghaei H, Paz-Ares L, Horn L, Spigel DR, Steins M, Ready NE et al (2015) Nivolumab versus docetaxel in advanced nonsquamous non–small-cell lung cancer. N Engl J Med 373(17):1627–1639

Braghiroli MI, Sabbaga J, Hoff PM (2012) Bevacizumab: overview of the literature. Expert Rev Anticancer Ther 12(5):567–580

Brahmer J, Reckamp KL, Baas P, Crinò L, Eberhardt WE, Poddubskaya E et al (2015) Nivolumab versus docetaxel in advanced squamous-cell non-small-cell lung cancer. N Engl J Med 373(2):123–135

Brandes AA, Bartolotti M, Tosoni A, Poggi R, Franceschi E (2015) Practical management of bevacizumab-related toxicities in glioblastoma. Oncologist 20(2):166–175

Bubien JK, Zhou L-J, Bell PD, Frizzell RA, Tedder TF (1993) Transfection of the CD20 cell surface molecule into ectopic cell types generates a Ca2+ conductance found constitutively in B lymphocytes. J Cell Biol 121(5):1121–1132

Burris HA, Rugo HS, Vukelja SJ, Vogel CL, Borson RA, Limentani S et al (2011) Phase II study of the antibody drug conjugate trastuzumab-DM1 for the treatment of human epidermal growth factor receptor 2 (HER2)–positive breast cancer after prior HER2-directed therapy. J Clin Oncol 29(4):398–405

Burstein HJ (2005) The distinctive nature of HER2-positive breast cancers. N Engl J Med 353(16):1652–1654

Buske C, Hoster E, Dreyling M, Eimermacher H, Wandt H, Metzner B et al (2009) The addition of rituximab to front-line therapy with CHOP (R-CHOP) results in a higher response rate and longer time to treatment failure in patients with lymphoplasmacytic lymphoma: results of a randomized trial of the German Low-Grade Lymphoma Study Group (GLSG). Leukemia 23(1):153–161

Camidge D, Heist R, Masters G, Scheff R, Starodub A, Messersmith W et al (eds) (2016) Therapy of metastatic, non-small cell lung cancer (mNSCLC) with the anti-Trop-2-SN-38 antibody-drug conjugate (ADC), sacituzumab govitecan (IMMU-132). In: ASCO meeting abstracts

Cardillo TM, Govindan SV, Sharkey RM, Trisal P, Goldenberg DM (2011) Humanized anti-Trop-2 IgG-SN-38 conjugate for effective treatment of diverse epithelial cancers: preclinical studies in human cancer xenograft models and monkeys. Clin Cancer Res 17(10):3157–3169

Cardillo TM, Govindan SV, Sharkey RM, Trisal P, Arrojo R, Liu D et al (2015) Sacituzumab govitecan (Immu-132), an anti-Trop-2/Sn-38 antibody–drug conjugate: characterization and efficacy in pancreatic, gastric, and other cancers. Bioconjug Chem 26(5):919–931

Cardillo TM, Sharkey RM, Rossi DL, Arrojo R, Mostafa A, Goldenberg DM (2017) Synthetic lethality exploitation by an anti-Trop-2-SN-38 antibody-drug conjugate, IMMU-132, plus PARP-inhibitors in BRCA1/2-wild-type triple-negative breast cancer. Clin Cancer Res. clincanres. 2401.016

Carlino MS, Atkinson V, Cebon JS, Jameson MB, Fitzharris BM, McNeil CM et al (2017) KEYNOTE-029: efficacy and safety of pembrolizumab (pembro) plus ipilimumab (ipi) for advanced melanoma. Am Soc Clin Oncol

Carmeliet P (2005) VEGF as a key mediator of angiogenesis in cancer. Oncology 69(Suppl 3):4–10

Carson KR, Evens AM, Richey EA, Habermann TM, Focosi D, Seymour JF et al (2009) Progressive multifocal leukoencephalopathy after rituximab therapy in HIV-negative patients: a report of 57 cases from the Research on Adverse Drug Events and Reports project. Blood 113 (20):4834–4840

Cella D, Grünwald V, Nathan P, Doan J, Dastani H, Taylor F et al (2016) Quality of life in patients with advanced renal cell carcinoma given nivolumab versus everolimus in CheckMate 025: a randomised, open-label, phase 3 trial. Lancet Oncol 17(7):994–1003

Chames P, Van Regenmortel M, Weiss E, Baty D (2009) Therapeutic antibodies: successes, limitations and hopes for the future. Br J Pharmacol 157(2):220–233

Chen R, Hou J, Newman E, Kim Y, Donohue C, Liu X et al (2015) CD30 downregulation, MMAE resistance, and MDR1 upregulation are all associated with resistance to brentuximab vedotin. Mol Cancer Ther 14(6):1376–1384

Chen R, Gopal AK, Smith SE, Ansell SM, Rosenblatt JD, Savage KJ et al (2016a) Five-year survival and durability results of brentuximab vedotin in patients with relapsed or refractory Hodgkin lymphoma. Blood. blood-2016-02-699850

Chen R, Zinzani P, Fanale M, Armand P, Johnson N, Ribrag V et al (2016b) Pembrolizumab for relapsed/refractory classical Hodgkin lymphoma (R/R cHL): phase 2 KEYNOTE-087 study. J Clin Oncol 34

Chinot OL, Wick W, Mason W, Henriksson R, Saran F, Nishikawa R et al (2014) Bevacizumab plus radiotherapy–temozolomide for newly diagnosed glioblastoma. N Engl J Med 370 (8):709–722

Choueiri TK, Hodi FS, Thompson JA, McDermott DF, Hwu W-J, Lawrence DP et al (2017) Pembrolizumab (pembro) plus low-dose ipilimumab (ipi) for patients (pts) with advanced renal cell carcinoma (RCC): phase 1 KEYNOTE-029 study. Am Soc Clin Oncol

Chow LQ, Haddad R, Gupta S, Mahipal A, Mehra R, Tahara M et al (2016) Antitumor activity of pembrolizumab in biomarker-unselected patients with recurrent and/or metastatic head and neck squamous cell carcinoma: results from the phase Ib KEYNOTE-012 expansion cohort. J Clin Oncol 34(32):3838–3845

Chowdhury S, McDermott DF, Voss MH, Hawkins RE, Aimone P, Voi M et al (2017) A phase I/II study to assess the safety and efficacy of pazopanib (PAZ) and pembrolizumab (PEM) in patients (pts) with advanced renal cell carcinoma (aRCC). Am Soc Clin Oncol

Chung CH, Mirakhur B, Chan E, Le Q-T, Berlin J, Morse M et al (2008) Cetuximab-induced anaphylaxis and IgE specific for galactose-α-1, 3-galactose. N Engl J Med 358(11):1109–1117

Cloughesy T, Vredenburgh J, Day B, Das A, Friedman H (2010) Updated safety and survival of patients with relapsed glioblastoma treated with bevacizumab in the BRAIN study. J Clin Oncol 28(15 Suppl):2008

Cobleigh MA, Vogel CL, Tripathy D, Robert NJ, Scholl S, Fehrenbacher L et al (1999) Multinational study of the efficacy and safety of humanized anti-HER2 monoclonal antibody in women who have HER2-overexpressing metastatic breast cancer that has progressed after chemotherapy for metastatic disease. J Clin Oncol 17(9):2639

Cohen SB, Emery P, Greenwald MW, Dougados M, Furie RA, Genovese MC et al (2006) Rituximab for rheumatoid arthritis refractory to anti–tumor necrosis factor therapy: results of a multicenter, randomized, double-blind, placebo-controlled, phase III trial evaluating primary efficacy and safety at twenty-four weeks. Arthritis Rheum 54(9):2793–2806

Coiffier B, Haioun C, Ketterer N, Engert A, Tilly H, Ma D et al (1998) Rituximab (anti-CD20 monoclonal antibody) for the treatment of patients with relapsing or refractory aggressive lymphoma: a multicenter phase II study. Blood 92(6):1927–1932

Coiffier B, Lepretre S, Pedersen LM, Gadeberg O, Fredriksen H, van Oers MH et al (2008) Safety and efficacy of ofatumumab, a fully human monoclonal anti-CD20 antibody, in patients with relapsed or refractory B-cell chronic lymphocytic leukemia: a phase 1-2 study. Blood 111(3): 1094–1100

Coiffier B, Thieblemont C, Van Den Neste E, Lepeu G, Plantier I, Castaigne S et al (2010) Long-term outcome of patients in the LNH-98.5 trial, the first randomized study comparing rituximab-CHOP to standard CHOP chemotherapy in DLBCL patients: a study by the Groupe d'Etudes des Lymphomes de l'Adulte. Blood 116(12):2040–2045

Corsello SM, Barnabei A, Marchetti P, De Vecchis L, Salvatori R, Torino F (2013) Endocrine side effects induced by immune checkpoint inhibitors. J Clin Endocrinol Metab 98(4):1361–1375

Damle RN, Wasil T, Fais F, Ghiotto F, Valetto A, Allen SL et al (1999) Ig V gene mutation status and CD38 expression as novel prognostic indicators in chronic lymphocytic leukemia. Blood 94(6):1840–1847

de Claro RA, McGinn K, Kwitkowski V, Bullock J, Khandelwal A, Habtemariam B et al (2012) US Food and Drug Administration approval summary: brentuximab vedotin for the treatment of relapsed Hodgkin lymphoma or relapsed systemic anaplastic large-cell lymphoma. Clin Cancer Res 18(21):5845–5849

Deaglio S, Mehta K, Malavasi F (2001) Human CD38: a (r) evolutionary story of enzymes and receptors. Leuk Res 25(1):1–12

Desjarlais JR, Lazar GA (2011) Modulation of antibody effector function. Exp Cell Res 317 (9):1278–1285

Desjarlais JR, Lazar GA, Zhukovsky EA, Chu SY (2007) Optimizing engagement of the immune system by anti-tumor antibodies: an engineer's perspective. Drug Discov Today 12(21–22):898–910

Dhomen NS, Mariadason J, Tebbutt N, Scott AM (2012) Therapeutic targeting of the epidermal growth factor receptor in human cancer. Crit Rev Oncog 17(1)

Dieras V, Harbeck N, Albain K, Burris H, Awada A, Crivellari D et al (2010) Abstract P3-14-01: a phase Ib/II trial of trastuzumab-DM1 with pertuzumab for patients with HER2-positive, locally advanced or metastatic breast cancer: interim efficacy and safety results. Cancer Res 70(24 Suppl):P3-14-01-P3-14-01

DiLillo DJ, Ravetch JV (2015) Differential Fc-receptor engagement drives an anti tumor vaccinal effect. Cell 161(5):1035–1045

Dimopoulos MA, Oriol A, Nahi H, San-Miguel J, Bahlis NJ, Usmani SZ et al (2016) Daratumumab, lenalidomide, and dexamethasone for multiple myeloma. N Engl J Med 375 (14):1319–1331

DiPippo VA, Olson WC, Nguyen HM, Brown LG, Vessella RL, Corey E (2015) Efficacy studies of an antibody-drug conjugate PSMA-ADC in patient-derived prostate cancer xenografts. Prostate 75(3):303–313

Dotan E, Cohen SJ, Starodub AN, Lieu CH, Messersmith WA, Guarino MJ et al (eds) (2016) Labetuzumab govitecan (IMMU-130), an anti-CEACAM5/SN-38 antibody-drug conjugate, is active in patients (pts) with heavily pretreated metastatic colorectal cancer (mCRC): phase II results. Cancer Res (Amer Assoc Cancer Research 615 Chestnut St, 17th Floor, Philadelphia, PA 19106-4404 USA)

Douillard J-Y, Siena S, Cassidy J, Tabernero J, Burkes R, Barugel M et al (2010) Randomized, phase III trial of panitumumab with infusional fluorouracil, leucovorin, and oxaliplatin (FOLFOX4) versus FOLFOX4 alone as first-line treatment in patients with previously untreated metastatic colorectal cancer: the PRIME study. J Clin Oncol 28(31):4697–4705

Douillard J-Y, Oliner KS, Siena S, Tabernero J, Burkes R, Barugel M et al (2013) Panitumumab–FOLFOX4 treatment and RAS mutations in colorectal cancer. N Engl J Med 369(11):1023–1034

Duncan AR, Winter G (1988) The binding site for C1q on IgG. Nature 332(6166):738–740

Dürkop H, Foss HD, Eitelbach F, Anagnostopoulos I, Latza U, Pileri S et al (2000) Expression of the CD30 antigen in non-lymphoid tissues and cells. J Pathol 190(5):613–618

Eggermont AM, Chiarion-Sileni V, Grob J-J, Dummer R, Wolchok JD, Schmidt H et al (2015) Adjuvant ipilimumab versus placebo after complete resection of high-risk stage III melanoma (EORTC 18071): a randomised, double-blind, phase 3 trial. Lancet Oncol 16(5):522–530

Eggermont AM, Chiarion-Sileni V, Grob J-J, Dummer R, Wolchok JD, Schmidt H et al (2016) Prolonged survival in stage III melanoma with ipilimumab adjuvant therapy. N Engl J Med 375 (19):1845–1855

Elinzano H, Hebda N, Luppe D (2016) PSMA ADC for progressive glioblastoma: phase II Brown University Oncology Research Group Study. J Clin Oncol 34

Ensslin CJ, Rosen AC, Wu S, Lacouture ME (2013) Pruritus in patients treated with targeted cancer therapies: systematic review and meta-analysis. J Am Acad Dermatol 69(5):708–720

Eremina V, Sood M, Haigh J, Nagy A, Lajoie G, Ferrara N et al (2003) Glomerular-specific alterations of VEGF-A expression lead to distinct congenital and acquired renal diseases. J Clin Investig 111(5):707–716

Escudier B, Bellmunt J, Négrier S, Bajetta E, Melichar B, Bracarda S et al (2010) Phase III trial of bevacizumab plus interferon alfa-2a in patients with metastatic renal cell carcinoma (AVOREN): final analysis of overall survival. J Clin Oncol 28(13):2144–2150

Estenfelder S, Tausch E, Robrecht S, Bahlo J, Goede V, Ritgen M et al (2016) Gene mutations and treatment outcome in the context of chlorambucil (Clb) without or with the addition of rituximab (R) or obinutuzumab (GA-101, G)-results of an extensive analysis of the phase III study CLL11 of the German CLL study group. Am Soc Hematol

Eve HE, Linch D, Qian W, Ross M, Seymour JF, Smith P et al (2009) Toxicity of fludarabine and cyclophosphamide with or without rituximab as initial therapy for patients with previously untreated mantle cell lymphoma: results of a randomised phase II study. Leuk Lymphoma 50 (2):211–215

Fakih M, Vincent M (2010) Adverse events associated with anti-EGFR therapies for the treatment of metastatic colorectal cancer. Curr Oncol 17(S1)

Fanning LJ, Connor AM, Wu GE (1996) Development of the immunoglobulin repertoire. Clin Immunol Immunopathol 79(1):1–14

Fehrenbacher L, Spira A, Ballinger M, Kowanetz M, Vansteenkiste J, Mazieres J et al (2016) Atezolizumab versus docetaxel for patients with previously treated non-small-cell lung cancer (POPLAR): a multicentre, open-label, phase 2 randomised controlled trial. Lancet 387 (10030):1837–1846

Ferrajoli A, O'Brien SM, Cortes JE, Giles FJ, Thomas DA, Faderl S et al (2003) Phase II study of alemtuzumab in chronic lymphoproliferative disorders. Cancer 98(4):773–778

Ferrara N (2010) Pathways mediating VEGF-independent tumor angiogenesis. Cytokine Growth Factor Rev 21(1):21–26

Ferrara N, Hillan KJ, Gerber H-P, Novotny W (2004) Discovery and development of bevacizumab, an anti-VEGF antibody for treating cancer. Nat Rev Drug Discov 3(5):391–400

Ferris RL, Jaffee EM, Ferrone S (2010) Tumor antigen-targeted, monoclonal antibody-based immunotherapy: clinical response, cellular immunity, and immunoescape. J Clin Oncol 28 (28):4390–4399

Ferris RL, Blumenschein G Jr, Fayette J, Guigay J, Colevas AD, Licitra L et al (2016) Nivolumab for recurrent squamous-cell carcinoma of the head and neck. N Engl J Med 2016(375):1856–1867

Feugier P, Van Hoof A, Sebban C, Solal-Celigny P, Bouabdallah R, Ferme C et al (2005) Long-term results of the R-CHOP study in the treatment of elderly patients with diffuse large B-cell lymphoma: a study by the Groupe d'Etude des Lymphomes de l'Adulte. J Clin Oncol 23 (18):4117–4126

Fischer K, Bahlo J, Fink A-M, Busch R, Böttcher S, Mayer J et al (2012) Extended follow up of the CLL8 protocol, a randomized phase-III trial of the German CLL Study Group (GCLLSG) comparing fludarabine and cyclophosphamide (FC) to FC plus rituximab (FCR) for previously untreated patients with chronic lymphocytic leukemia (CLL): results on survival, progression-free survival, delayed neutropenias and secondary malignancies confirm superiority of the FCR regimen. Am Soc Hematol

Flanagan RJ, Jones AL (2004) Fab antibody fragments: some applications in clinical toxicology. Drug Saf 27(14):1115–1133

Flavell DJ, Noss A, Pulford KA, Ling N, Flavell SU (1997) Systemic therapy with 3BIT, a triple combination cocktail of anti-CD19,-CD22, and-CD38-saporin immunotoxins, is curative of human B-cell lymphoma in severe combined immunodeficient mice. Can Res 57(21):4824–4829

Francisco JA, Cerveny CG, Meyer DL, Mixan BJ, Klussman K, Chace DF et al (2003) cAC10-vcMMAE, an anti-CD30–monomethyl auristatin E conjugate with potent and selective antitumor activity. Blood 102(4):1458–1465

Fraser G, Smith C, Imrie K, Meyer R (2007) Care HDSGoCCOsPiE-B. Alemtuzumab in chronic lymphocytic leukemia. Curr Oncol 14(3):96 (Toronto)

Frattini M, Saletti P, Romagnani E, Martin V, Molinari F, Ghisletta M et al (2007) PTEN loss of expression predicts cetuximab efficacy in metastatic colorectal cancer patients. Br J Cancer 97 (8):1139–1145

Freudenberg JA, Wang Q, Katsumata M, Drebin J, Nagatomo I, Greene MI (2009) The role of HER2 in early breast cancer metastasis and the origins of resistance to HER2-targeted therapies. Exp Mol Pathol 87(1):1–11

Friedman HS, Prados MD, Wen PY, Mikkelsen T, Schiff D, Abrey LE et al (2009) Bevacizumab alone and in combination with irinotecan in recurrent glioblastoma. J Clin Oncol 27(28):4733–4740

Fuchs CS, Tomasek J, Yong CJ, Dumitru F, Passalacqua R, Goswami C et al (2014) Ramucirumab monotherapy for previously treated advanced gastric or gastro-oesophageal junction adeno-carcinoma (REGARD): an international, randomised, multicentre, placebo-controlled, phase 3 trial. Lancet 383(9911):31–39

Gan HK, Burgess AW, Clayton AH, Scott AM (2012) Targeting of a conformationally exposed, tumor-specific epitope of EGFR as a strategy for cancer therapy. Can Res 72(12):2924–2930

Garnock-Jones KP (2013) Brentuximab vedotin: a review of its use in patients with Hodgkin lymphoma and systemic anaplastic large cell lymphoma following previous treatment failure. Drugs 73(4):371–381

Garon EB, Ciuleanu T-E, Arrieta O, Prabhash K, Syrigos KN, Goksel T et al (2014) Ramucirumab plus docetaxel versus placebo plus docetaxel for second-line treatment of stage IV non-small-cell lung cancer after disease progression on platinum-based therapy (REVEL): a multicentre, double-blind, randomised phase 3 trial. Lancet 384(9944):665–673

Garon EB, Rizvi NA, Hui R, Leighl N, Balmanoukian AS, Eder JP et al (2015) Pembrolizumab for the treatment of non-small-cell lung cancer. N Engl J Med 372(21):2018–2028

Garrett JT, Arteaga CL (2011) Resistance to HER2-directed antibodies and tyrosine kinase inhibitors: mechanisms and clinical implications. Cancer Biol Ther 11(9):793–800

Garrett TP, McKern NM, Lou M, Elleman TC, Adams TE, Lovrecz GO et al (2002) Crystal structure of a truncated epidermal growth factor receptor extracellular domain bound to transforming growth factor α. Cell 110(6):763–773

Gerena-Lewis M, Crawford J, Bonomi P, Maddox AM, Hainsworth J, McCune DE et al (2009) A phase II trial of Denileukin Diftitox in patients with previously treated advanced non-small cell lung cancer. Am J Clin Oncol 32(3):269–273

Ghielmini M, Rufibach K, Salles G, Leoncini-Franscini L, Leger-Falandry C, Cogliatti S et al (2005) Single agent rituximab in patients with follicular or mantle cell lymphoma: clinical and biological factors that are predictive of response and event-free survival as well as the effect of rituximab on the immune system: a study of the Swiss Group for Clinical Cancer Research (SAKK). Ann Oncol 16(10):1675–1682

Gianni L, Pienkowski T, Im Y-H, Roman L, Tseng L-M, Liu M-C et al (2012) Efficacy and safety of neoadjuvant pertuzumab and trastuzumab in women with locally advanced, inflammatory, or early HER2-positive breast cancer (NeoSphere): a randomised multicentre, open-label, phase 2 trial. Lancet Oncol 13(1):25–32

Giantonio BJ, Catalano PJ, Meropol NJ, O'Dwyer PJ, Mitchell EP, Alberts SR et al (2007) Bevacizumab in combination with oxaliplatin, fluorouracil, and leucovorin (FOLFOX4) for previously treated metastatic colorectal cancer: results from the Eastern Cooperative Oncology Group Study E3200. J Clin Oncol 25(12):1539–1544

Ginaldi L, De Martinis M, Matutes E, Farahat N, Morilla R, Dyer MJ et al (1998) Levels of expression of CD52 in normal and leukemic B and T cells: correlation with in vivo therapeutic responses to Campath-1H. Leuk Res 22(2):185–191

Goede V, Fischer K, Busch R, Engelke A, Eichhorst B, Wendtner CM et al (2014) Obinutuzumab plus chlorambucil in patients with CLL and coexisting conditions. N Engl J Med 370 (12):1101–1110

Goede V, Fischer K, Bosch F, Follows G, Frederiksen H, Cuneo A et al (2015) Updated survival analysis from the CLL11 study: obinutuzumab versus rituximab in chemoimmunotherapy-treated patients with chronic lymphocytic leukemia. Blood 126(23):1733

Goldenberg DM, Cardillo TM, Govindan SV, Rossi EA, Sharkey RM (2015) Trop-2 is a novel target for solid cancer therapy with sacituzumab govitecan (IMMU-132), an antibody-drug conjugate (ADC). Oncotarget 6(26):22496

Gopal AK, Press OW (1999) Clinical applications of anti-CD20 antibodies. J Lab Clin Med 134 (5):445–450

Gopal AK, Chen R, Smith SE, Ansell SM, Rosenblatt JD, Savage KJ et al (2014) Durable remissions in a pivotal phase 2 study of brentuximab vedotin in relapsed or refractory Hodgkin lymphoma. Blood. blood-2014-08-595801

Gordon LI, Molina A, Witzig T, Emmanouilides C, Raubtischek A, Darif M et al (2004) Durable responses after ibritumomab tiuxetan radioimmunotherapy for CD20+ B-cell lymphoma: long-term follow-up of a phase 1/2 study. Blood 103(12):4429–4431

Govindan SV, Cardillo TM, Rossi EA, McBride WJ, Sharkey RM, Goldenberg DM (2015) IMMU-130, a unique antibody-drug conjugate (ADC) of SN-38 targeting CEACAM5 antigen: preclinical basis for clinical activity in metastatic colorectal cancer (mCRC). Am Soc Clin Oncol

Gowryshankar A, Nagaraja V, Eslick GD (2013) HER2 status in Barrett's esophagus & esophageal cancer: a meta analysis. J Gastrointest Oncol 5(1):25–35

Grazette LP, Boecker W, Matsui T, Semigran M, Force TL, Hajjar RJ et al (2004) Inhibition of ErbB2 causes mitochondrial dysfunction in cardiomyocytes. J Am Coll Cardiol 44(11):2231–2238

Grushko T, Filiaci V, Mundt A, Ridderstråle K, Olopade O, Fleming G (2008) An exploratory analysis of HER-2 amplification and overexpression in advanced endometrial carcinoma: a Gynecologic Oncology Group study. Gynecol Oncol 108(1):3–9

Guidetti A, Carlo-Stella C, Ruella M, Miceli R, Devizzi L, Locatelli SL et al (2011) Myeloablative doses of yttrium-90-ibritumomab tiuxetan and the risk of secondary myelodysplasia/acute myelogenous leukemia. Cancer 117(22):5074–5084

Habermann TM, Weller EA, Morrison VA, Gascoyne RD, Cassileth PA, Cohn JB et al (2006) Rituximab-CHOP versus CHOP alone or with maintenance rituximab in older patients with diffuse large B-cell lymphoma. J Clin Oncol 24(19):3121–3127

Haense N, Atmaca A, Pauligk C, Steinmetz K, Marmé F, Haag G-M et al (2016) A phase I trial of the trifunctional anti Her2 × anti CD3 antibody ertumaxomab in patients with advanced solid tumors. BMC Cancer 16(1):420

Hagenbeek A, Bischof-Delaloye A, Radford JA, Rohatiner A, Salles G, Van Hoof A et al (2007) 90Y-Ibritumomab Tiuxetan (Zevalin®) consolidation of first remission in advanced stage follicular non-Hodgkin's lymphoma: first results of the international randomized phase 3 first-line indolent trial (FIT) in 414 patients. Am Soc Hematol

Hainsworth JD, Spigel DR, Markus TM, Shipley D, Thompson D, Rotman R et al (2009) Rituximab plus short-duration chemotherapy followed by Yttrium-90 Ibritumomab tiuxetan as first-line treatment for patients with follicular non-Hodgkin lymphoma: a phase II trial of the Sarah Cannon Oncology Research Consortium. Clin Lymphoma Myeloma 9(3):223–228

Halim A, Bagley RG, Keler T (2016) Glycoprotein NMB (gpNMB) overexpression is prevalent in human cancers: pancreatic cancer, non-small cell lung cancer, head and neck cancer, and osteosarcoma. AACR

Hallek M, Fischer K, Fingerle-Rowson G, Fink A, Busch R, Mayer J et al (2010) Addition of rituximab to fludarabine and cyclophosphamide in patients with chronic lymphocytic leukaemia: a randomised, open-label, phase 3 trial. Lancet 376(9747):1164–1174

Hamid O, Robert C, Daud A, Hodi FS, Hwu W-J, Kefford R et al (2013) Safety and tumor responses with lambrolizumab (anti–PD-1) in melanoma. N Engl J Med 369(2):134–144

Hamid O, Puzanov I, Dummer R, Schachter J, Daud A, Schadendorf D et al (2016) Final overall survival for KEYNOTE-002: pembrolizumab (pembro) versus investigator-choice chemotherapy (chemo) for ipilimumab (ipi)-refractory melanoma. Ann Oncol 27(suppl 6):1107O

Hammers H, Plimack E, Infante J, Ernstoff M, Rini B, Mcdermott D et al (2014) Phase I study of nivolumab in combination with ipilimumab (ipi) in metastatic renal cell carcinoma (mrcc). BJU Int 114:8

Hansen HJ, Jones AL, Sharkey RM, Grebenau R, Blazejewski N, Kunz A et al (1990) Preclinical evaluation of an "instant" 99mTc-labeling kit for antibody imaging. Can Res 50(3 Suppl):794s–798s

Hapani S, Chu D, Wu S (2009) Risk of gastrointestinal perforation in patients with cancer treated with bevacizumab: a meta-analysis. Lancet Oncol 10(6):559–568

Hapani S, Sher A, Chu D, Wu S (2010) Increased risk of serious hemorrhage with bevacizumab in cancer patients: a meta-analysis. Oncology 79(1–2):27–38

Heiss MM, Murawa P, Koralewski P, Kutarska E, Kolesnik OO, Ivanchenko VV et al (2010) The trifunctional antibody catumaxomab for the treatment of malignant ascites due to epithelial cancer: results of a prospective randomized phase II/III trial. Int J Cancer 127(9):2209–2221

Hellmann MD, Rizvi NA, Goldman JW, Gettinger SN, Borghaei H, Brahmer JR et al (2017) Nivolumab plus ipilimumab as first-line treatment for advanced non-small-cell lung cancer (CheckMate 012): results of an open-label, phase 1, multicohort study. Lancet Oncol 18(1):31–41

Herbst RS, Baas P, Kim D-W, Felip E, Pérez-Gracia JL, Han J-Y et al (2016) Pembrolizumab versus docetaxel for previously treated, PD-L1-positive, advanced non-small-cell lung cancer (KEYNOTE-010): a randomised controlled trial. Lancet 387(10027):1540–1550

Heresi GA, Farver CF, Stoller JK (2008) Interstitial pneumonitis and alveolar hemorrhage complicating use of rituximab. Respiration 76(4):449–453

Herrera L, Farah R, Pellegrini V, Aquino D, Sandler E, Buchanan G et al (2000) Immunotoxins against CD19 and CD22 are effective in killing precursor-B acute lymphoblastic leukemia cells in vitro. Leukemia 14(5):853–858

Hillen F, Griffioen AW (2007) Tumour vascularization: sprouting angiogenesis and beyond. Cancer Metastasis Rev 26(3–4):489–502

Hillmen P, Skotnicki AB, Robak T, Jaksic B, Dmoszynska A, Wu J et al (2007) Alemtuzumab compared with chlorambucil as first-line therapy for chronic lymphocytic leukemia. J Clin Oncol 25(35):5616–5623

Hillmen P, Robak T, Janssens A, Babu KG, Kloczko J, Grosicki S et al (2015) Chlorambucil plus ofatumumab versus chlorambucil alone in previously untreated patients with chronic lymphocytic leukaemia (COMPLEMENT 1): a randomised, multicentre, open-label phase 3 trial. Lancet 385(9980):1873–1883

Hobor S, Van Emburgh BO, Crowley E, Misale S, Di Nicolantonio F, Bardelli A (2014) TGFα and amphiregulin paracrine network promotes resistance to EGFR blockade in colorectal cancer cells. Clin Cancer Res 20(24):6429–6438

Hodi FS, O'Day SJ, McDermott DF, Weber RW, Sosman JA, Haanen JB et al (2010a) Improved survival with ipilimumab in patients with metastatic melanoma. N Engl J Med 363(8):711–723

Hodi FS, O'day SJ, McDermott DF, Weber RW, Sosman JA, Haanen JB et al (2010b) Improved survival with ipilimumab in patients with metastatic melanoma. N Engl J Med 2010(363):711–723

Hodi FS, Chesney J, Pavlick AC, Robert C, Grossmann KF, McDermott DF et al (2016) Combined nivolumab and ipilimumab versus ipilimumab alone in patients with advanced melanoma: 2-year overall survival outcomes in a multicentre, randomised, controlled, phase 2 trial. Lancet Oncol 17(11):1558–1568

Hogarth PM, Pietersz GA (2012) Fc receptor-targeted therapies for the treatment of inflammation, cancer and beyond. Nat Rev Drug Discov 11(4):311–331

Holliger P, Hudson PJ (2005) Engineered antibody fragments and the rise of single domains. Nat Biotechnol 23(9):1126–1136

Holmes K, Roberts OL, Thomas AM, Cross MJ (2007) Vascular endothelial growth factor receptor-2: structure, function, intracellular signalling and therapeutic inhibition. Cell Signal 19 (10):2003–2012

Holmgaard RB, Zamarin D, Munn DH, Wolchok JD, Allison JP (2013) Indoleamine 2, 3-dioxygenase is a critical resistance mechanism in antitumor T cell immunotherapy targeting CTLA-4. J Exp Med jem. 20130066

Horn L, Brahmer J, Reck M, Borghaei H, Spigel D, Steins M et al (2015) 417OPhase 3, randomized trial (CheckMate 057) of nivolumab vs docetaxel in advanced non-squamous (non-SQ) non-small cell lung cancer (NSCLC): subgroup analyses and patient reported outcomes (PROs). Ann Oncol 26(suppl 9):ix125-ix

Horning SJ, Younes A, Jain V, Kroll S, Lucas J, Podoloff D et al (2005) Efficacy and safety of tositumomab and iodine-131 tositumomab (Bexxar) in B-cell lymphoma, progressive after rituximab. J Clin Oncol 23(4):712–719

Hsi ED, Steinle R, Balasa B, Szmania S, Draksharapu A, Shum BP et al (2008) CS1, a potential new therapeutic antibody target for the treatment of multiple myeloma. Clin Cancer Res 14 (9):2775–2784

Hudis CA (2007) Trastuzumab—mechanism of action and use in clinical practice. N Engl J Med 357(1):39–51

Hugo W, Zaretsky JM, Sun L, Song C, Moreno BH, Hu-Lieskovan S et al (2016) Genomic and transcriptomic features of response to anti-PD-1 therapy in metastatic melanoma. Cell 165 (1):35–44

Hurvitz SA, Dirix L, Kocsis J, Bianchi GV, Lu J, Vinholes J et al (2013) Phase II randomized study of trastuzumab emtansine versus trastuzumab plus docetaxel in patients with human epidermal growth factor receptor 2–positive metastatic breast cancer. J Clin Oncol JCO. 2012.44. 9694

Hurwitz H, Fehrenbacher L, Novotny W, Cartwright T, Hainsworth J, Heim W et al (2004) Bevacizumab plus irinotecan, fluorouracil, and leucovorin for metastatic colorectal cancer. N Engl J Med 350(23):2335–2342

Iida M, Brand TM, Starr MM, Li C, Huppert EJ, Luthar N et al (2013) Sym004, a novel EGFR antibody mixture, can overcome acquired resistance to cetuximab. Neoplasia 15(10):1196–1206

Jacobs SA, Swerdlow SH, Kant J, Foon KA, Jankowitz R, Land SR et al (2008) Phase II trial of short-course CHOP-R followed by 90Y-ibritumomab tiuxetan and extended rituximab in previously untreated follicular lymphoma. Clin Cancer Res 14(21):7088–7094

Jawa Z, Perez RM, Garlie L, Singh M, Qamar R, Khandheria BK et al (2016) Risk factors of trastuzumab-induced cardiotoxicity in breast cancer: a meta-analysis. Medicine 95(44):e5195

Johns TG, Stockert E, Ritter G, Jungbluth AA, Huang HJS, Cavenee WK et al (2002) Novel monoclonal antibody specific for the de2-7 epidermal growth factor receptor (EGFR) that also recognizes the EGFR expressed in cells containing amplification of the EGFR gene. Int J Cancer 98(3):398–408

Johnson DH, Fehrenbacher L, Novotny WF, Herbst RS, Nemunaitis JJ, Jablons DM et al (2004) Randomized phase II trial comparing bevacizumab plus carboplatin and paclitaxel with carboplatin and paclitaxel alone in previously untreated locally advanced or metastatic non-small-cell lung cancer. J Clin Oncol 22(11):2184–2191

Jonker DJ, O'callaghan CJ, Karapetis CS, Zalcberg JR, Tu D, Au H-J et al (2007) Cetuximab for the treatment of colorectal cancer. N Engl J Med 357(20):2040–2048

Junttila TT, Li G, Parsons K, Phillips GL, Sliwkowski MX (2011) Trastuzumab-DM1 (T-DM1) retains all the mechanisms of action of trastuzumab and efficiently inhibits growth of lapatinib insensitive breast cancer. Breast Cancer Res Treat 128(2):347–356

Kang HJ, Park JS, Kim D-W, Lee J, Jeong YJ, Choi SM et al (2012) Adverse pulmonary reactions associated with the use of monoclonal antibodies in cancer patients. Respir Med 106(3):443–450

Karapetis CS, Khambata-Ford S, Jonker DJ, O'callaghan CJ, Tu D, Tebbutt NC et al (2008) K-ras mutations and benefit from cetuximab in advanced colorectal cancer. New Engl J Med 359 (17):1757–1765

Kasi PM, Tawbi HA, Oddis CV, Kulkarni HS (2012) Clinical review: serious adverse events associated with the use of rituximab-a critical care perspective. Crit Care 16(4):231

Kataoka Y, Mukohara T, Shimada H, Saijo N, Hirai M, Minami H (2010) Association between gain-of-function mutations in PIK3CA and resistance to HER2-targeted agents in HER2-amplified breast cancer cell lines. Ann Oncol 21(2):255–262

Kaufman HL, Russell J, Hamid O, Bhatia S, Terheyden P, D'Angelo SP et al (2016) Avelumab in patients with chemotherapy-refractory metastatic Merkel cell carcinoma: a multicentre, single-group, open-label, phase 2 trial. Lancet Oncol 17(10):1374–1385

Kawashima O, Kamiyoshihara M, Sakata S, Endo K, Saito R, Morishita Y (2000) The clinicopathological significance of preoperative serum-soluble interleukin-2 receptor concentrations in operable non-small-cell lung cancer patients. Ann Surg Oncol 7(3):239–245

Keating MJ, Flinn I, Jain V, Binet J-L, Hillmen P, Byrd J et al (2002) Therapeutic role of alemtuzumab (Campath-1H) in patients who have failed fludarabine: results of a large international study. Blood 99(10):3554–3561

Kerbel RS (2008) Tumor angiogenesis. N Engl J Med 358(19):2039–2049

Kim KW, Ramaiya NH, Krajewski KM, Jagannathan JP, Tirumani SH, Srivastava A et al (2013) Ipilimumab associated hepatitis: imaging and clinicopathologic findings. Invest New Drugs 31 (4):1071–1077

Klapper LN, Glathe S, Vaisman N, Hynes NE, Andrews GC, Sela M et al (1999) The ErbB-2/HER2 oncoprotein of human carcinomas may function solely as a shared coreceptor for multiple stroma-derived growth factors. Proc Natl Acad Sci 96(9):4995–5000

Kleptish A, Gilles L, Ioannis K, Eliezer R, Ami S (2009) Enhancing the action of rituximab in chronic lymphocytic leukemia by adding fresh frozen plasma. Ann N Y Acad Sci 1173 (1):865–873

Klos KS, Zhou X, Lee S, Zhang L, Yang W, Nagata Y et al (2003) Combined trastuzumab and paclitaxel treatment better inhibits ErbB-2-mediated angiogenesis in breast carcinoma through a more effective inhibition of Akt than either treatment alone. Cancer 98(7):1377–1385

Knox SJ, Goris ML, Trisler K, Negrin R, Davis T, Liles T-M et al (1996) Yttrium-90-labeled anti-CD20 monoclonal antibody therapy of recurrent B-cell lymphoma. Clin Cancer Res 2 (3):457–470

Kobayashi Y, Komatsu Y, Yuki S, Fukushima H, Sasaki T, Iwanaga I et al (2015) Randomized controlled trial on the skin toxicity of panitumumab in Japanese patients with metastatic colorectal cancer: HGCSG1001 study; J-STEPP. Future Oncol 11(4):617–627

Kohler G, Milstein C (1975) Continuous cultures of fused cells secreting antibody of predefined specificity. Nature 256(5517):495–497

Kosmas C, Stamatopoulos K, Stavroyianni N, Tsavaris N, Papadaki T (2002) Anti-CD20-based therapy of B cell lymphoma: state of the art. Leukemia 16(10):2004

Kreitman RJ (2009) Recombinant immunotoxins containing truncated bacterial toxins for the treatment of hematologic malignancies. BioDrugs 23(1):1–13

Kruser TJ, Wheeler DL (2010) Mechanisms of resistance to HER family targeting antibodies. Exp Cell Res 316(7):1083–1100

Kumaresan PR, Lai WC, Chuang SS, Bennett M, Mathew PA (2002) CS1, a novel member of the CD2 family, is homophilic and regulates NK cell function. Mol Immunol 39(1):1–8

Kuramochi Y, Guo X, Sawyer DB (2006) Neuregulin activates erbB2-dependent src/FAK signaling and cytoskeletal remodeling in isolated adult rat cardiac myocytes. J Mol Cell Cardiol 41(2):228–235

Lacouture ME, Mitchell EP, Piperdi B, Pillai MV, Shearer H, Iannotti N et al (2010) Skin toxicity evaluation protocol with panitumumab (STEPP), a phase II, open-label, randomized trial evaluating the impact of a pre-Emptive Skin treatment regimen on skin toxicities and quality of life in patients with metastatic colorectal cancer. J Clin Oncol 28(8):1351–1357

Laffleur B, Pascal V, Sirac C, Cogne M (2012) Production of human or humanized antibodies in mice. Methods Mol Biol 901:149–159 (Clifton, NJ)

Larkin J, Chiarion-Sileni V, Gonzalez R, Grob JJ, Cowey CL, Lao CD et al (2015) Combined nivolumab and ipilimumab or monotherapy in untreated melanoma. N Engl J Med 2015 (373):23–34

Larkin J, Minor D, D'Angelo S, Neyns B, Smylie M, Miller WH Jr et al (2016) Overall survival in patients with advanced melanoma who received nivolumab versus investigator's choice chemotherapy in CheckMate 037: a randomized, controlled, open-label phase III trial. J Clin Oncol 0(0):JCO.2016.71.8023

Lassman A, Gan H, Fichtel L, Merrell R, Van Den Bent M, Kumthekar P et al (2015) A phase 1 study evaluating ABT-414 with temozolomide (TMZ) or concurrent radiotherapy (RT) and TMZ in glioblastoma (GBM) (S43. 006). Neurology 84(14 Suppl):S43. 006

Lassman A, van den Bent M, Gan H, Reardon D, Kumthekar P, Butowski N et al (2016) Efficacy of a novel antibody-drug conjugate (ADC), ABT-414, with temozolomide (TMZ) in recurrent glioblastoma (rGBM). Ann Oncol 27(Suppl 6):326PD

Laurent-Puig P, Cayre A, Manceau G, Buc E, Bachet J-B, Lecomte T et al (2009) Analysis of PTEN, BRAF, and EGFR status in determining benefit from cetuximab therapy in wild-type KRAS metastatic colon cancer. J Clin Oncol 27(35):5924–5930

Leach DR, Krummel MF, Allison JP (1996) Enhancement of antitumor immunity by CTLA-4 blockade. Science 271(5256):1734–1736 (New York, NY)

Lemarié CA, Paradis P, Schiffrin EL (2008) New insights on signaling cascades induced by cross-talk between angiotensin II and aldosterone. J Mol Med 86(6):673–678

Li G, Fields C, Parsons K, Guo J, Phillips GL (2010) 223 Trastuzumab-DM1: mechanisms of action and mechanisms of resistance. Eur J Cancer Suppl 8(7):73

Liggett W, Hainsworth J, Spigel D, Meluch A, Raefsky E, Kennedy S et al (2005) Fludarabine/rituximab (FR) followed by alemtuzumab as first-line treatment for patients with chronic lymphocytic leukemia (CLL) or small lymphocytic lymphoma (SLL): a Minnie Pearl Cancer Research Network phase II trial. J Clin Oncol 23(16 Suppl):6556

Lin P, Owens R, Tricot G, Wilson CS (2004) Flow cytometric immunophenotypic analysis of 306 cases of multiple myeloma. Am J Clin Pathol 121(4):482–488

Liu L, Shao X, Gao W, Bai J, Wang R, Huang P et al (2010a) The role of human epidermal growth factor receptor 2 as a prognostic factor in lung cancer: a meta-analysis of published data. J Thorac Oncol 5(12):1922–1932

Liu JJ, Lin B, Hao YY, Li FF, Liu DW, Qi Y et al (2010b) Lewis(y) antigen stimulates the growth of ovarian cancer cells via regulation of the epidermal growth factor receptor pathway. Oncol Rep 23(3):833–841

Loi S, Michiels S, Lambrechts D, Fumagalli D, Claes B, Kellokumpu-Lehtinen P-L et al (2013) Somatic mutation profiling and associations with prognosis and trastuzumab benefit in early breast cancer. J Nat Cancer Instit djt121

Lonberg N, Huszar D (1995) Human antibodies from transgenic mice. Int Rev Immunol 13(1):65–93

Long G, Mcneil C, Schachter J, Robert C, Ribas A, Arance A et al (2016) Pembrolizumab versus ipilimumab for advanced melanoma: final overall survival analysis of Keynote-006. Asia-Pac J Clin Oncol 12:61–62

Lonial S, Vij R, Harousseau J-L, Facon T, Moreau P, Mazumder A et al (2012) Elotuzumab in combination with lenalidomide and low-dose dexamethasone in relapsed or refractory multiple myeloma. J Clin Oncol 30(16):1953–1959

Lonial S, Dimopoulos M, Palumbo A, White D, Grosicki S, Spicka I et al (2015) Elotuzumab therapy for relapsed or refractory multiple myeloma. N Engl J Med 373(7):621–631

Lonial S, Richardson PG, Mateos M-V, Weisel K, Dimopoulos MA, Moreau P, Sy O, Katz J, Gupta M, Palumbo A (2016) ELOQUENT-2 update: phase III study of elotuzumab plus lenalidomide/dexamethasone (ELd) vs Ld in relapsed/refractory multiple myeloma (RRMM)—identifying responders by subset analysis. J Clin Oncol 34

Lonser RR, Glenn GM, Walther M, Chew EY, Libutti SK, Linehan WM et al (2003) von Hippel-Lindau disease. Lancet 361(9374):2059–2067

Loupakis F, Pollina L, Stasi I, Ruzzo A, Scartozzi M, Santini D et al (2009) PTEN expression and KRAS mutations on primary tumors and metastases in the prediction of benefit from cetuximab plus irinotecan for patients with metastatic colorectal cancer. J Clin Oncol 27(16):2622–2629

Lu Y, Zi X, Zhao Y, Mascarenhas D, Pollak M (2001) Insulin-like growth factor-I receptor signaling and resistance to trastuzumab (Herceptin). J Natl Cancer Inst 93(24):1852–1857

Lundin J, Kimby E, Björkholm M, Broliden P-A, Celsing F, Hjalmar V et al (2002) Phase II trial of subcutaneous anti-CD52 monoclonal antibody alemtuzumab (Campath-1H) as first-line treatment for patients with B-cell chronic lymphocytic leukemia (B-CLL). Blood 100(3):768–773

Luwor RB, Johns TG, Murone C, Huang HS, Cavenee WK, Ritter G et al (2001) Monoclonal antibody 806 inhibits the growth of tumor xenografts expressing either the de2–7 or amplified epidermal growth factor receptor (EGFR) but not wild-type EGFR. Can Res 61(14):5355–5361

Malavasi F, Funaro A, Roggero S, Horenstein A, Calosso L, Mehta K (1994) Human CD38: a glycoprotein in search of a function. Immunol Today 15(3):95–97

Maloney DG, Grillo-López AJ, White CA, Bodkin D, Schilder RJ, Neidhart JA et al (1997) IDEC-C2B8 (Rituximab) anti-CD20 monoclonal antibody therapy in patients with relapsed low-grade non-Hodgkin's lymphoma. 2188–2195. 1997-09-15 00:00:00

Manders P, Joshua A, Kefford R, Robert C, Ribas A, Hamid O et al (2016) Three-year overall survival for patients with advanced melanoma treated with pembrolizumab in Keynote-001. Asia-Pac J Clin Oncol 12:47–48

Marcus R, Imrie K, Belch A, Cunningham D, Flores E, Catalano J et al (2005) CVP chemotherapy plus rituximab compared with CVP as first-line treatment for advanced follicular lymphoma. Blood 105(4):1417–1423

Maric G, Rose A, Annis MG, Siegel PM (2013) Glycoprotein non-metastatic b (GPNMB): a metastatic mediator and emerging therapeutic target in cancer. OncoTargets Ther 6:839–852

McDermott D, Motzer R, Atkins M, Plimack E, Sznol M, George S (2016) Long-term overall survival (OS) with nivolumab in previously treated patients with advanced renal cell carcinoma (aRCC) from phase I and II studies. J Clin Oncol 34(Suppl):abstr 4507

Merino AG (2011) Monoclonal antibodies. Basic features. Neurologia 26(5):301–306

Mineo J-F, Bordron A, Baroncini M, Maurage C-A, Ramirez C, Siminski R-M et al (2007) Low HER2-expressing glioblastomas are more often secondary to anaplastic transformation of low-grade glioma. J Neurooncol 85(3):281–287

Misale S, Di Nicolantonio F, Sartore-Bianchi A, Siena S, Bardelli A (2014) Resistance to anti-EGFR therapy in colorectal cancer: from heterogeneity to convergent evolution. Cancer Discov 4(11):1269–1280

Mitchell EP, Perez-Soler R, Van Cutsem E, Lacouture ME (2007) Clinical presentation and pathophysiology of EGFRI dermatologic toxicities. Oncology 21(11 Suppl 5):4–9 (Williston Park, NY)

Moja L, Tagliabue L, Balduzzi S, Parmelli E, Pistotti V, Guarneri V et al (2012) Trastuzumab containing regimens for early breast cancer. Cochrane Libr

Morrison SL (1985) Transfectomas provide novel chimeric antibodies. Science 229(4719):1202–1207 (New York, NY)

Morrison C, Zanagnolo V, Ramirez N, Cohn DE, Kelbick N, Copeland L et al (2006) HER-2 is an independent prognostic factor in endometrial cancer: association with outcome in a large cohort of surgically staged patients. J Clin Oncol 24(15):2376–2385

Morschhauser F, Radford J, Van Hoof A, Vitolo U, Soubeyran P, Tilly H et al (2008) Phase III trial of consolidation therapy with yttrium-90–ibritumomab tiuxetan compared with no additional therapy after first remission in advanced follicular lymphoma. J Clin Oncol 26 (32):5156–5164

Morschhauser F, Radford J, Van Hoof A, Botto B, Rohatiner AZ, Salles G et al (2013) [90]Yttrium-ibritumomab tiuxetan consolidation of first remission in advanced-stage follicular non-Hodgkin lymphoma: updated results after a median follow-up of 7.3 years from the international, randomized, phase III first-line indolent trial. J Clin Oncol 31(16):1977–1983

Moskowitz CH, Nademanee A, Masszi T, Agura E, Holowiecki J, Abidi MH et al (2015) Brentuximab vedotin as consolidation therapy after autologous stem-cell transplantation in patients with Hodgkin's lymphoma at risk of relapse or progression (AETHERA): a randomised, double-blind, placebo-controlled, phase 3 trial. Lancet 385(9980):1853–1862

Moskowitz CH, Zinzani PL, Fanale MA, Armand P, Johnson NA, Radford JA et al (2016) Pembrolizumab in relapsed/refractory classical Hodgkin lymphoma: primary end point analysis of the phase 2 Keynote-087 study. Am Soc Hematol

Motzer RJ, Rini BI, McDermott DF, Redman BG, Kuzel TM, Harrison MR et al (2014) Nivolumab for metastatic renal cell carcinoma: results of a randomized phase II trial. J Clin Oncol 33(13):1430–1437

Motzer RJ, Escudier B, McDermott DF, George S, Hammers HJ, Srinivas S et al (2015) Nivolumab versus everolimus in advanced renal-cell carcinoma. N Engl J Med 373(19):1803–1813

Nagaraja V, Shaw N, Morey A, Cox M, Eslick G (2016) HER2 expression in oesophageal carcinoma and Barrett's oesophagus associated adenocarcinoma: an Australian study. Eur J Surg Oncol (EJSO) 42(1):140–148

Nagata Y, Lan K-H, Zhou X, Tan M, Esteva FJ, Sahin AA et al (2004) PTEN activation contributes to tumor inhibition by trastuzumab, and loss of PTEN predicts trastuzumab resistance in patients. Cancer Cell 6(2):117–127

Nahta R (2012) Pharmacological strategies to overcome HER2 cross-talk and Trastuzumab resistance. Curr Med Chem 19(7):1065–1075

Nahta R, Esteva FJ (2006) Molecular mechanisms of trastuzumab resistance. Breast Cancer Res 8 (6):667–674

Naidoo J, Page D, Li B, Connell L, Schindler K, Lacouture M et al (2015) Toxicities of the anti-PD-1 and anti-PD-L1 immune checkpoint antibodies. Ann Oncol 26(12):2375–2391

Naumnik W, Chyczewska E (2000) The clinical significance of serum soluble interleukin 2 receptor (sIL-2R) concentration in lung cancer. Folia Histochemica Cytobiol 39:185–186 (Polish Academy of Sciences, Polish Histochemical and Cytochemical Society)

Neuberger MS, Williams GT, Mitchell EB, Jouhal SS, Flanagan JG, Rabbitts TH (1985) A hapten-specific chimaeric IgE antibody with human physiological effector function. Nature 314 (6008):268–270

Nguyen DD, Cao TM, Dugan K, Starcher SA, Fechter RL, Coutre SE (2002) Cytomegalovirus viremia during Campath-1H therapy for relapsed and refractory chronic lymphocytic leukemia and prolymphocytic leukemia. Clin Lymphoma 3(2):105–110

Nijhof I, Groen R, Lokhorst H, Van Kessel B, Bloem A, Van Velzen J et al (2015) Upregulation of CD38 expression on multiple myeloma cells by all-trans retinoic acid improves the efficacy of daratumumab. Leukemia 29(10):2039–2049

Nijhof IS, Casneuf T, van Velzen J, van Kessel B, Axel AE, Syed K et al (2016) CD38 levels are associated with response and complement inhibitors contribute to resistance in myeloma patients treated with daratumumab. Blood. blood-2016-03-703439

Nimmerjahn F, Ravetch JV (2008) Fcγ receptors as regulators of immune responses. Nat Rev Immunol 8(1):34–47

Norderhaug L, Olafsen T, Michaelsen TE, Sandlie I (1997) Versatile vectors for transient and stable expression of recombinant antibody molecules in mammalian cells. J Immunol Methods 204(1):77–87

O'Brien NA, Browne BC, Chow L, Wang Y, Ginther C, Arboleda J et al (2010) Activated phosphoinositide 3-kinase/AKT signaling confers resistance to trastuzumab but not lapatinib. Mol Cancer Ther 9(6):1489–1502

Olayioye MA, Neve RM, Lane HA, Hynes NE (2000) The ErbB signaling network: receptor heterodimerization in development and cancer. EMBO J 19(13):3159–3167

Olsen E, Duvic M, Frankel A, Kim Y, Martin A, Vonderheid E et al (2001) Pivotal phase III trial of two dose levels of denileukin diftitox for the treatment of cutaneous T-cell lymphoma. J Clin Oncol 19(2):376–388

Oostendorp M, Lammerts van Bueren JJ, Doshi P, Khan I, Ahmadi T, Parren PW et al (2015) When blood transfusion medicine becomes complicated due to interference by monoclonal antibody therapy. Transfusion 55(6pt2):1555–1562

Osterborg A, Dyer M, Bunjes D, Pangalis GA, Bastion Y, Catovsky D et al (1997) Phase II multicenter study of human CD52 antibody in previously treated chronic lymphocytic leukemia. European study group of CAMPATH-1H treatment in chronic lymphocytic leukemia. J Clin Oncol 15(4):1567–1574

Ott P, Pavlick A, Johnson D, Hart L, Infante J, Luke J et al (2016) A phase 2 study of glembatumumab vedotin (GV), an antibody-drug conjugate (ADC) targeting gpNMB, in advanced melanoma. Ann Oncol 27(Suppl 6):1147P

Palumbo A, Chanan-Khan A, Weisel K, Nooka AK, Masszi T, Beksac M et al (2016) Daratumumab, bortezomib, and dexamethasone for multiple myeloma. N Engl J Med 375 (8):754–766

Parakh S, Parslow AC, Gan HK, Scott AM (2016a) Antibody-mediated delivery of therapeutics for cancer therapy. Expert Opin Drug Deliv 13(3):401–419

Parakh S, Nguyen R, Opie JM, Andrews MC (2016b) Late presentation of generalised bullous pemphigoid-like reaction in a patient treated with pembrolizumab for metastatic melanoma. Australas J Dermatol

Paz-Ares L, Mezger J, Ciuleanu TE, Fischer JR, von Pawel J, Provencio M et al (2015) Necitumumab plus pemetrexed and cisplatin as first-line therapy in patients with stage IV non-squamous non-small-cell lung cancer (INSPIRE): an open-label, randomised, controlled phase 3 study. Lancet Oncol 16(3):328–337

Paz-Ares L, Socinski M, Shahidi J, Hozak R, Soldatenkova V, Kurek R et al (2016) Correlation of EGFR-expression with safety and efficacy outcomes in SQUIRE: a randomized, multicenter, open-label, phase III study of gemcitabine-cisplatin plus necitumumab versus gemcitabine-cisplatin alone in the first-line treatment of patients with stage IV squamous non-small cell lung cancer. Ann Oncol mdw214

Peacock N, Saleh M, Bendell J, Rose A, Dong Z, Siegel P et al (2009) A phase I/II study of CR011-vcMMAE, an antibody-drug conjugate, in patients (pts) with locally advanced or metastatic breast cancer (MBC). J Clin Oncol 27(15S):1067

Peeters M, Siena S, Van Cutsem E, Sobrero A, Hendlisz A, Cascinu S et al (2009) Association of progression-free survival, overall survival, and patient-reported outcomes by skin toxicity and KRAS status in patients receiving panitumumab monotherapy. Cancer 115(7):1544–1554

Peeters M, Price TJ, Cervantes A, Sobrero AF, Ducreux M, Hotko Y et al (2010) Randomized phase III study of panitumumab with fluorouracil, leucovorin, and irinotecan (FOLFIRI) compared with FOLFIRI alone as second-line treatment in patients with metastatic colorectal cancer. J Clin Oncol 28(31):4706–4713

Peng W, Chen JQ, Liu C, Malu S, Creasy C, Tetzlaff MT et al (2016) Loss of PTEN promotes resistance to T cell-mediated immunotherapy. Cancer Discov 6(2):202–216

Perez EA, Romond EH, Suman VJ, Jeong J-H, Davidson NE, Geyer CE et al (2011) Four-year follow-up of trastuzumab plus adjuvant chemotherapy for operable human epidermal growth factor receptor 2–positive breast cancer: joint analysis of data from NCCTG N9831 and NSABP B-31. J Clin Oncol 29(25):3366–3373

Perez EA, Dueck AC, McCullough AE, Chen B, Geiger XJ, Jenkins RB et al (2013) Impact of PTEN protein expression on benefit from adjuvant trastuzumab in early-stage human epidermal growth factor receptor 2–positive breast cancer in the North Central Cancer Treatment Group N9831 trial. J Clin Oncol 31(17):2115–2122

Perez EA, Romond EH, Suman VJ, Jeong J-H, Sledge G, Geyer CE et al (2014) Trastuzumab plus adjuvant chemotherapy for human epidermal growth factor receptor 2–positive breast cancer: planned joint analysis of overall survival from NSABP B-31 and NCCTG N9831. J Clin Oncol 32(33):3744–3752

Perrone F, Lampis A, Orsenigo M, Di Bartolomeo M, Gevorgyan A, Losa M et al (2009) PI3KCA/PTEN deregulation contributes to impaired responses to cetuximab in metastatic colorectal cancer patients. Ann Oncol 20(1):84–90

Petrylak D, Kantoff P, Rotshteyn Y, Israel R, Olson W, Ramakrishna T et al (2011) Prostate-specific membrane antigen antibody drug conjugate (PSMA ADC): a phase I trial in taxane-refractory prostate cancer. J Clin Oncol 29(7 Suppl):158

Petrylak DP, Vogelzang NJ, Chatta GS, Fleming MT, Smith DC, Appleman LJ et al (2015) A phase 2 study of prostate specific membrane antigen antibody drug conjugate (PSMA ADC) in patients (pts) with progressive metastatic castration-resistant prostate cancer (mCRPC) following abiraterone and/or enzalutamide (abi/enz). Am Soc Clin Oncol

Pfreundschuh M, Kuhnt E, Trümper L, Osterborg A, Trneny M, Shepherd L et al (2010) Randomised intergroup trial of first line treatment for young low-risk patients (<61 years) with diffuse large B-cell non-Hodgkin's lymphoma (DLBCL) with a CHOP-like Regimen with or without the anti-CD20 antibody rituximab–6-year follow-up of the mint study of the Mabthera International Trial (MInT) group. Blood 116(21):111

Plesner T, Arkenau H-T, Lokhorst HM, Gimsing P, Krejcik J, Lemech C et al (2014) Safety and efficacy of daratumumab with lenalidomide and dexamethasone in relapsed or relapsed, refractory multiple myeloma. Blood 124(21):84

Pogue-Geile KL, Song N, Jeong J-H, Gavin PG, Kim S-R, Blackmon NL et al (2015) Intrinsic subtypes, PIK3CA mutation, and the degree of benefit from adjuvant trastuzumab in the NSABP B-31 trial. J Clin Oncol 33(12):1340–1347

Pollack VA, Alvarez E, Tse KF, Torgov MY, Xie S, Shenoy SG et al (2007) Treatment parameters modulating regression of human melanoma xenografts by an antibody–drug conjugate (CR390-vcMMAE) targeting GPNMB. Cancer Chemother Pharmacol 60(3):423–435

Postow MA (ed) (2015) Managing immune checkpoint-blocking antibody side effects. Am Soc Clin Oncol

Postow MA, Chesney J, Pavlick AC, Robert C, Grossmann K, McDermott D et al (2015) Nivolumab and ipilimumab versus ipilimumab in untreated melanoma. N Engl J Med 2015 (372):2006–2017

Provencio M, Cruz Mora MÁ, Gómez-Codina J, Quero Blanco C, Llanos M, García-Arroyo FR et al (2014) Consolidation treatment with Yttrium-90 ibritumomab tiuxetan after new induction regimen in patients with intermediate-and high-risk follicular lymphoma according to the follicular lymphoma international prognostic index: a multicenter, prospective phase II trial of the Spanish Lymphoma Oncology Group. Leuk Lymphoma 55(1):51–55

Pujade-Lauraine E, Hilpert F, Weber B, Reuss A, Poveda A, Kristensen G et al (2014) Bevacizumab combined with chemotherapy for platinum-resistant recurrent ovarian cancer: the AURELIA open-label randomized phase III trial. J Clin Oncol 32(13):1302–1308

Queen C, Schneider WP, Selick HE, Payne PW, Landolfi NF, Duncan JF et al (1989) A humanized antibody that binds to the interleukin 2 receptor. Proc Natl Acad Sci 86(24):10029–10033

Rai K, Freter C, Mercier R, Cooper M, Mitchell B, Stadtmauer E et al (2002) Alemtuzumab in previously treated chronic lymphocytic leukemia patients who also had received fludarabine. J Clin Oncol 20(18):3891–3897

Ranpura V, Pulipati B, Chu D, Zhu X, Wu S (2010) Increased risk of high-grade hypertension with bevacizumab in cancer patients: a meta-analysis. Am J Hypertens 23(5):460–468

Re GG, Waters C, Poisson L, Willingham MC, Sugamura K, Frankel AE (1996) Interleukin 2 (IL-2) receptor expression and sensitivity to diphtheria fusion toxin DAB389IL-2 in cultured hematopoietic cells. Can Res 56(11):2590–2595

Reck M, Rodríguez-Abreu D, Robinson AG, Hui R, Csőszi T, Fülöp A et al (2016) Pembrolizumab versus chemotherapy for PD-L1-positive non-small-cell lung cancer. N Engl J Med 375(19):1823–1833

Reichelt U, Duesedau P, Tsourlakis MC, Quaas A, Link BC, Schurr PG et al (2007) Frequent homogeneous HER-2 amplification in primary and metastatic adenocarcinoma of the esophagus. Mod Pathol 20(1):120–129

Rettig WJ, Old LJ (1989) Immunogenetics of human cell surface differentiation. Annu Rev Immunol 7(1):481–511

Ribas A, Puzanov I, Dummer R, Schadendorf D, Hamid O, Robert C et al (2015) Pembrolizumab versus investigator-choice chemotherapy for ipilimumab-refractory melanoma (KEYNOTE-002): a randomised, controlled, phase 2 trial. Lancet Oncol 16(8):908–918

Ribas A, Hamid O, Daud A, Hodi FS, Wolchok JD, Kefford R et al (2016) Association of pembrolizumab with tumor response and survival among patients with advanced melanoma. JAMA 315(15):1600–1609

Richards JO, Karki S, Lazar GA, Chen H, Dang W, Desjarlais JR (2008) Optimization of antibody binding to FcγRIIa enhances macrophage phagocytosis of tumor cells. Mol Cancer Ther 7 (8):2517–2527

Richardson PG, Jagannath S, Moreau P, Jakubowiak AJ, Raab MS, Facon T et al (2015) Elotuzumab in combination with lenalidomide and dexamethasone in patients with relapsed multiple myeloma: final phase 2 results from the randomised, open-label, phase 1b–2 dose-escalation study. Lancet Haematol 2(12):e516–e527

Ricklin D, Hajishengallis G, Yang K, Lambris JD (2010) Complement: a key system for immune surveillance and homeostasis. Nat Immunol 11(9):785–797

Riechmann L, Foote J, Winter G (1988) Expression of an antibody Fv fragment in myeloma cells. J Mol Biol 203(3):825–828

Rini BI, Halabi S, Rosenberg JE, Stadler WM, Vaena DA, Ou S-S et al (2008) Bevacizumab plus interferon alfa compared with interferon alfa monotherapy in patients with metastatic renal cell carcinoma: CALGB 90206. J Clin Oncol 26(33):5422–5428

Rini BI, Halabi S, Rosenberg JE, Stadler WM, Vaena DA, Archer L et al (2010) Phase III trial of bevacizumab plus interferon alfa versus interferon alfa monotherapy in patients with metastatic renal cell carcinoma: final results of CALGB 90206. J Clin Oncol 28(13):2137–2143

Ritchie M, Tchistiakova L, Scott N (eds) (2013) Implications of receptor-mediated endocytosis and intracellular trafficking dynamics in the development of antibody drug conjugates. MAbs. Taylor & Francis

Ritter CA, Perez-Torres M, Rinehart C, Guix M, Dugger T, Engelman JA et al (2007) Human breast cancer cells selected for resistance to trastuzumab in vivo overexpress epidermal growth factor receptor and ErbB ligands and remain dependent on the ErbB receptor network. Clin Cancer Res 13(16):4909–4919

Rittmeyer A, Barlesi F, Waterkamp D, Park K, Ciardiello F, Von Pawel J et al (2017) Atezolizumab versus docetaxel in patients with previously treated non-small-cell lung cancer (OAK): a phase 3, open-label, multicentre randomised controlled trial. Lancet 389(10066):255–265

Rizvi NA, Brahmer JR, Ou S-HI, Segal NH, Khleif S, Hwu W-J et al (2015) Safety and clinical activity of MEDI4736, an anti-programmed cell death-ligand 1 (PD-L1) antibody, in patients with non-small cell lung cancer (NSCLC). Am Soc Clin Oncol

Rizzieri D (2016) Zevalin®(ibritumomab tiuxetan): after more than a decade of treatment experience, what have we learned? Crit Rev Oncol/Hematol 105:5–17

Robak T, Dmoszynska A, Solal-Céligny P, Warzocha K, Loscertales J, Catalano J et al (2010) Rituximab plus fludarabine and cyclophosphamide prolongs progression-free survival compared with fludarabine and cyclophosphamide alone in previously treated chronic lymphocytic leukemia. J Clin Oncol 28(10):1756–1765

Robak T, Warzocha K, Govind Babu K, Kulyaba Y, Kuliczkowski K, Abdulkadyrov K et al (2017) Ofatumumab plus fludarabine and cyclophosphamide in relapsed chronic lymphocytic leukemia: results from the COMPLEMENT 2 trial. Leuk Lymphoma 58(5):1084–1093

Robert C, Long GV, Brady B, Dutriaux C, Maio M, Mortier L et al (2015a) Nivolumab in previously untreated melanoma without BRAF mutation. N Engl J Med 372(4):320–330

Robert C, Schachter J, Long GV, Arance A, Grob JJ, Mortier L et al (2015b) Pembrolizumab versus ipilimumab in advanced melanoma. N Engl J Med 372(26):2521–2532

Rose AA, Grosset A-A, Dong Z, Russo C, MacDonald PA, Bertos NR et al (2010) Glycoprotein nonmetastatic B is an independent prognostic indicator of recurrence and a novel therapeutic target in breast cancer. Clin Cancer Res 16(7):2147–2156

Rosenberg JE, Hoffman-Censits J, Powles T, Van Der Heijden MS, Balar AV, Necchi A et al (2016) Atezolizumab in patients with locally advanced and metastatic urothelial carcinoma who have progressed following treatment with platinum-based chemotherapy: a single-arm, multicentre, phase 2 trial. Lancet 387(10031):1909–1920

Rossi D, Khiabanian H, Spina V, Ciardullo C, Bruscaggin A, Famà R et al (2014) Clinical impact of small TP53 mutated subclones in chronic lymphocytic leukemia. Blood 123(14):2139–2147

Ruf P, Gires O, Jäger M, Fellinger K, Atz J, Lindhofer H (2007) Characterisation of the new EpCAM-specific antibody HO-3: implications for trifunctional antibody immunotherapy of cancer. Br J Cancer 97(3):315–321

Salles G, Seymour JF, Offner F, López-Guillermo A, Belada D, Xerri L et al (2011) Rituximab maintenance for 2 years in patients with high tumour burden follicular lymphoma responding to rituximab plus chemotherapy (PRIMA): a phase 3, randomised controlled trial. Lancet 377 (9759):42–51

Sanchez L, Wang Y, Siegel DS, Wang ML (2016) Daratumumab: a first-in-class CD38 monoclonal antibody for the treatment of multiple myeloma. J Hematol Oncol 9(1):51

Sandler A, Gray R, Perry MC, Brahmer J, Schiller JH, Dowlati A et al (2006) Paclitaxel–carboplatin alone or with bevacizumab for non-small-cell lung cancer. N Engl J Med 355 (24):2542–2550

Santin AD, Bellone S, Van Stedum S, Bushen W, Palmieri M, Siegel ER et al (2005) Amplification of c-erbB2 oncogene. Cancer 104(7):1391–1397

Santin AD, Bellone S, Roman JJ, McKenney JK, Pecorelli S (2008) Trastuzumab treatment in patients with advanced or recurrent endometrial carcinoma overexpressing HER2/neu. Int J Gynecol Obstet 102(2):128–131

Scappaticci FA, Skillings JR, Holden SN, Gerber H-P, Miller K, Kabbinavar F et al (2007) Arterial thromboembolic events in patients with metastatic carcinoma treated with chemotherapy and bevacizumab. J Natl Cancer Inst 99(16):1232–1239

Schneeweiss A, Chia S, Hickish T, Harvey V, Eniu A, Hegg R et al (2013) Pertuzumab plus trastuzumab in combination with standard neoadjuvant anthracycline-containing and anthracycline-free chemotherapy regimens in patients with HER2-positive early breast cancer: a randomized phase II cardiac safety study (TRYPHAENA). Ann Oncol 24(9):2278–2284

Scott LJ (2017) Brentuximab vedotin: a review in CD30-positive Hodgkin lymphoma. Drugs 77 (4):435–445

Scott AM, Wolchok JD, Old LJ (2012) Antibody therapy of cancer. Nat Rev Cancer 12(4):278–287

Segaert S, Van Cutsem E (2005) Clinical signs, pathophysiology and management of skin toxicity during therapy with epidermal growth factor receptor inhibitors. Ann Oncol 16(9):1425–1433

Segal NH, Verghis J, Govindan S, Maliakal P, Sharkey RM, Wegener WA et al (2013) Abstract LB-159: a phase I study of IMMU-130 (labetuzumab-SN38) anti-CEACAM5 antibody-drug conjugate (ADC) in patients with metastatic colorectal cancer (mCRC). AACR

Sehn LH, Chua N, Mayer J, Dueck G, Trněný M, Bouabdallah K et al (2016) Obinutuzumab plus bendamustine versus bendamustine monotherapy in patients with rituximab-refractory indolent non-Hodgkin lymphoma (GADOLIN): a randomised, controlled, open-label, multicentre, phase 3 trial. Lancet Oncol 17(8):1081–1093

Seiwert TY, Burtness B, Mehra R, Weiss J, Berger R, Eder JP et al (2016) Safety and clinical activity of pembrolizumab for treatment of recurrent or metastatic squamous cell carcinoma of the head and neck (KEYNOTE-012): an open-label, multicentre, phase 1b trial. Lancet Oncol 17(7):956–965

Semrad TJ, O'Donnell R, Wun T, Chew H, Harvey D, Zhou H et al (2007) Epidemiology of venous thromboembolism in 9489 patients with malignant glioma. J Neurosurg 106(4):601–608

Shaked Y, Bertolini F, Man S, Rogers MS, Cervi D, Foutz T et al (2005) Genetic heterogeneity of the vasculogenic phenotype parallels angiogenesis: implications for cellular surrogate marker analysis of antiangiogenesis. Cancer Cell 7(1):101–111

Sharma P, Callahan MK, Bono P, Kim J, Spiliopoulou P, Calvo E et al (2016) Nivolumab monotherapy in recurrent metastatic urothelial carcinoma (CheckMate 032): a multicentre, open-label, two-stage, multi-arm, phase 1/2 trial. Lancet Oncol 17(11):1590–1598

Sharma P, Retz M, Siefker-Radtke A, Baron A, Necchi A, Bedke J et al (2017) Nivolumab in metastatic urothelial carcinoma after platinum therapy (CheckMate 275): a multicentre, single-arm, phase 2 trial. Lancet Oncol 18(3):312–322

Shattuck DL, Miller JK, Carraway KL, Sweeney C (2008) Met receptor contributes to trastuzumab resistance of Her2-overexpressing breast cancer cells. Can Res 68(5):1471–1477

Siena S, Sartore-Bianchi A, Lonardi S, Trusolino L, Martino C, Bencardino K et al (2015) Trastuzumab and lapatinib in HER2-amplified metastatic colorectal cancer patients (mCRC): the HERACLES trial. Am Soc Clin Oncol

Slamon DJ, Clark GM, Wong SG, Levin WJ, Ullrich A, McGuire WL (1987) Human breast cancer: correlation of relapse and survival with amplification of the HER-2/neu oncogene. Science 235(4785):177–182

Slamon DJ, Leyland-Jones B, Shak S, Fuchs H, Paton V, Bajamonde A et al (2001) Use of chemotherapy plus a monoclonal antibody against HER2 for metastatic breast cancer that overexpresses HER2. N Engl J Med 344(11):783–792

Slamon D, Eiermann W, Robert N, Pienkowski T, Martin M, Rolski J et al (2009) Phase III randomized trial comparing doxorubicin and cyclophosphamide followed by docetaxel (AC → T) with doxorubicin and cyclophosphamide followed by docetaxel and trastuzumab (AC → TH) with docetaxel, carboplatin and trastuzumab (TCH) in HER2 positive early breast cancer patients: BCIRG 006 study. Cancer Res 69(24 Suppl):62

Smith GP (1985) Filamentous fusion phage: novel expression vectors that display cloned antigens on the virion surface. Science 228(4705):1315–1317 (New York, NY)

Socinski M, Creelan B, Horn L, Reck M, Paz-Ares L, Steins M et al (2016) NSCLC, metastaticCheckMate 026: a phase 3 trial of nivolumab vs investigator's choice (IC) of platinum-based doublet chemotherapy (PT-DC) as first-line therapy for stage iv/recurrent programmed death ligand 1 (PD-L1)-positive NSCLC. Ann Oncol 27(Suppl 6):LBA7_PR

Soria J-C, Mauguen A, Reck M, Sandler A, Saijo N, Johnson D et al (2012) Systematic review and meta-analysis of randomised, phase II/III trials adding bevacizumab to platinum-based chemotherapy as first-line treatment in patients with advanced non-small-cell lung cancer. Ann Oncol mds590

Sorich M, Wiese M, Rowland A, Kichenadasse G, McKinnon R, Karapetis C (2015) Extended RAS mutations and anti-EGFR monoclonal antibody survival benefit in metastatic colorectal cancer: a meta-analysis of randomized, controlled trials. Ann Oncol 26(1):13–21

Spector NL, Blackwell KL (2009) Understanding the mechanisms behind trastuzumab therapy for human epidermal growth factor receptor 2–positive breast cancer. J Clin Oncol 27(34):5838–5847

Spratlin JL, Cohen RB, Eadens M, Gore L, Camidge DR, Diab S et al (2010) Phase I pharmacologic and biologic study of ramucirumab (IMC-1121B), a fully human immunoglobulin G1 monoclonal antibody targeting the vascular endothelial growth factor receptor-2. J Clin Oncol 28(5):780–787

Starodub A, Ocean AJ, Messersmith WA, Picozzi VJ, Guarino MJ, Bardia A et al (2015) Therapy of gastrointestinal malignancies with an anti-Trop-2-SN-38 antibody drug conjugate (ADC) (sacituzumab govitecan): phase I/II clinical experience. Am Soc Clin Oncol

Stish B, Oh S, Chen H, Dudek A, Kratzke R, Vallera D (2009) Design and modification of EGF4KDEL 7Mut, a novel bispecific ligand-directed toxin, with decreased immunogenicity and potent anti-mesothelioma activity. Br J Cancer 101(7):1114–1123

Sugimoto H, Hamano Y, Charytan D, Cosgrove D, Kieran M, Sudhakar A et al (2003) Neutralization of circulating vascular endothelial growth factor (VEGF) by anti-VEGF antibodies and soluble VEGF receptor 1 (sFlt-1) induces proteinuria. J Biol Chem 278 (15):12605–12608

Swain SM, Ewer MS, Cortés J, Amadori D, Miles D, Knott A et al (2013) Cardiac tolerability of pertuzumab plus trastuzumab plus docetaxel in patients with HER2-positive metastatic breast cancer in CLEOPATRA: a randomized, double-blind, placebo-controlled phase III study. Oncologist 18(3):257–264

Swain SM, Baselga J, Kim S-B, Ro J, Semiglazov V, Campone M et al (2015) Pertuzumab, trastuzumab, and docetaxel in HER2-positive metastatic breast cancer. N Engl J Med 372 (8):724–734

Taal W, Oosterkamp HM, Walenkamp AM, Dubbink HJ, Beerepoot LV, Hanse MC et al (2014) Single-agent bevacizumab or lomustine versus a combination of bevacizumab plus lomustine in patients with recurrent glioblastoma (BELOB trial): a randomised controlled phase 2 trial. Lancet Oncol 15(9):943–953

Tabernero J, Yoshino T, Cohn AL, Obermannova R, Bodoky G, Garcia-Carbonero R et al (2015) Ramucirumab versus placebo in combination with second-line FOLFIRI in patients with metastatic colorectal carcinoma that progressed during or after first-line therapy with bevacizumab, oxaliplatin, and a fluoropyrimidine (RAISE): a randomised, double-blind, multicentre, phase 3 study. Lancet Oncol 16(5):499–508

Tagawa ST, Ocean AJ, Lam ET, Saylor PJ, Bardia A, Hajdenberg J et al (2017) Therapy for chemopretreated metastatic urothelial cancer (mUC) with the antibody-drug conjugate (ADC) sacituzumab govitecan (IMMU-132). Am Soc Clin Oncol

Tai Y-T, Dillon M, Song W, Leiba M, Li X-F, Burger P et al (2008) Anti-CS1 humanized monoclonal antibody HuLuc63 inhibits myeloma cell adhesion and induces antibody-dependent cellular cytotoxicity in the bone marrow milieu. Blood 112(4):1329–1337

Takei K, Yamazaki T, Sawada U, Ishizuka H, Aizawa S (2006) Analysis of changes in CD20, CD55, and CD59 expression on established rituximab-resistant B-lymphoma cell lines. Leuk Res 30(5):625–631

Tanner M, Hollmen M, Junttila T, Kapanen A, Tommola S, Soini Y et al (2005) Amplification of HER-2 in gastric carcinoma: association with Topoisomerase IIα gene amplification, intestinal type, poor prognosis and sensitivity to trastuzumab. Ann Oncol 16(2):273–278

Teicher BA, Chari RV (2011) Antibody conjugate therapeutics: challenges and potential. Clin Cancer Res 17(20):6389–6397

Teicher BA, Ellis LM (2008) Antiangiogenic agents in cancer therapy. Springer Science & Business Media

Telang S, Rasku MA, Clem AL, Carter K, Klarer AC, Badger WR et al (2011) Phase II trial of the regulatory T cell-depleting agent, denileukin diftitox, in patients with unresectable stage IV melanoma. BMC Cancer 11(1):515

Thatcher N, Hirsch FR, Luft AV, Szczesna A, Ciuleanu TE, Dediu M et al (2015) Necitumumab plus gemcitabine and cisplatin versus gemcitabine and cisplatin alone as first-line therapy in patients with stage IV squamous non-small-cell lung cancer (SQUIRE): an open-label, randomised, controlled phase 3 trial. Lancet Oncol 16(7):763–774

Thompson PA, Tam CS, O'Brien SM, Wierda WG, Stingo F, Plunkett W et al (2016) Fludarabine, cyclophosphamide, and rituximab treatment achieves long-term disease-free survival in IGHV-mutated chronic lymphocytic leukemia. Blood 127(3):303–309

Timmerman JM, Engert A, Younes A, Santoro A, Armand P, Fanale MA et al (2016) Checkmate 205 update with minimum 12-month follow up: a phase 2 study of nivolumab in patients with relapsed/refractory classical Hodgkin lymphoma. Am Soc Hematol

Tol J, Nagtegaal ID, Punt CJ (2009) BRAF mutation in metastatic colorectal cancer. N Engl J Med 361(1):98–99

Tonelli AR, Lottenberg R, Allan RW, Sriram P (2009) Rituximab-induced hypersensitivity pneumonitis. Respiration 78(2):225–229

Tonini G, Vincenzi B, Santini D, Olzi D, Lambiase A, Bonini S (2005) Ocular toxicity related to cetuximab monotherapy in an advanced colorectal cancer patient. J Natl Cancer Inst 97 (8):606–607

Topalian SL, Sznol M, McDermott DF, Kluger HM, Carvajal RD, Sharfman WH et al (2014) Survival, durable tumor remission, and long-term safety in patients with advanced melanoma receiving nivolumab. J Clin Oncol 32(10):1020–1030

Topp MS, Gökbuget N, Stein AS, Zugmaier G, O'Brien S, Bargou RC et al (2015) Safety and activity of blinatumomab for adult patients with relapsed or refractory B-precursor acute lymphoblastic leukaemia: a multicentre, single-arm, phase 2 study. Lancet Oncol 16(1):57–66

Trastuzumab FDA label (version approved on 01/18/2008). Available from: http://www.fda.gov/cder/foi/label/2008/103792s5175lbl.pdf

Tse KF, Jeffers M, Pollack VA, McCabe DA, Shadish ML, Khramtsov NV et al (2006) CR389, a fully human monoclonal antibody-auristatin E conjugate, for the treatment of melanoma. Clin Cancer Res 12(4):1373–1382

Tuefferd M, Couturier J, Penault-Llorca F, Vincent-Salomon A, Broët P, Guastalla J-P et al (2007) HER2 status in ovarian carcinomas: a multicenter GINECO study of 320 patients. PLoS ONE 2 (11):e1138

Untch M, Rezai M, Loibl S, Fasching PA, Huober J, Tesch H et al (2010) Neoadjuvant treatment with trastuzumab in HER2-positive breast cancer: results from the GeparQuattro study. J Clin Oncol 28(12):2024–2031

Usmani S, Sexton R, Ailawadhi S, Shah J, Valent J, Rosenzweig M et al (2015) Phase I safety data of lenalidomide, bortezomib, dexamethasone, and elotuzumab as induction therapy for newly diagnosed symptomatic multiple myeloma: SWOG S1211. Blood Cancer J 5:e334

Vallera DA, Todhunter DA, Kuroki DW, Shu Y, Sicheneder A, Chen H (2005) A bispecific recombinant immunotoxin, DT2219, targeting human CD19 and CD22 receptors in a mouse xenograft model of B-cell leukemia/lymphoma. Clin Cancer Res 11(10):3879–3888

Van Beijnum JR, Nowak-Sliwinska P, Huijbers EJ, Thijssen VL, Griffioen AW (2015) The great escape; the hallmarks of resistance to antiangiogenic therapy. Pharmacol Rev 67(2):441–461

Van Cutsem E, Peeters M, Siena S, Humblet Y, Hendlisz A, Neyns B et al (2007a) Open-label phase III trial of panitumumab plus best supportive care compared with best supportive care alone in patients with chemotherapy-refractory metastatic colorectal cancer. J Clin Oncol 25 (13):1658–1664

Van Cutsem E, Siena S, Humblet Y, Canon J, Maurel J, Bajetta E et al (2007b) An open-label, single-arm study assessing safety and efficacy of panitumumab in patients with metastatic colorectal cancer refractory to standard chemotherapy. Ann Oncol mdm399

Van Cutsem E, Köhne C-H, Hitre E, Zaluski J, Chang Chien C-R, Makhson A et al (2009) Cetuximab and chemotherapy as initial treatment for metastatic colorectal cancer. N Engl J Med 360(14):1408–1417

Van Cutsem E, Köhne C-H, Láng I, Folprecht G, Nowacki MP, Cascinu S et al (2011) Cetuximab plus irinotecan, fluorouracil, and leucovorin as first-line treatment for metastatic colorectal cancer: updated analysis of overall survival according to tumor KRAS and BRAF mutation status. J Clin Oncol 29(15):2011–2019

van Rhee F, Szmania SM, Dillon M, van Abbema AM, Li X, Stone MK et al (2009) Combinatorial efficacy of anti-CS1 monoclonal antibody elotuzumab (HuLuc63) and bortezomib against multiple myeloma. Mol Cancer Ther 8(9):2616–2624

Verma S, Miles D, Gianni L, Krop IE, Welslau M, Baselga J et al (2012) Trastuzumab emtansine for HER2-positive advanced breast cancer. N Engl J Med 367(19):1783–1791

Vermorken JB, Mesia R, Rivera F, Remenar E, Kawecki A, Rottey S et al (2008) Platinum-based chemotherapy plus cetuximab in head and neck cancer. N Engl J Med 359(11):1116–1127

Vermorken J, Psyrri A, Mesia R, Peyrade F, Beier F, De Blas B et al (2014) Impact of tumor HPV status on outcome in patients with recurrent and/or metastatic squamous cell carcinoma of the head and neck receiving chemotherapy with or without cetuximab: retrospective analysis of the phase III EXTREME trial. Ann Oncol mdt574

Vogel CL, Cobleigh MA, Tripathy D, Gutheil JC, Harris LN, Fehrenbacher L et al (2002) Efficacy and safety of trastuzumab as a single agent in first-line treatment of HER2-overexpressing metastatic breast cancer. J Clin Oncol 20(3):719–726

Von Minckwitz G, Procter MJ, De Azambuja E, Zardavas D, Knott A, Viale G et al (2017) APHINITY trial (BIG 4-11): a randomized comparison of chemotherapy (C) plus trastuzumab (T) plus placebo (Pla) versus chemotherapy plus trastuzumab (T) plus pertuzumab (P) as adjuvant therapy in patients (pts) with HER2-positive early breast cancer (EBC). Am Soc Clin Oncol

Wang Y, Liu Y, Du Y, Yin W, Lu J (2013) The predictive role of phosphatase and tensin homolog (PTEN) loss, phosphoinositol-3 (PI3) kinase (PIK3CA) mutation, and PI3K pathway activation in sensitivity to trastuzumab in HER2-positive breast cancer: a meta-analysis. Curr Med Res Opin 29(6):633–642

Watanabe T, Masuyama J, Sohma Y, Inazawa H, Horie K, Kojima K et al (2006) CD52 is a novel costimulatory molecule for induction of CD4+ regulatory T cells. Clin Immunol 120(3):247–259

Weber JS, Kähler KC, Hauschild A (2012) Management of immune-related adverse events and kinetics of response with ipilimumab. J Clin Oncol 30(21):2691–2697

Weber JS, D'Angelo SP, Minor D, Hodi FS, Gutzmer R, Neyns B et al (2015a) Nivolumab versus chemotherapy in patients with advanced melanoma who progressed after anti-CTLA-4 treatment (CheckMate 037): a randomised, controlled, open-label, phase 3 trial. Lancet Oncol 16(4):375–384

Weber JS, Yang JC, Atkins MB, Disis ML (2015b) Toxicities of immunotherapy for the practitioner. J Clin Oncol 33(18):2092–2099

Wierda WG, Kipps TJ, Mayer J, Stilgenbauer S, Williams CD, Hellmann A et al (2010) Ofatumumab as single-agent CD20 immunotherapy in fludarabine-refractory chronic lympho-cytic leukemia. J Clin Oncol 28(10):1749–1755

Wildiers H, Kim S, Gonzalez-Martin A, LoRusso P, Ferrero J, Smitt M et al (eds) (2013) T-DM1 for HER2-positive metastatic breast cancer (MBC): primary results from TH3RESA, a phase 3 study of T-DM1 vs treatment of physician's choice. Eur J Cancer (Elsevier Sci Ltd the Boulevard, Langford Lane, Kidlington, Oxford OX5 1GB, Oxon, England)

Wilke H, Muro K, Van Cutsem E, Oh S-C, Bodoky G, Shimada Y et al (2014) Ramucirumab plus paclitaxel versus placebo plus paclitaxel in patients with previously treated advanced gastric or gastro-oesophageal junction adenocarcinoma (RAINBOW): a double-blind, randomised phase 3 trial. Lancet Oncol 15(11):1224–1235

Willett CG, Boucher Y, di Tomaso E, Duda DG, Munn LL, Tong RT et al (2004) Direct evidence that the VEGF-specific antibody bevacizumab has antivascular effects in human rectal cancer. Nat Med 10(2):145–147

Winter G, Milstein C (1991) Man-made antibodies. Nature 349(6307):293–299

Winter JN, Weller EA, Horning SJ, Krajewska M, Variakojis D, Habermann TM et al (2006) Prognostic significance of Bcl-6 protein expression in DLBCL treated with CHOP or R-CHOP: a prospective correlative study. Blood 107(11):4207–4213

Wiseman GA, Gordon LI, Multani PS, Witzig TE, Spies S, Bartlett NL et al (2002) Ibritumomab tiuxetan radioimmunotherapy for patients with relapsed or refractory non-Hodgkin lymphoma and mild thrombocytopenia: a phase II multicenter trial. Blood 99(12):4336–4342

Witzig TE (2002) Zevalin™. Drugs Future 27(6):563–568

Witzig TE, White CA, Wiseman GA, Gordon LI, Emmanouilides C, Raubitschek A et al (1999) Phase I/II trial of IDEC-Y2B8 radioimmunotherapy for treatment of relapsed or refractory CD20⁺ B-cell non-Hodgkin's lymphoma. J Clin Oncol 17(12):3793–3803

Wolchok JD, Neyns B, Linette G, Negrier S, Lutzky J, Thomas L et al (2010) Ipilimumab monotherapy in patients with pretreated advanced melanoma: a randomised, double-blind, multicentre, phase 2, dose-ranging study. Lancet Oncol 11(2):155–164

Wolchok JD, Kluger H, Callahan MK, Postow MA, Rizvi NA, Lesokhin AM et al (2013) Nivolumab plus ipilimumab in advanced melanoma. N Engl J Med 369(2):122–133

Wolchok J, Chiarion-Sileni V, Gonzalez R, Rutkowski P, Grob J, Cowey C et al (2016) Updated results from a phase III trial of nivolumab (NIVO) combined with ipilimumab (IPI) in treatment-naive patients (pts) with advanced melanoma (MEL) (CheckMate 067). J Clin Oncol 34(Suppl; abstr 9505)

Wu S, Kim C, Baer L, Zhu X (2010) Bevacizumab increases risk for severe proteinuria in cancer patients. J Am Soc Nephrol 21(8):1381–1389

Wuerkenbieke D, Wang J, Li Y, Ma C (2015) miRNA-150 downregulation promotes pertuzumab resistance in ovarian cancer cells via AKT activation. Arch Gynecol Obstet 292(5):1109–1116

Xia MQ, Tone M, Packman L, Hale G, Waldmann H (1991) Characterization of the CAMPATH-1 (CDw52) antigen: biochemical analysis and cDNA cloning reveal an unusually small peptide backbone. Eur J Immunol 21(7):1677–1684

Xu W, Miao KR, Zhu DX, Fang C, Zhu HY, Dong HJ et al (2011) Enhancing the action of rituximab by adding fresh frozen plasma for the treatment of fludarabine refractory chronic lymphocytic leukemia. Int J Cancer 128(9):2192–2201

Yakes FM, Chinratanalab W, Ritter CA, King W, Seelig S, Arteaga CL (2002) Herceptin-induced inhibition of phosphatidylinositol-3 kinase and Akt Is required for antibody-mediated effects on p27, cyclin D1, and antitumor action. Can Res 62(14):4132–4141

Yang X-D, Jia X-C, Corvalan JR, Wang P, Davis CG (2001) Development of ABX-EGF, a fully human anti-EGF receptor monoclonal antibody, for cancer therapy. Crit Rev Oncol/Hematol 38(1):17–23

Yang JC, Haworth L, Sherry RM, Hwu P, Schwartzentruber DJ, Topalian SL et al (2003) A randomized trial of bevacizumab, an anti-vascular endothelial growth factor antibody, for metastatic renal cancer. N Engl J Med 349(5):427–434

YERVOY™ (ipilimumab) (2011) US prescribing information: risk evaluation and mitigation strategy (REMS). Bristol-Myers Squibb Company, Princeton, NJ, USA. Available from: http://www.hcp.yervoy.com/

Yonemura Y, Ninomiya I, Yamaguchi A, Fushida S, Kimura H, Ohoyama S et al (1991) Evaluation of immunoreactivity for erbB-2 protein as a marker of poor short term prognosis in gastric cancer. Can Res 51(3):1034–1038

Yonesaka K, Zejnullahu K, Okamoto I, Satoh T, Cappuzzo F, Souglakos J et al (2011) Activation of ERBB2 signaling causes resistance to the EGFR-directed therapeutic antibody cetuximab. Sci Transl Med 3(99):99ra86–99ra86

Younes A, Kadin ME (2003) Emerging applications of the tumor necrosis factor family of ligands and receptors in cancer therapy. J Clin Oncol 21(18):3526–3534

Younes A, Gopal AK, Smith SE, Ansell SM, Rosenblatt JD, Savage KJ et al (2012) Results of a pivotal phase II study of brentuximab vedotin for patients with relapsed or refractory Hodgkin's lymphoma. J Clin Oncol 30(18):2183–2189

Zaretsky JM, Garcia-Diaz A, Shin DS, Escuin-Ordinas H, Hugo W, Hu-Lieskovan S et al (2016) Mutations associated with acquired resistance to PD-1 blockade in melanoma. N Engl J Med 375(9):819–829

Zeidler R, Reisbach G, Wollenberg B, Lang S, Chaubal S, Schmitt B et al (1999) Simultaneous activation of T cells and accessory cells by a new class of intact bispecific antibody results in efficient tumor cell killing. J Immunol 163(3):1246–1252

Zeidler R, Mysliwietz J, Csanady M, Walz A, Ziegler I, Schmitt B et al (2000) The Fc-region of a
    new class of intact bispecific antibody mediates activation of accessory cells and NK cells and
    induces direct phagocytosis of tumour cells. Br J Cancer 83(2):261
Zent CS, Bone ND, Geyer SM, Kay NE (2005) Tumor cells resistant to alemtuzumab complement
    mediated cytotoxicity in patients with high risk previously untreated early stage CLL: a
    possible mechanism of treatment failure. Blood 106(11):2973
Zhuang G, Brantley-Sieders DM, Vaught D, Yu J, Xie L, Wells S et al (2010) Elevation of
    receptor tyrosine kinase EphA2 mediates resistance to trastuzumab therapy. Can Res 70
    (1):299–308
Zonder JA, Mohrbacher AF, Singhal S, Van Rhee F, Bensinger WI, Ding H et al (2012) A phase 1,
    multicenter, open-label, dose escalation study of elotuzumab in patients with advanced
    multiple myeloma. Blood 120(3):552–559

Clinical Experience with Bispecific T Cell Engagers

Nicola Gökbuget

1 Construction and Mechanism of Action

Bispecific T cell engager (BiTE) antibodies consist of two different single-chain Fv fragments, being specific for a target on a malignant cell on one arm and for CD3 on the other arm (Dahlen et al. 2018). CD3 is a characteristic T cell antigen, which is part of the T cell receptor signaling complex (Krshnan et al. 2016). Cytotoxic T cells are especially important effectors in this scenario. If the linker molecule is very small, T cells are brought very close to the target cells, leading to cell lysis. In principle, different target antigens in hematologic malignancies or solid tumors can be addressed by these constructs such as EpCAM, HER2/neu, EGFR, CEA, CD33, CD19, EPHA2, PSMA, BCMA, and MCSP (or HMW-MAA) (Frankel and Baeuerle 2013).

Most clinical experience has been obtained with the bispecific antibody construct blinatumomab (Loffler et al. 2000; Bargou et al. 2008). The following review will therefore focus mainly on this specific compound.

The malignant target-specific arm of blinatumomab binds to any CD19-positive B lymphocyte. CD19 is a B-lineage surface antigen, which is expressed throughout B cell development except for the terminally differentiated plasma cell (Carter and Fearon 1992; Nadler et al. 1983). The other part of the antibody binds to CD3-positive T cells (Loffler et al. 2003). Both fragments are joined by a glycine–serine linker (Loffler et al. 2000). This design allows for optimal rotation and thereby enables a close interaction between the T cell and leukemia cells. Through binding, T cells are activated, start cytokine excretion, and direct cytotoxicity without co-stimulation (Dreier et al. 2002). Thus, the compound is able to induce a

N. Gökbuget (✉)
Department of Medicine II, University Hospital Goethe University, Theodor Stern Kai 7, 60590 Frankfurt, Germany
e-mail: goekbuget@em.uni-frankfurt.de

© Springer Nature Switzerland AG 2020   71
M. Theobald (ed.), *Current Immunotherapeutic Strategies in Cancer*,
Recent Results in Cancer Research 214,
https://doi.org/10.1007/978-3-030-23765-3_2

T cell response in an MHC-independent manner and thereby circumvents a number of frequent escape mechanisms. Importantly, T cell activation appears only in the presence of CD19-positive target cells (Kufer et al. 2001). Blinatumomab has a higher affinity to CD19 compared to CD3. Therefore, the antibody construct preferably binds to CD19 and T cells can move from one B cell to another, performing an effective serial lysis (Dreier et al. 2002; Hoffmann et al. 2005, 2011). Blinatumomab is able to establish tight cytolytic synapses between effector cells and target cells (Offner et al. 2006). This leads to a perforin-/granzyme-mediated destruction of the target cells (Gruen et al. 2004; Conter et al. 2010). T cell activation and proliferation is polyclonal and involves CD8- and CD4-positive cells. T cells express activation markers as well as adhesion molecules on their surface (Nagorsen and Baeuerle 2011; Wolf et al. 2005). The activated T cells release inflammatory cytokines such as IL-6, IL-10, and Interferon-γ with dose-dependent peak concentrations (Hoffmann et al. 2005; Brandl et al. 2007; Brischwein et al. 2006). T cell activation markers such as CD69 and CD25 are increased in the T cell fraction upon recovery (Bargou et al. 2008). Overall, the mechanism of action relies on the presence of at least a low number of functional T cells of the patient.

2 Pharmacokinetics and Pharmacodynamics of Blinatumomab

Blinatumomab is a small molecule with a molecular weight of 55 kDa (Loffler et al. 2000; Nagorsen and Baeuerle 2011; Nagorsen et al. 2009) [reviewed in (Goebeler and Bargou 2016)]. The half-life is approximately 2 h. It is cleaved in circulation into amino acids and does not undergo renal or hepatic clearance (Klinger et al. 2016a). Due to its short half-life, blinatumomab has to be administered as a continuous infusion in order to maintain constant activity. The usual current application mode is a four-week continuous infusion, followed by a two-week treatment-free interval. Patients are usually monitored as inpatients for at least 3–7 days at the start of therapy or at dose escalation. In the outpatient setting, the continuous infusion usually requires implanted port and mini-pump systems.

Mean steady-state concentration (Css) of blinatumomab depends on dose (9 µg/d vs. 28 µg/d) and ranges between 211 pg/ml versus 621 pg/ml. At the start of infusion, inflammatory cytokines such as Interferon-γ, TNF, IL-2, IL6, and IL-10 increase. In parallel, a depletion of B cells is observed (Bargou et al. 2008).

Dosing in earlier trials was based on body surface with 5 µg/m^2/d as starting dose and 15 µg/m^2/d as final dose (Topp et al. 2015a). Later, a fixed schedule with corresponding doses of 9 and 28 µg/d was used (Kantarjian et al. 2017) in adults. In children, the dosing based on body surface was maintained. In non-Hodgkin's lymphoma (NHL), 5–60 µg/m^2/d or dosing regimes up to 112 µg/d were tested with stepwise dose escalation (Goebeler and Bargou 2016; Viardot et al. 2016).

3 Clinical Efficacy of Blinatumomab

Clinical activity of blinatumomab was first tested in relapsed or refractory (R/R) NHL, where it showed efficacy in very low doses. The observed activity in NHL cases with bone marrow involvement was of specific interest. Subsequent clinical development focused on acute lymphoblastic leukemia (ALL). B-precursor ALL constitutes 70–80% of all ALL cases, and CD19 is expressed on the blast cells in more than 95% of the cases. Therefore, blinatumomab was tested for R/R B-precursor ALL and B-precursor ALL with persistent minimal residual disease (MRD), and the first experience was gained in newly diagnosed ALL [reviewed in Goebeler and Bargou (2016), Wilke and Gökbuget (2017), DasGupta et al. (2018)].

3.1 Relapsed/Refractory Non-Hodgkin's Lymphoma

The first application of blinatumomab took place in patients with R/R NHL (Bargou et al. 2008). The trial included patients with different lymphoma entities. Thirty-eight patients received blinatumomab at doses from 0.0005 to 0.06 mg/m^2 per day. Eleven major responses were observed including four complete responses. Partial and complete tumor regressions were first observed at a dose level of 0.015 mg (Table 1). Responses were reported for all lymphoma entities (Bargou et al. 2008).

Overall, 76 patients with different entities of R/R NHL were treated in an extended phase I trial between 2004 and 2011. Dose levels of 0.5–90 µg/m^2/d for 4–8 weeks were tested during the dose-finding phase of the trial which included 42 patients. The maximum tolerated dose (MTD) was defined as 60 µg/m^2/d, i.e., 112 µg/d flat dose. Additional 34 patients were treated with the dose of 60 µg/m^2/d, and stepwise dosing in different variations was tested such as single-step, double-step, and the use of pentosan polysulfate as a potential strategy to mitigate neurologic effects. Thus, the target dose of 60 µg/m^2/d was administered as a constant (flat) dose, single-step (starting with 5 µg/m^2/d for 7 days) or double-step dose escalation (starting with 5 µg/m^2/d for 7 days, then 15 µg/m^2/d for 7 days until reaching 60 µg/m^2/d). Most patients, however, were treated with the latter dose escalation schedule.

At a dose of 60 µg/m^2/day, the overall response rate was 69% in 34 evaluable patients (37% CR/CRu and 31% PR). Notably, no responses were observed at doses lower than 15 µg/m^2/day (corresponding to 30 µg/day). Neurologic events of grade 3 were observed in 22% of the patients (Goebeler and Bargou 2016).

A phase II trial included patients with R/R diffuse large B cell lymphoma (DLBCL). Again, the definition of a tolerable and effective dosing schedule was one major goal of the trial. The target dose was 112 µg/d as a continuous infusion for up to 8 weeks, followed by a four-week treatment-free interval. Patients in cohort I were treated with 9 µg/d during week 1, followed by 28 µg/d for week 2 and 112 µg/d thereafter. In a second cohort, patients were treated with a flat dose of

N. Gökbuget

Table 1 Results from clinical trials with blinatumomab in ALL and NHL

Author	Year	No. of patients	Median age	Indication	Treatment regimen	Response	Overall survival in months
Bargou et al. (2008)	2008	38	Adult	Adult relapsed NHL	0.0005–0.06 mg/m²/d	29% major responses	Not available
Topp et al. (2011)	2011	21	47 (20–77)	Adult MRD-positive B-prec ALL	15 µg/m²/d × 4 wk, q6wk	80% MRD response	Not available
Topp et al. (2014)	2014	36	32 (18–77)	Adult R/R B-prec ALL	5–30 µg/m²/d × 4 wk, q6wk	69% CR and CRh, 88% MRD response within cycle 1	9.8
Topp et al. (2015b)	2015	189	39 (18–79)	Adult R/R Ph-negative B-prec ALL	9 µg/d for the first wk, 28 µg/d for 3 wk, q6wk, subsequent cycles 28 µg/d for 4 wk, q6wk	43% CR or CRh within two cycles, 82% MRD response	6.1
Viardot et al. (2016)	2016	25	66 (34–85)	Adult R/R DLBCL	9–112 µg/d × 8 wk (stepwise dose escalation 9–28–112 µg/d, flat dosing 112 µg/d)	43% ORR	5.0
Goebeler et al. (2016)	2016	76	65 (20–80)	Adult relapsed NHL	0.5–90 µg/m²/d × 4–8 wk with seven starting dose levels and continuous dose	At 60 µg/day: 69% ORR, 37% CR/Cru, 31% PR	Not available
Von Stackelberg et al. (2016)	2016	70 (at recommended dosage)	8 (<1–17)	Pediatric R/R B-prec ALL	In phase I: stepwise dosage 5/15 µg/m²/d for 7 days each, 30 µg/m²/d thereafter, for 4 wks q6wks. In phase II: 5 µg/m²/d for 7 days, 15 µg/m²/d thereafter, for 4 wks q6wks	38.6% CR rate	7.5
Kantarjian et al. (2017)	2017	405 B: 271 SOC: 134	41 (18–80)	Adult Ph-negative R/R B-prec ALL	9 µg/d for the first wk, 28 µg/d for 3 wk, q6wk, subsequent cycles 28 µg/d for 4 wk, q6wk; comparative arm: standard of care chemotherapy	B: 46% CR/CRi SOC: 28% CR/CRi	B: 7.8 SOC: 4.0
Martinelli et al. (2017)	2017	45	55 (23–78)	Adult Ph-positive R/R ALL	9 µg/d for the first wk, 28 µg/d for 3 wk, q6wk, subsequent cycles 28 µg/d for 4 wk, q6wk	CR/CRh rate 36% within the first two cycles, of those 86% with complete MRD response	7.1
Gökbuget et al. (2018a)	2018	116	45 (18–76)	Adult MRD-positive B-prec ALL	15 µg/m²/d for 4 wk, for up to four cycles	Mol CR rate 80% within 103 evaluable patients	36.5

Adapted from Wilke and Gökbuget (2017)

112 µg/d from day 1. Nine patients were included in cohort I. Cohort II was stopped after the inclusion of two patients since both patients had developed grade III neurologic events. Fourteen patients were treated with the dosing schedule defined in cohort I in the third cohort. Patients had been heavily pretreated with a median of three prior treatment lines. Twenty-one patients were evaluable for response with an overall response rate of 43 and 19% complete remissions after one cycle (Viardot et al. 2016).

Overall in NHL with predominantly extramedullary involvement, higher doses appear to be required compared to ALL with bone marrow involvement. For tolerability, several dose steps were required. The delay until the achievement of target dose could be a disadvantage in aggressive disease subtypes. Treatment discontinuations due to neurologic events and the prolonged period to reach effective dose remained the major issues for practicability of blinatumomab treatment in R/R NHL. After promising data have been reported for CAR T cells in NHL and the marketing authorization for two compounds, the role of blinatumomab will have to be newly defined in the lymphoma setting [reviews in Watkins and Bartlett (2018), Sanders and Stewart (2017)].

3.2 Relapsed/Refractory Acute Lymphoblastic Leukemia

R/R ALL is characterized by a very poor prognosis. This applies particularly to early relapses during ongoing chemotherapy and refractory relapses, i.e., non-response to a first salvage approach (Gökbuget 2017). According to the current standard, patients with R/R ALL receive a remission induction therapy and then become candidates for an allogeneic stem cell transplantation (SCT) as ultimate curative treatment. SCT is a treatment consisting of a conditioning regimen and the donor cell transfer which is not well standardized. It is associated with a considerable procedure-related mortality depending on age, duration of follow-up, and several other factors.

The obvious medical need and the promising results in NHL with bone marrow involvement encouraged the evaluation of blinatumomab in R/R ALL with particularly poor prognostic features. The initial goal was to induce a complete remission (CR) without the persistent minimal residual disease (MRD) in order to offer the patients a subsequent SCT. More recently, the need for subsequent SCT has been debated due to the high mortality.

The optimal dosing schedule was defined in a phase II study with three cohorts and different schedules for dose increase. Overall, 36 patients were treated. In this trial also patients with late relapses, characterized by a more favorable prognosis, were included. For patients with higher leukemia burden, a prephase treatment with dexamethasone and cyclophosphamide was recommended. Whereas a starting dose of 15 µg/m²/d (corresponds to 28 µg/d flat dose) was associated with the highest rate of adverse events, a stepwise increase with a starting dose of 5 µg/m²/d and increase to 15 µg/m²/d after one week showed the lowest rate of adverse events. A further dose increase in the third step to 30 µg/m²/d did not appear to improve the response rates. The overall rate of complete hematologic remission (CR) and CR with incomplete recovery (CRi) was 69%. The median overall survival was around 9 months (Topp et al. 2014). Selected patients, who achieved an MRD-negative remission in this trial, achieved long-term survival (Zugmaier et al. 2015).

A large international phase II study was conducted subsequently and focused on patients with unfavorable relapse characteristics only, i.e., early relapses or refractory diseases and relapses after SCT. The CR/CRi rate was 43% in 189 patients a median age of 39 years (Topp et al. 2015a). The median survival was 6.1 months. 82–88% of the patients with CR/CRi reached a negative MRD status. 40–52% of the patients with CR/CRi proceeded to SCT. In an attempt to analyze the impact of SCT on long-term outcome, censoring of patients at the time point of SCT was performed in the Kaplan–Meier analysis. There was no difference in terms of outcome for whether SCT was censored or not (Topp et al. 2015a). Based on the promising response rates in a phase II trial, the regulatory authorities in USA, Europe, and other countries provided marketing authorization for blinatumomab in relapsed/refractory Ph-/BCR-ABL-negative B-precursor ALL.

Ph-/BCR-ABL-positive ALL is the most frequent molecularly defined subgroup of adult ALL and contributes approximately 25% of the cases. Although treatment options have been improved considerably in the past decade after the introduction of tyrosine kinase inhibitors directed to the BCR-ABL gene fusion, still patients relapse, e.g., due to resistance-inducing mutations. Ph-/BCR-ABL-positive ALL is a subgroup of B-precursor ALL and usually CD19-positive. Thus, immunotherapy is an attractive additional targeted treatment approach. Blinatumomab was tested in a patient population mostly resistant to several lines of tyrosine kinase inhibitors. The CR/CRi rate was 36 with 86% complete MRD response in CR/CRi patients and thus similar to Ph-negative ALL; the overall survival was 7.1 months (Martinelli et al. 2017).

Blinatumomab was also evaluated in a phase I/II trial for relapsed pediatric B-precursor ALL. Again, the patient population was characterized by specifically unfavorable prognostic features. 61% of the patients had a relapse after prior SCT. The phase I part of the trial with 49 patients confirmed the maximum tolerated dose of 15 $\mu g/m^2/d$ with a starting dose of 5 $\mu g/m^2/d$ and a dose increase to 15 $\mu g/m^2/d$ after one week of treatment. Forty-four patients were treated in the phase II part of the trial accounting for a total of 70 patients treated with the recommended dose. 39% achieved a CR within the first two cycles. 52% of the CR patients achieved a complete MRD response, and the median overall survival was 7.5 months (Von Stackelberg et al. 2016).

In the next development phase, blinatumomab was evaluated in adult ALL in a randomized large international trial for R/R ALL in comparison with standard of care chemotherapy. The options for standard of care (SOC) included a number of different regimens (FLAG ± anthracycline, high-dose cytarabine, high-dose methotrexate, or clofarabine-based regimens). The randomization was 2:1 for blinatumomab without option for cross-over. Again, the patient population was characterized by prognostically unfavorable features, e.g., around 40% patients with prior SCT and 60% patients beyond first salvage. Overall, 405 patients (271 for blinatumomab and 134 for standard of care) were included. CR/CRi rates were 46% for blinatumomab versus 28% for SOC. The median survival time for the blinatumomab-treated patients was significantly superior with 7.8 months compared to 4.0 months for SOC (Kantarjian et al. 2017). Thus, the trial confirmed the very poor outcome with SOC therapy and yielded similar results for blinatumomab as reported in the earlier phase trials.

Additional background data were provided in a retrospective trial with historical data on R/R ALL compiled from several adult ALL study groups and large centers. With different statistical methods such as weighted analysis and propensity score analysis, an advantage for patients treated with blinatumomab compared to SOC was detected in terms of response rate and overall survival (Gökbuget et al. 2016).

Overall, blinatumomab yielded promising CR/CRi rates in poor prognostic subgroups of adult and pediatric R/R ALL. In most cases, responses occurred quickly within one cycle of therapy and were deep remissions with an MRD response in around 80% of the cases. For many patients, the achievement of CR offered a bridge to transplantation. However, overall median survival was still around 6–7 months, which is due to relapses without SCT or after SCT and also to mortality after SCT; the latter is most probably not correlated to blinatumomab treatment.

More recently, the combination strategies have been tested in R/R ALL. In one trial, the low-dose chemotherapy was combined with the CD22 antibody, inotuzumab ozogamicin (Kantarjian et al. 2016), at different dose levels and schedules in first salvage of R/R ALL. After an amendment, blinatumomab was added to this backbone and replaced four consolidation cycles with chemotherapy. Due to the different schedules, the interim results of this approach are difficult to interpret (Jabbour et al. 2018). Other combination strategies are ongoing in clinical trials for adult and pediatric ALL (Table 2).

Table 2 Active or planned interventional clinical trials with blinatumomab[a]

NCT number[b]	Regimen	Stage	Age (yrs)	Planned number	Planned period
02744768	Dasatinib, prednisone, Blina (Ph+)	de novo	≥ 18	60	2017–2021
02877303	Hyper CVAD and Blina	de novo	≥ 14	60	2016–2020
02458014	Blina in MRD-positive ALL	de novo	≥ 18	40	2015–2020
03114865	Blina maintenance after SCT	de novo	≥ 18	12	2017–2020
03109093	Blina in MRD-positive ALL	de novo	≥ 18	60	2017–2021
[a]03751709	Blina and haploidentical mismatch cell therapy	–	≥ 18	10	2018–2022
03523429	Chemotherapy and Blina consolidation in HR ALL	de novo	18–55	38	2018–2025

(continued)

Table 2 (continued)

NCT number[b]	Regimen	Stage	Age (yrs)	Planned number	Planned period
02807883	Blina maintenance after SCT	de novo	18–70	30	2016–2021
03709719	Blina in HR ALL	de novo	18–59	95	2018–2028
03367299	Sequential chemotherapy and Blina	de novo	18–65	149	2018–2023
02003222	Chemotherapy versus Blina in consolidation	de novo	30–70	509	2015–2020
03541083	Blina prephase and chemotherapy	de novo	18–70	80	2018–2026
01371630	Chemotherapy, inotuzumab, and Blina	de novo	56–74	256	2011–2019
[a]03480438	Chemotherapy and Blina	de novo	56–74	50	2018–2021
03263572	Blina and ponatinib (Ph+)	de novo	≥ 60	60	2017–2023
02143414	Blina and chemotherapy or Blina and dasatinib (Ph+)	de novo	≥ 65	44	2015–2021
03643276	Chemotherapy and Blina consolidation (randomized)	de novo	<18	5000	2012–2028
03117751	Chemotherapy and Blina or others	de novo	<18	1000	2017–2026
02877303	Blina and inotuzumab	R/R de novo	≥ 18	64	2018–2021
03476239	Blina in Chinese ALL patients	R/R	≥ 18	120	2017–2021
[a]03628053	Tisagenlecleucel versus Blina or inotuzumab (randomized)	R/R	≥ 18	220	2019–2022
03160079	Blina and pembrolizumab in ALL with high marrow count	R/R	≥ 18	24	2017–2022
02997761	Ibrutinib and Blina	R/R	≥ 18	20	2017–2021
03518112	Chemotherapy and Blina	R/R	≥ 18	44	2018–2029
02879695	Blina and nivolumab w/o ipilimumab	R/R	≥ 16	30	2017–2021
02101853	Blina versus chemotherapy (randomized)	R/R	1–30	598	2014–2022
02393859	Blina versus chemotherapy (randomized)	R/R	<18	202	2015–2023

Blina—blinatumomab; Ph+—Ph-/BCR-ABL-positive ALL; R/R—relapsed/refractory; yrs—years; MRD—minimal residual disease

[a]In preparation

[b]Available through clinicaltrials.gov

3.3 Minimal Residual Disease of Acute Lymphoblastic Leukemia

The minimal residual disease can be evaluated by quantitative assays in more than 90% of the cases of ALL (Campana and Pui 2017). In patients with complete hematologic remission after the initial treatment phase, the persistence of MRD is the most unfavorable prognostic factor for relapse (Campana and Pui 2017; Gökbuget et al. 2012; Berry et al. 2017). This means that patients with persistent or recurrent MRD are prone to relapse due to their highly chemotherapy-resistant disease despite continued treatment. Even SCT may not abrogate completely the negative impact of MRD. Many groups and guidelines define an indication for SCT in this high-risk situation. Fortunately, patients are still in hematologic remission, with a low leukemia burden and generally in good condition. Therefore, the treatment of upcoming ALL relapse in the stage of the minimal residual disease could be a promising new approach.

The first trial with blinatumomab in ALL was conducted in MRD-positive ALL. Patients were in complete hematologic remission with detectable disease above a level of 10^{-4}, i.e., 0.01%. MRD testing was performed in a reference laboratory with quantitative PCR according to standardized criteria. The primary endpoint was complete MRD response defined as a negative MRD status confirmed with a sensitivity of at least 10^{-4}. In 20 evaluable patients with MRD above 10^{-4}, 80% achieved a complete MRD response (Topp et al. 2011). Three responses were observed in five evaluable patients with Ph-/BCR-ABL-positive ALL. Long-term follow-up confirmed a relapse-free survival of 61%. Overall, four patients with complete MRD response remained in long-term remission without SCT or further therapy (Topp et al. 2012).

Subsequently, a larger international trial was conducted in MRD-positive ALL. In contrast to the first trial, the MRD level had to be above 10^{-3}, i.e., 0.1%. The trial included patients in the first remission but also one-third of patients with persistent MRD after salvage therapy for a prior hematologic relapse. Dosing was different compared to the R/R setting. The starting dose was 15 µg/m^2/d without dose increase after one week but with the option for a dose reduction to 5 µg/m^2/d in case of toxicities. 78% showed complete MRD response (Gökbuget et al. 2018a). The median survival was 36.5 months compared to approximately 6 months in R/R ALL. The median relapse-free survival was superior in patients treated in first CR (24.6 months) compared to second or later CR (11 months). The study also demonstrated a significant advantage in terms of the overall survival for those patients who achieved a complete MRD response after one cycle (35.2 months) compared to those without (7.1 months). Overall, 67% of the patients received an SCT during follow-up in ongoing CR (Gökbuget et al. 2018a).

A recent follow-up of these data confirmed the promising data with a median overall survival of 36.5 months after a median follow-up of 36.5 months. The median survival was not reached in patients with a complete MRD response compared to 12.5 months in MRD non-responders. Comparing patients with and without subsequent SCT, the proportion of survivors was 40% in transplanted and 33% in non-transplanted patients (Gökbuget et al. 2018b).

Overall, the use of blinatumomab in the MRD setting yielded favorable results in terms of responses, survival, and duration of remission, particularly if compared to the R/R setting. Based on these data, the regulatory authorities in the USA and Europe granted marketing authorization for blinatumomab in MRD-positive ALL.

Whereas the majority of patients received a subsequent SCT, preliminary results indicate that some patients stayed in long-term remission without any further therapy after blinatumomab. However, currently, there is no approach to predict long-term response to blinatumomab only. A prerequisite for this treatment approach is to establish an MRD assay in all patients with newly diagnosed ALL and to follow up for MRD regularly.

3.4 Newly Diagnosed Acute Lymphoblastic Leukemia

Based on the promising data from R/R and MRD-positive ALL, the first trials have been started for newly diagnosed ALL (Table 2). A US phase III trial in older patients with de novo ALL tests the impact of blinatumomab consolidation independent of MRD status and/or subsequent SCT in a randomized design (NCT02003222). The approach to administer blinatumomab in patients who remain MRD-positive during first-line treatment is further evaluated by several groups (NCT02458014; NCT03109093). Other trials with blinatumomab in combination with chemotherapy, i.e., consolidation in high-risk patients with de novo ALL or other sequential strategies, are underway (NCT02877303; NCT03523429; NCT03709719; NCT03367299). In a trial for younger patients, four alternating cycles of the intensive hyper-CVAD regimen were followed by four consecutive cycles of blinatumomab and a maintenance phase. The number of evaluable patients was still low ($N = 14$) and follow-up short. Preliminary data indicate that the regimen was tolerable and effective (Richard-Carpentier et al. 2018).

One ongoing trial evaluates the use of blinatumomab in prephase treatment (NCT03541083). Maintenance after SCT is addressed in clinical trials as well (NCT02807883; NCT03114865). A large pediatric first-line trial compares blinatumomab and chemotherapy in defined high-risk subgroups in consolidation (NCT03643276), and another non-randomized trial combines blinatumomab with other targeted agents (NCT03117751; NCT02807883). In older patients with ALL, the sequential application of dose-reduced chemotherapy and blinatumomab may be a promising approach (NCT01371630; NCT03480438). The first interim results were reported for a trial in patients older than 65 years. Treatment was based on blinatumomab for 1–2 cycles of induction until the achievement of CR. Patients received then three additional consolidation cycles with blinatumomab, followed by 18 months of intensified maintenance therapy. The rate of CR/CRi in 29 eligible patients with a median age of 75 years was 66%, whereas the treatment was tolerable and no induction death occurred. These results look promising for a difficult-to-treat patient population, but follow-up data have to be awaited (Advani et al. 2018).

In Ph-positive ALL, studies with sequential application of tyrosine kinase inhibitors and blinatumomab are of interest (NCT02744768; NCT03263572; NCT02143414). Overall, a variety of approaches is evaluated in de novo ALL. It remains open whether and how advantages can be demonstrated compared to standard therapies, since most trials are not randomized and too small in terms of patient number to allow reasonable comparisons.

4 Safety and Tolerability of Blinatumomab

The most frequent adverse events with grade III or more observed with blinatumomab result most probably from cytokine release such as febrile neutropenia, infection, pyrexia, and hematological toxicities (Topp et al. 2015a; Kantarjian et al. 2017; Viardot et al. 2016; Goebeler et al. 2016; Gökbuget et al. 2018a). Peripheral edema and fatigue were also common, but these events never exceeded grade 2 (Topp et al. 2015a; Kantarjian et al. 2017; Viardot et al. 2016; Goebeler et al. 2016; Gökbuget et al. 2018a). Fever and asthenia are known effects of cytokine release. At infusion start and in correlation with cytokine release, patients may develop considerable increases of C-reactive protein without the presence of infection. Other transient effects may be due to redistribution of cells such as thrombocytopenia. Liver enzymes may show a transient increase as well and usually do not require infusion interruptions. Fatal adverse events described in clinical trials were mostly attributed to progressive disease or relapse or to events after subsequent SCT or due to infections. The latter are in most cases due to preexisting cytopenias in heavily pretreated patient populations, cytopenias induced by blinatumomab, or caused by lack of response. In case of long-term use, blinatumomab is important to consider that lymphopenia as well as decrease of immunoglobulin serum levels may be induced. Central venous line or infusion devices may also be the cause of an infection and should be inspected regularly by healthcare professionals [reviewed in Wilke and Gökbuget (2017)]. For clinical handling, neurologic events and cytokine release are of greatest importance.

Cytokine Release Syndrome
Cytokine release syndrome (CRS) is a frequent effect of immunotherapies and was observed in early trials with blinatumomab in ALL (Topp et al. 2014). With pre-phase treatment in patients with higher leukemia load, dose step, and pretreatment with dexamethasone, the incidence of CRS is less than 5% (Topp et al. 2015a; Kantarjian et al. 2017). In case of signs and symptoms despite the above-mentioned approaches, treatment can be discontinued immediately. The IL6 antibody tocilizumab, which is frequently used in the context of CAR T cell therapy (Neelapu et al. 2018), may be applied in severe cases, although this is rarely needed. There is one report of hemophagocytic lymphohistiocytosis in a pediatric patient during

blinatumomab treatment, which could be controlled by tocilizumab infusion (Teachey et al. 2013).

Neurologic Adverse Events

Throughout all disease entities and treatment schedules 52–71% of all patients developed neurologic events (Topp et al. 2015a; Kantarjian et al. 2017; Viardot et al. 2016; Goebeler et al. 2016; Gökbuget et al. 2018a). They ranged from mild disorders like tremor, headache, and dizziness to severe symptoms of encephalopathy and seizures. Encephalopathies may start with early signs like an increasing tremor and aphasia and can have a variety of clinical manifestations such as confusion, ataxia, dysarthria, aphasia, cognitive disorders, somnolence, and coma. The syndrome is often associated with several symptoms. In most cases, the symptoms are completely reversible. Often, early intervention with dexamethasone can be helpful. In other cases, treatment is interrupted and started after reconstitution at a lower dose [reviewed in Wilke and Gökbuget (2017)].

Neurotoxicities have been observed with other CD19-directed therapies, particularly with chimeric antigen receptor-modified (CAR) T cells (Neelapu et al. 2018). After these therapies, even fatal brain edema has been observed (Torre et al. 2018). For blinatumomab, the highest incidences of neurotoxicities have been observed in NHL patients at higher doses (Viardot et al. 2016; Goebeler et al. 2016).

The pathogenetic mechanisms are probably similar to those observed with CAR T cell therapies, though less frequent and less severe, and still not fully understood. In a recent survey on 133 adults treated with CD19 CAR T cells, a number of factors were associated with increased risk of neurologic events such as ALL versus other malignancies, high CD19+ cells in bone marrow, high CAR T cell dose, cytokine release syndrome, and preexisting neurologic comorbidities. Further investigations revealed that patients with severe neurotoxicity demonstrated evidence of endothelial activation, including disseminated intravascular coagulation, capillary leak, and increased blood–brain barrier permeability. The latter was associated with higher concentrations of systemic cytokines in the cerebrovascular fluid (Gust et al. 2017).

Thus, most probably neurologic events are correlated to a cytokine release by activated T cells within the CNS. This effect may be induced by an altered blood–brain barrier, which may occur after the adhesion of activated T cells to the endothelium of brain vessels. It may also be induced by the presence of target cells in the CSF, which may be submicroscopic. In patients with NHL, the risk of neurologic events was associated with a low peripheral blood B/T cell ratio leading to the hypothesis that in the presence of less target cells in circulation more activated T cells migrate to tissues (Viardot et al. 2016).

The use of dexamethasone may limit the T cell cytokine activity. In NHL, pentosan polysulfate (PPS) was tested (Smits and Sentman 2016). PPS is a P-selectin antagonist which may decrease the adhesion of circulating T cells to the blood vessel endothelium and thereby reduce the migration of activated T cells into the CSF.

In a pathogenetic model for neurologic events, the mechanisms and potential mitigation strategies were tested (Klinger et al. 2016b). In this flow chamber model, the addition of blinatumomab induced reduced T cell rolling velocity and increased T cell adhesion to the endothelial cells by upregulation of P-selectin and ICAM-1 adhesion molecules on endothelial cells. The effect was reversed by the addition of substances interfering with this interaction, e.g., PPS, minocycline (Klinger et al. 2016b). Overall, the authors suggested a stepwise model for the pathogenesis of neurologic adverse events starting with increased endothelial adhesiveness of activated T cells, activation of endothelium by these T cells, extravasation of T cells and attraction of further circulating leukocytes, cytokine release by extravasated T cells in the brain including further transient neuroinflammation which may be increased by attracted other leukocytes (Klinger et al. 2016b).

Neurologic adverse events are usually quickly reversible after interruption of treatment, and the reoccurrence of seizures may be prohibited by seizure prophylaxis. Encephalopathies may reoccur even after dose reduction and lead to permanent discontinuation in some patients. Therefore, the identification of risk factors and mitigation strategies for neurologic adverse events is of utmost importance for all T cell-activating therapies.

5 Prognostic Factors and Potential Mechanisms of Resistance

So far, the potential mechanisms of primary resistance or relapse after blinatumomab are poorly understood. In the setting of MRD, no pretreatment factor was associated with non-response. Long-term outcome was poorer in patients who did not respond to blinatumomab and in patients treated in a more advanced disease stage, i.e., later complete remission compared to first remission (Gökbuget et al. 2018a). In R/R ALL, several trials showed a lower rate of CR/CRh in patients with a higher degree of bone marrow blast infiltration, i.e., >50%. In the large phase II trial, the CR/CRh rate was 29% compared to 73% in patients with more or less than 50% bone marrow infiltration, respectively (Topp et al. 2015a). In the randomized trial of blinatumomab, the CR/CRi rates were 34% versus 65% and the median survival times 5.0 versus 11 months, respectively (Kantarjian et al. 2017). As another sign of higher leukemia load, increased LDH levels at relapse were found to be unfavorable (Duell et al. 2017). Lower leukemia load can also contribute to better tolerability, particularly lower incidence of cytokine release syndrome. Similar observations were also described for other immunotherapies. It remains open to discussion, whether the higher efficacy in lower level disease is a result of a more favorable effector-to-target cell ratio or due to different disease biology. At least in relapse after SCT, the effector-to-target ratio may have a role for efficacy (Schlegel et al. 2014).

The outcome with blinatumomab in the R/R setting is also better in less advanced stages of disease. Thus, the CR/CRi rates were 40% versus 53% in patients treated in first compared to second salvage of R/R ALL, and the corresponding median survival rates were 11 versus 5 months (Kantarjian et al. 2017). The reason is probably that with each line of salvage additional mutations are induced and that these mutations induce not only drug resistance but also general resistance mechanisms as inhibition of apoptosis.

A larger retrospective analysis of 65 patients with R/R confirmed high leukemia burden (bone marrow blasts >50%), history of prior extramedullary ALL, and current extramedullary ALL as predictors of lower CR rate. 41% of the refractory patients showed evidence of extramedullary progression and negative or dim expression of CD19 in 41% of the cases. Also, 40% of the relapses were located in the extramedullary compartment and CD19 was negative or dim in 41% of the relapse cases (Aldoss et al. 2017). Thus, another potential mechanism is the origin of relapses from 'sanctuary' sites, i.e., regions less accessible to cells of the immune system as relapses in CNS, testis, and other extramedullary sites were observed (Topp et al. 2012, 2015b). It can be debated whether a better control of extramedullary sites of ALL might be achieved by the use of higher doses such as in NHL trials.

Data on immunologic factors for the prediction of response and resistance are scarce. A higher rate of T cell expansion was observed in long-term survivors after blinatumomab treatment (Zugmaier et al. 2015). A higher percentage of CD3-positive T cells and lower levels of regulatory T cells (Treg) were described as well (Duell et al. 2017).

PD-L1 expression and upregulation on lymphoblasts and the bone marrow microenvironment at baseline and in response to cytokines including those released upon blinatumomab exposure may inhibit T cell function through the PD-1 receptor and lead to resistance to blinatumomab (Feucht et al. 2016). The efficacy of blinatumomab may thus be increased by approaches to reduce the number of Tregs, e.g., by the use of immunosuppressive compounds like cyclophosphamide (Le and Jaffee 2012). Prephase treatment with dexamethasone and cyclophosphamide was part of an early trial with blinatumomab (Topp et al. 2014).

There is also some evidence that inhibition of PD-1/PD-L1 might increase the efficacy and reduce the primary and secondary resistance of blinatumomab (Kobold et al. 2018). Blockade of PD-1 and/or PD-L1 has improved T cell responsiveness in vitro (Feucht et al. 2016; Laszlo et al. 2015). A case report on a pediatric nonresponder to blinatumomab demonstrated a reduction of leukemic burden from 45 to 1% after a combination of blinatumomab and pembrolizumab (Feucht et al. 2016). Consequently, the combination with nivolumab, ipilimumab (NCT02879695), or pembrolizumab (NCT03160079) is currently under investigation.

Secondary resistance may also be induced by disease correlated mechanisms. Thus, continued treatment directed to only one target may induce clonal selection such as CD19 loss (Ruella and Maus 2016) due to different mechanisms such as loss of the extracellular domain of CD19 (Sotillo et al. 2015), conformational changes of the extracellular domain of CD19 due to mutations (Yu et al. 2017), and intracellular accumulation of CD19 after the loss of a chaperone molecule (CD81) (Braig et al. 2017). Interestingly, relapse in MLL-rearranged B-precursor ALL, which is associated with a very early immature phenotype, may be associated with a lineage shift to acute myeloid leukemia (Gardner et al. 2016; Rayes and Abdu-elkarem 2016).

Further analyses on the impact of genetic aberrations on response and resistance to blinatumomab are ongoing. One trial of 29 patients with pediatric or adult ALL showed high response rates (83%) in Ph-like ALL with CRLF2 aberrations and 60% in other cases of Ph-like ALL, which is a molecular subtype of ALL with reported poor prognosis. Further analysis revealed that reduced infiltration of cytotoxic CD8+ T cells was correlated with non-response to blinatumomab (Zhao et al. 2018).

Generally, the use of single-target treatments in an aggressive and biologically unstable disease like ALL bears a high risk for different types of resistance. Therefore, the combination of different targeted strategies, e.g., with other antibody treatments such as the conjugated CD22 antibody inotuzumab (NCT02877303) or with tyrosine kinase inhibitors in Ph-/BCR-ABL-positive ALL (NCT02744768, NCT03263572) or the sequential treatment with chemotherapy are suitable approaches. This includes the use of conventional maintenance chemotherapy after treatment with blinatumomab in order to use the relapse risk.

In the majority of patients with R/R ALL, an SCT in complete remission is considered as standard of care, and in many cases, blinatumomab was administered for remission induction and bridge to transplantation. However, the mortality of SCT in patient cohorts with a median age of 45 and more is considerable. As a result at the current follow-up of the trials, a clear advantage of subsequent SCT is difficult to detect; this may change with longer follow-up.

6 Summary and Outlook

Bispecific T cell engagers represent a new class of promising compounds for malignant disease. They represent a hybrid approach between antibody treatment and cell therapy. Experience is most prominent with blinatumomab in R/R and MRD-positive ALL, but the treatment principle may be suitable for a variety of malignancies.

Immunotherapy in general and the redirection of T cells to CD19-positive leukemia cells provide an alternative mechanism of action, which can yield antileukemic activity even in patients with chemotherapy-refractory disease. This applies for different subtypes of ALL such as unfavorable relapses of Ph-/BCR-ABL-negative ALL, Ph-/BCR-ABL-positive ALL, and pediatric ALL.

Response rates were lower in patients in later stages of disease and in patients with higher tumor load. Resistance may be due to intrinsic inhibition of T cell expansion and escape mechanisms such as target loss. Survival rates after treatment with blinatumomab in R/R ALL are superior to chemotherapy but not satisfactory.

The best results were achieved in MRD-positive ALL, i.e., a lower leukemia load. The current development goes into the direction of first-line therapy, where blinatumomab is integrated in a multi-drug multi-target treatment backbone. In R/R ALL, the reduction of leukemia burden by a prephase treatment is currently investigated.

The application of blinatumomab as a continuous infusion and risk of adverse events such as infection, neurotoxicity, and cytokine release syndrome make it advisable that patients are treated in centers with experience of blinatumomab treatment. Usability may in the future be improved by other ways of applications—instead of a four-week continuous infusion. It is important, however, that prolonged half-life compounds would also reduce the flexibility of treatment steering in case of toxicities.

One major unsolved question refers to the role of SCT after remission induction with blinatumomab either in R/R setting or in MRD-positive ALL. The transplant-associated mortality is considerable particularly in older patients, whereas relapse risk is high in patients without subsequent SCT. Overall, it may be reasonable to avoid high-risk transplant procedures such as mismatch transplantations or full conditioning regimens in older patients on the one hand. On the other hand, the treatment should be continued in patients who do not qualify for SCT, e.g., sequential multi-agent consolidation and maintenance treatments.

The available data on the activity of blinatumomab in high-risk subpopulations such as Ph-positive ALL, Ph-like ALL, or MLL-rearranged ALL are still scarce and of great interest.

In newly diagnosed ALL, it remains to be demonstrated whether blinatumomab in combination with dose-reduced chemotherapy yields similar or better results in older ALL patients compared to standard chemotherapy. Even for younger patients, the potential to reduce cytotoxic chemotherapy by the use of blinatumomab or other antibodies is of great interest. Given the promising potential of the compound, it will be a challenge to design convincing clinical trials for the first-line treatment. This is essential, because blinatumomab is a drug with an extraordinary high price. Further expansion of use will also depend on the results of controlled clinical trials in earlier lines of treatment and probably on pricing policy.

The future will also show whether results in R/R ALL or other treatment situations can be further improved by the combination of different antibody treatments, e.g., inotuzumab ozogamicin. Furthermore, the position of blinatumomab in treatment algorithm will also be compared to other approaches including inotuzumab ozogamicin and CAR T cells.

The development of reliable biomarkers will be essential not only for prediction of response but also for further treatment optimization.

Further optimization of bispecific T cell engagers may take place in several directions [reviewed in Velasquez et al. (2018)] with the particular goal to overcome potential limitations of these treatments such as the development of antigen-loss variants, limited T cell activation, or immunosuppressive effects of tumor environment. The risk of target loss may be reduced by combination therapies with other antibodies or by the development of trispecifics. Limited T cell activation may be induced by the secretion of inhibitory molecules by malignant cells such as TGFβ or PD-L1 and/or the attraction of Tregs (Velasquez et al. 2018). The blockade of PD-1 and/or PD-L1 may be an option (Feucht et al. 2016; Laszlo et al. 2015). Due to the potentially severe adverse events, this approach should be tested in clinical trials. The accumulation of Tregs may be addressed by the application of low doses of cyclophosphamide (Le and Jaffee 2012).

The future will show whether the current compounds can be further optimized and whether the treatment principle can be successfully translated to other malignant diseases including solid tumors. Current ongoing trials for different targets such as EpCAM, HER2, or Mucin 1 are summarized in Runcie et al. (2018). In acute myeloid leukemia, CD123- and CD33-directed T cell engagers are tested in clinical trials (NCT02715011; NCT02520427).

References

Advani AS, Moseley A, O'Dwyer KM, Wood B, Fang M, Wieduwilt MJ et al (2018) Results of SWOG 1318: a phase 2 trial of blinatumomab followed by pomp (prednisone, vincristine, methotrexate, 6-mercaptopurine) maintenance in elderly patients with newly diagnosed philadelphia chromosome negative B-cell acute lymphoblastic leukemia. Blood 132

Aldoss I, Song J, Stiller T, Nguyen T, Palmer J, O'Donnell M et al (2017) Correlates of resistance and relapse during blinatumomab therapy for relapsed/refractory acute lymphoblastic leukemia. Am J Hematol 92(9):858–865

Bargou R, Leo E, Zugmaier G, Klinger M, Goebeler M, Knop S et al (2008) Tumor regression in cancer patients by very low doses of a T cell-engaging antibody. Science 321(5891):974–977

Berry DA, Zhou S, Higley H, Mukundan L, Fu S, Reaman GH et al (2017) Association of minimal residual disease with clinical outcome in pediatric and adult acute lymphoblastic leukemia: a meta-analysis. JAMA Oncol 3(7):e170580

Braig F, Brandt A, Goebeler M, Tony HP, Kurze AK, Nollau P et al (2017) Resistance to anti-CD19/CD3 BiTE in acute lymphoblastic leukemia may be mediated by disrupted CD19 membrane trafficking. Blood 129(1):100–104

Brandl C, Haas C, d'Argouges S, Fisch T, Kufer P, Brischwein K et al (2007) The effect of dexamethasone on polyclonal T cell activation and redirected target cell lysis as induced by a CD19/CD3-bispecific single-chain antibody construct. Cancer Immunol Immunother 56 (10):1551–1563

Brischwein K, Schlereth B, Guller B, Steiger C, Wolf A, Lutterbuese R et al (2006) MT110: a novel bispecific single-chain antibody construct with high efficacy in eradicating established tumors. Mol Immunol 43(8):1129–1143

Campana D, Pui CH (2017) Minimal residual disease-guided therapy in childhood acute lymphoblastic leukemia. Blood 129(14):1913–1918

Carter RH, Fearon DT (1992) CD19: lowering the threshold for antigen receptor stimulation of B lymphocytes. Science 256(5053):105–107

Conter V, Bartram CR, Valsecchi MG, Schrauder A, Panzer-Grumayer R, Moricke A et al (2010) Molecular response to treatment redefines all prognostic factors in children and adolescents with B-cell precursor acute lymphoblastic leukemia: results in 3184 patients of the AIEOP-BFM ALL 2000 study. Blood 115(16):3206–3214

Dahlen E, Veitonmaki N, Norlen P (2018) Bispecific antibodies in cancer immunotherapy. Ther Adv Vaccines Immunother 6(1):3–17

DasGupta RK, Marini BL, Rudoni J, Perissinotti AJ (2018) A review of CD19-targeted immunotherapies for relapsed or refractory acute lymphoblastic leukemia. J Oncol Pharm Pract 24(6):453–467

Dreier T, Lorenczewski G, Brandl C, Hoffmann P, Syring U, Hanakam F et al (2002) Extremely potent, rapid and costimulation-independent cytotoxic T-cell response against lymphoma cells catalyzed by a single-chain bispecific antibody. Int J Cancer 100(6):690–697

Duell J, Dittrich M, Bedke T, Mueller T, Eisele F, Rosenwald A et al (2017) Frequency of regulatory T cells determines the outcome of the T-cell-engaging antibody blinatumomab in patients with B-precursor ALL. Leukemia 31(10):2181–2190

Feucht J, Kayser S, Gorodezki D, Hamieh M, Doring M, Blaeschke F et al (2016) T-cell responses against CD19+ pediatric acute lymphoblastic leukemia mediated by bispecific T-cell engager (BiTE) are regulated contrarily by PD-L1 and CD80/CD86 on leukemic blasts. Oncotarget 7 (47):76902–76919

Frankel SR, Baeuerle PA (2013) Targeting T cells to tumor cells using bispecific antibodies. Curr Opin Chem Biol 17(3):385–392

Gardner R, Wu D, Cherian S, Fang M, Hanafi LA, Finney O et al (2016) Acquisition of a CD19-negative myeloid phenotype allows immune escape of MLL-rearranged B-ALL from CD19 CAR-T-cell therapy. Blood 127(20):2406–2410

Goebeler ME, Bargou R (2016) Blinatumomab: a CD19/CD3 bispecific T cell engager (BiTE) with unique anti-tumor efficacy. Leuk Lymphoma 57(5):1021–1032

Goebeler ME, Knop S, Viardot A, Kufer P, Topp MS, Einsele H et al (2016) Bispecific T-cell engager (BiTE) antibody construct blinatumomab for the treatment of patients with relapsed/refractory non-hodgkin lymphoma: final results from a phase I study. J Clin Oncol 34(10):1104–1111

Gökbuget N (2017) How should we treat a patient with relapsed Ph-negative B-ALL and what novel approaches are being investigated? Best Pract Res Clin Haematol 30(3):261–274

Gökbuget N, Kneba M, Raff T, Trautmann H, Bartram CR, Arnold R et al (2012) Adult patients with acute lymphoblastic leukemia and molecular failure display a poor prognosis and are candidates for stem cell transplantation and targeted therapies. Blood 120(9):1868–1876

Gökbuget N, Kelsh M, Chia V, Advani A, Bassan R, Dombret H et al (2016) Blinatumomab vs historical standard therapy of adult relapsed/refractory acute lymphoblastic leukemia. Blood Cancer J 6(9):e473

Gökbuget N, Dombret H, Bonifacio M, Reichle A, Graux C, Faul C ct al (2018a) Blinatumomab for minimal residual disease in adults with B-precursor acute lymphoblastic leukemia. Blood

Gökbuget N, Dombret H, Zugmaier G, Bonifacio M, Graux C, Faul C et al (2018b) Blinatumomab for minimal residual disease (MRD) in adults with B-cell precursor acute lymphoblastic leukemia (BCP-ALL): median overall survival (OS) is not reached in complete MRD responders at a median follow-up of 53.1 months. Blood 132:554

Gruen M, Bommert K, Bargou RC (2004) T-cell-mediated lysis of B cells induced by a CD19×CD3 bispecific single-chain antibody is perforin dependent and death receptor independent. Cancer Immunol Immunother 53(7):625–632

Gust J, Hay KA, Hanafi LA, Li D, Myerson D, Gonzalez-Cuyar LF et al (2017) Endothelial activation and blood-brain barrier disruption in neurotoxicity after adoptive immunotherapy with CD19 CAR-T cells. Cancer Discov 7(12):1404–1419

Hoffmann P, Hofmeister R, Brischwein K, Brandl C, Crommer S, Bargou R et al (2005) Serial killing of tumor cells by cytotoxic T cells redirected with a CD19-/CD3-bispecific single-chain antibody construct. Int J Cancer 115(1):98–104

Hoffmann SC, Wabnitz GH, Samstag Y, Moldenhauer G, Ludwig T (2011) Functional analysis of bispecific antibody (EpCAMxCD3)-mediated T-lymphocyte and cancer cell interaction by single-cell force spectroscopy. Int J Cancer 128(9):2096–2104

Jabbour E, Sasaki K, Ravandi F, Huang X, Short NJ, Khouri M et al (2018) Chemoimmunotherapy with inotuzumab ozogamicin combined with mini-hyper-CVD, with or without blinatumomab, is highly effective in patients with Philadelphia chromosome-negative acute lymphoblastic leukemia in first salvage. Cancer 124(20):4044–4055

Kantarjian HM, DeAngelo DJ, Stelljes M, Martinelli G, Liedtke M, Stock W et al (2016) Inotuzumab ozogamicin versus standard therapy for acute lymphoblastic leukemia. N Engl J Med 375(8):740–753

Kantarjian H, Stein A, Gökbuget N, Fielding AK, Schuh AC, Ribera JM et al (2017) Blinatumomab versus chemotherapy for advanced acute lymphoblastic leukemia. N Engl J Med 376(9):836–847

Klinger M, Benjamin J, Kischel R, Stienen S, Zugmaier G (2016a) Harnessing T cells to fight cancer with BiTE(R) antibody constructs–past developments and future directions. Immunol Rev 270(1):193–208

Klinger M, Zugmaier G, Naegele V, Goebeler M, Brandl C, Bargou RC et al (2016b) Pathogenesis-based development of potential mitigation strategies for blinatumomab-associated neurologic events (NEs). Blood 128

Kobold S, Pantelyushin S, Rataj F, Vom Berg J (2018) Rationale for combining bispecific T cell activating antibodies with checkpoint blockade for cancer therapy. Front Oncol 8:285

Krshnan L, Park S, Im W, Call MJ, Call ME (2016) A conserved αβ transmembrane interface forms the core of a compact T-cell receptor-CD3 structure within the membrane. Proc Natl Acad Sci U S A 113(43):E6649–E6658

Kufer P, Zettl F, Borschert K, Lutterbuse R, Kischel R, Riethmuller G (2001) Minimal costimulatory requirements for T cell priming and TH1 differentiation: activation of naive human T lymphocytes by tumor cells armed with bifunctional antibody constructs. Cancer Immun 1:10

Laszlo GS, Gudgeon CJ, Harrington KH, Walter RB (2015) T-cell ligands modulate the cytolytic activity of the CD33/CD3 BiTE antibody construct, AMG 330. Blood Cancer J 5:e340

Le DT, Jaffee EM (2012) Regulatory T-cell modulation using cyclophosphamide in vaccine approaches: a current perspective. Cancer Res 72(14):3439–3444

Loffler A, Kufer P, Lutterbuse R, Zettl F, Daniel PT, Schwenkenbecher JM et al (2000) A recombinant bispecific single-chain antibody, CD19×CD3, induces rapid and high lymphoma-directed cytotoxicity by unstimulated T lymphocytes. Blood 95(6):2098–2103

Loffler A, Gruen M, Wuchter C, Schriever F, Kufer P, Dreier T et al (2003) Efficient elimination of chronic lymphocytic leukaemia B cells by autologous T cells with a bispecific anti-CD19/anti-CD3 single-chain antibody construct. Leukemia 17(5):900–909

Martinelli G, Boissel N, Chevallier P, Ottmann O, Gökbuget N, Topp MS et al (2017) Complete hematologic and molecular response in adult patients with relapsed/refractory philadelphia chromosome-positive B-precursor acute lymphoblastic leukemia following treatment with blinatumomab: results from a phase II, single-arm, multicenter study. J Clin Oncol 35(16):1795–1802

Nadler LM, Anderson KC, Marti G, Bates M, Park E, Daley JF et al (1983) B4, a human B lymphocyte-associated antigen expressed on normal, mitogen-activated, and malignant B lymphocytes. J Immunol 131(1):244–250

Nagorsen D, Baeuerle PA (2011) Immunomodulatory therapy of cancer with T cell-engaging BiTE antibody blinatumomab. Exp Cell Res 317(9):1255–1260

Nagorsen D, Bargou R, Ruttinger D, Kufer P, Baeuerle PA, Zugmaier G (2009) Immunotherapy of lymphoma and leukemia with T-cell engaging BiTE antibody blinatumomab. Leuk Lymphoma 50(6):886–891

Neelapu SS, Tummala S, Kebriaei P, Wierda W, Gutierrez C, Locke FL et al (2018) Chimeric antigen receptor T-cell therapy—assessment and management of toxicities. Nat Rev Clin Oncol 15(1):47–62

Offner S, Hofmeister R, Romaniuk A, Kufer P, Baeuerle PA (2006) Induction of regular cytolytic T cell synapses by bispecific single-chain antibody constructs on MHC class I-negative tumor cells. Mol Immunol 43(6):763–771

Rayes IK, Abduelkarem AR (2016) A qualitative study exploring physicians' perceptions on the role of community pharmacists in Dubai. Pharm Pract (Granada) 14(3):738

Richard-Carpentier G, Kantarjian HM, Short NJ, Ravandi F, Ferrajoli A, Schroeder HM et al (2018) A phase II study of the hyper-CVAD regimen in sequential combination with blinatumomab as frontline therapy for adults with B-cell acute lymphoblastic leukemia (B-ALL). Blood 132(32)

Ruella M, Maus MV (2016) Catch me if you can: leukemia escape after CD19-directed T cell immunotherapies. Comput Struct Biotechnol J 14:357–362

Runcie K, Budman DR, John V, Seetharamu N (2018) Bi-specific and tri-specific antibodies—the next big thing in solid tumor therapeutics. Mol Med 24(1):50

Sanders S, Stewart DA (2017) Targeting non-Hodgkin lymphoma with blinatumomab. Expert Opin Biol Ther 17(8):1013–1017

Schlegel P, Lang P, Zugmaier G, Ebinger M, Kreyenberg H, Witte KE et al (2014) Pediatric posttransplant relapsed/refractory B-precursor acute lymphoblastic leukemia shows durable remission by therapy with the T-cell engaging bispecific antibody blinatumomab. Haematologica 99(7):1212–1219

Smits NC, Sentman CL (2016) Bispecific T-cell engagers (BiTEs) as treatment of B-cell lymphoma. J Clin Oncol 34(10):1131–1133

Sotillo E, Barrett DM, Black KL, Bagashev A, Oldridge D, Wu G et al (2015) Convergence of acquired mutations and alternative splicing of CD19 enables resistance to CART-19 immunotherapy. Cancer Discov 5(12):1282–1295

Teachey DT, Rheingold SR, Maude SL, Zugmaier G, Barrett DM, Seif AE et al (2013) Cytokine release syndrome after blinatumomab treatment related to abnormal macrophage activation and ameliorated with cytokine-directed therapy. Blood 121(26):5154–5157

Topp MS, Kufer P, Gökbuget N, Goebeler M, Klinger M, Neumann S et al (2011) Targeted therapy with the T-cell-engaging antibody blinatumomab of chemotherapy-refractory minimal residual disease in B-lineage acute lymphoblastic leukemia patients results in high response rate and prolonged leukemia-free survival. J Clin Oncol: Off J Am Soc Clin Oncol 29 (18):2493–2498

Topp M, Gökbuget N, Zugmaier G, Viardot A, Stelljes M, Neumann S et al (2012) Anti-CD19 BiTE blinatumomab induces high complete remission rate and prolongs overall survival in adult patients with relapsed/refractory B-precursor acute lymphoblastic leukemia (ALL). Blood 120(21):#670

Topp MS, Gökbuget N, Zugmaier G, Klappers P, Stelljes M, Neumann S et al (2014) Phase II trial of the anti-CD19 bispecific T cell-engager blinatumomab shows hematologic and molecular remissions in patients with relapsed or refractory B-precursor acute lymphoblastic leukemia. J Clin Oncol 32(36):4134–4140

Topp MS, Gökbuget N, Stein AS, Zugmaier G, O'Brien S, Bargou RC et al (2015a) Safety and activity of blinatumomab for adult patients with relapsed or refractory B-precursor acute lymphoblastic leukaemia: a multicentre, single-arm, phase 2 study. Lancet Oncol 16(1):57–66

Topp MS, Gökbuget N, Stein AS, Zugmaier G, O'Brien S, Bargou RC et al (2015b) Safety and activity of blinatumomab for adult patients with relapsed or refractory B-precursor acute lymphoblastic leukaemia: a multicentre, single-arm, phase 2 study. Lancet Oncol

Torre M, Solomon IH, Sutherland CL, Nikiforow S, DeAngelo DJ, Stone RM et al (2018) Neuropathology of a case with fatal CAR T-cell-associated cerebral edema. J Neuropathol Exp Neurol 77(10):877–882

Velasquez MP, Bonifant CL, Gottschalk S (2018) Redirecting T cells to hematological malignancies with bispecific antibodies. Blood 131(1):30–38

Viardot A, Goebeler ME, Hess G, Neumann S, Pfreundschuh M, Adrian N et al (2016) Phase 2 study of the bispecific T-cell engager (BiTE) antibody blinatumomab in relapsed/refractory diffuse large B-cell lymphoma. Blood 127(11):1410–1416

Von Stackelberg A, Locatelli F, Zugmaier G, Handgretinger R, Trippett T, Rizzari C et al (2016) Phase I/Phase II study of blinatumomab in pediatric patients with relapsed/refractory acute lymphoblastic leukemia. J Clin Oncol. Published online ahead of print at http://www.jco.org on 3 Oct 2016

Watkins MP, Bartlett NL (2018) CD19-targeted immunotherapies for treatment of patients with non-Hodgkin B-cell lymphomas. Expert Opin Investig Drugs 27(7):601–611

Wilke AC, Gökbuget N (2017) Clinical applications and safety evaluation of the new CD19 specific T-cell engager antibody construct blinatumomab. Expert Opin Drug Saf 16(10):1191–1202

Wolf E, Hofmeister R, Kufer P, Schlereth B, Baeuerle PA (2005) BiTEs: bispecific antibody constructs with unique anti-tumor activity. Drug Discov Today 10(18):1237–1244

Yu H, Sotillo E, Harrington C, Wertheim G, Paessler M, Maude SL et al (2017) Repeated loss of target surface antigen after immunotherapy in primary mediastinal large B cell lymphoma. Am J Hematol 92(1):E11–E13

Zhao Y, Aldoss I, Qu C, Marcucci G, Stein AS, Bhatia R et al (2018) Genomic determinants of response to blinatumomab in relapsed/refractory (R/R) B-cell precursor acute lymphoblastic leukemia in adults. Blood 132(1552)

Zugmaier G, Gökbuget N, Klinger M, Viardot A, Stelljes M, Neumann S et al (2015) Long-term survival and T-cell kinetics in relapsed/refractory ALL patients who achieved MRD response after blinatumomab treatment. Blood 126(24):2578–2584

Advances and Challenges of CAR T Cells in Clinical Trials

Astrid Holzinger and Hinrich Abken

Abbreviations

CAR	Chimeric antigen receptor
CRS	Cytokine release syndrome
CTLA-4	Cytotoxic T lymphocyte-associated antigen-4
EGFR	Epithelial growth factor receptor
GMP	Good manufacturing practice
IFN	Interferon
Ig	Immunoglobulin
IL	Interleukin
MHC	Major histocompatibility complex
PD-1	Programmed cell death-1
scFv	Single-chain fragment of variable region
TCR	T cell receptor

---

1 Introduction

The concept of adoptive cell therapy with specifically redirected T cells is based on the observation that the immune system can control malignant diseases in the long term. In particular, tumor-infiltrating lymphocytes isolated from melanoma lesions,

---

A. Holzinger · H. Abken (✉)
RCI Regensburg Center for Interventional Immunology,
Franz-Josef-Strauss Allee 11, 93053 Regensburg, Germany
e-mail: hinrich.abken@ukr.de

A. Holzinger · H. Abken
Chair Genetic Immunotherapy, RCI c/o University Hospital Regensburg,
Regensburg, Germany

© Springer Nature Switzerland AG 2020
M. Theobald (ed.), *Current Immunotherapeutic Strategies in Cancer*,
Recent Results in Cancer Research 214,
https://doi.org/10.1007/978-3-030-23765-3_3

extensively amplified ex vivo, and re-administered to the patient are capable to induce tumor regression and even long-term remission in a substantial number of patients (Dudley et al. 2002). However, the antigen specificity of such isolated and amplified T cells is assumed to be predominantly tumor-specific, although frequently not known. To provide defined specificity in targeting cancer cells, patient's T cells are engineered with a transgenic chimeric antigen receptor (CAR), as discussed herein, or with T cell receptor (TCR) chains. The CAR is a recombinant composite transmembrane molecule which consists in the extracellular moiety of an antigen-binding domain and in the intracellular moiety of signaling domains capable to initiate T cell activation upon antigen engagement. The redirected activation of T cells and their therapeutic efficacy against cancer depend on multiple parameters including the CAR design, the CAR signaling, the binding affinity, the number of antigens on target cells, the spatial accessibility of the targeted antigen epitope, the maturation stage of T cells, and preconditioning of the patient's immune system. In the following, we summarize the major aspects and discuss developments in addressing the challenges of adoptive CAR T cell therapy in the clinical context.

2 The Evolution of the Prototype Chimeric Antigen Receptor

Adoptive cell therapy of cancer aims at redirecting T cells specifically toward the tumor lesion. Due to the limited number of available TCRs with known specificity for tumors and the frequent loss of major histocompatibility complex (MHC) presented antigen by cancer cells, a strategy was needed to overcome the limitations and to adapt the concept to a variety of targets. In this situation, Zelig Eshhar and colleagues (Weizmann Institute of Science) demonstrated that a composite receptor molecule with an antibody-derived binding domain in the extracellular domain and a TCR-derived signaling domain in the intracellular domain is capable of both recognizing a specific antigen on target cells and activating engineered T cells upon antigen engagement (Gross et al. 1989). Such modularly composed chimeric antigen receptor (CAR), at first named "T-body" or "immunoreceptor," allows targeting of a broad variety of antigens and signaling through various domains and combinations thereof initiating defined T cell functions. The prototype CAR is composed of a single-chain fragment of variable region (scFv) antibody for binding in the extracellular domain, a spacer of various lengths bridging to the transmembrane domain, and a signaling moiety mostly derived from the TCR CD3ζ intracellular chain with or without linked costimulatory domain. The scFv is engineered by joining the heavy and light chain variable (V) regions of an antibody by a linker, which provides some flexibility, in the order V_H-linker-V_L or V_L-linker-V_H. The primary activating domain is mostly the CD3ζ intracellular chain or a downstream kinase of the TCR; the Fc ε receptor-I (FcεRI) signaling chain is also used. The "first-generation" CARs contain only the primary signal (signal-1), while the "second-generation" CARs in addition contain a costimulatory domain (signal-2), like CD28, 4-1BB, OX40, ICOS, or CD27. The CD28 and 4-1BB domain are usually at the membrane proximal position followed by CD3ζ in the distal position; OX40 is also active in the membrane distal position. The first-generation CAR T cells have limited activation potential, while both signal-1 and signal-2 are required for inducing full T cell activation (Alvarez-Vallina and Hawkins 1996; Finney et al. 1998; Hombach et al. 2001); the second-generation CAR T cells show durable in cytokine release, amplification, and anti-tumor activity and are currently in clinical exploration. The "third-generation" CARs contain a combination of costimulatory domains along with the primary signal and provide benefit for T cells progressed in terminal maturation (Hombach et al. 2013).

The different costimulatory domains impact T cell activity and persistence in a different fashion. In particular, CD28 costimulation increases glucose uptake and ATP generation, while 4-1BB increases catabolism and mitochondrial respiratory chain capacities (Kawalekar et al. 2016). The differences in metabolic addiction are due to different signaling pathways initiated by CD28 and 4-1BB costimulation. CD28 activates the PI3K/Akt/mTOR signaling pathway which stimulates aerobic glycolysis (Frauwirth et al. 2002), and 4-1BB stimulates the Wnt/β-catenin pathway which is linked to oxidative phosphorylation and fatty acid oxidation (Kawalekar et al. 2016). Canonical Wnt/β-catenin favors the formation of central memory cells and long-term survival of T cells, while CD28-induced PI3K/Akt signaling sustains the immediate response effector cell phenotype (van der Windt and Pearce 2012; van der Windt et al. 2012, Pearce et al. 2009; Sukumar et al. 2013; Gattinoni et al. 2009). Accordingly, Akt inhibition during ex vivo priming and expansion triggers a central memory T cell phenotype with high levels of fatty acid oxidation and finally improved anti-tumor activities (van der Waart et al. 2014). After repetitive stimulation, CD28 CAR T cells are converted to CD45RO$^+$ CCR7$^-$ effector memory cells, while 4-1BB CAR T cells predominantly show a CD45RO$^+$ CCR7$^+$ central memory phenotype (Kawalekar et al. 2016) with extended persistence in the blood (Hombach and Abken 2007; Zhang et al. 2015; Wang et al. 2016).

The modular composition of the prototype CAR has advantages for the use in adoptive cell therapy of various diseases.

(a) As a consequence of targeting by an antibody, the target recognition is independent of MHC presentation of antigen which is frequently deficient in cancer cells. Any antigen can basically be targeted including non-classical T cell antigens like carbohydrates, lipids, or structural variants of an antigen as far as a binding molecule is available.

(b) The CAR-recognized antigen needs to be on the surface of the target cell; intracellular antigens are usually not visible to CAR T cells. However, the CAR T cell can gain TCR-like specificity by binding to MHC-presented peptide through an antibody and thereby sense intracellular antigens, e.g., NY-ESO-1 peptide presented by HLA-A2 (Stewart-Jones et al. 2009; Ma et al. 2016).

(c) The use of a scFv single-chain antibody with linked heavy and light chain variable regions allows the design of a one-polypeptide-chain CAR. Since a number of scFvs loose specificity and affinity compared with the native antibody, an alternative CAR is composed of two chains, i.e., the Ig heavy chain with the variable and constant region is linked to the transmembrane and signaling CAR moieties, while the Ig light chain is co-expressed and spontaneously associates with the heavy chain forming a fully functional antibody for CAR targeting (Faitschuk et al. 2016a).

(d) Naturally occurring binding domains or ligands are alternatively used for CAR targeting, including mutated IL-13 for targeting IL-13 receptor-α2 which is overexpressed by a broad variety of solid tumors but less by healthy tissues (Kahlon et al. 2004; Kong et al. 2012; Krebs et al. 2014). Alternatively, recombinant binding domains can be integrated into the CAR-like designed ankyrin repeat proteins (DARPins), which are composed of 33 amino acids ankyrin repeats and form a β-turn followed by two antiparallel α-helices and a loop reaching the β-turn of the next repeat (Hammill et al. 2015). Adnectin, derived from fibronectin, was used for CAR targeting epithelial growth factor receptor (EGFR) with high selectivity for high versus low expressing cells (Han et al. 2017).

(e) The spacer in the extracellular CAR moiety between the scFv and the transmembrane domain requires empiric optimization with respect to antigen binding and T cell activation. Assumed the optimal CAR T cell activation requires a distance of about 15 nm to the target cell as does the TCR (Grakoui et al. 1999), a longer spacer is capable to target an epitope near the target cell membrane, while a smaller spacer is optimal for a more distal epitope. The distance of the binding domain to the membrane can substantially be varied by using spacer of various lengths, e.g., IgG1 CH1–CH2–CH3 or CH2–CH3 or CH3 (Srivastava and Riddell 2015).

(f) CARs comprising the CD3ζ transmembrane domain engage signaling components of the TCR/CD3 complex and further downstream kinases which makes CAR T cell activation highly efficient (Bridgeman et al. 2010). However, the CAR is also functional in TCR knockout cells (Torikai et al. 2012) and in non-T cells like NK cells indicating that the signaling domain alone is sufficient to associate with kinases and to initiate a productive signaling cascade.

3 The Growing Family of CARs

(a) *TRUCK: a CAR T cell releasing a transgenic product*

CAR T cells can be used as "living factories" to release a transgenic polypeptide product "on demand" upon CAR signaling. The so-called TRUCKs (Chmielewski et al. 2014), the "fourth-generation" of CAR cells, are CAR T cells engineered with a constitutive or inducible expression cassette aiming at delivering the transgenic protein in therapeutic concentrations in the targeted tissue, while the concentrations in the periphery remain low. The strategy is of particular interest to combine the redirected CAR T cell attack with the action of a locally deposited, biologically active protein while avoiding systemic toxicity. Technically, the induced protein expression is under control of the $NFAT_6$-IL-2 minimal promoter which is activated upon CAR signaling. So far, the release of transgenic cytokines by CAR T cells was reported, for instance, IL-12 or IL-18 (Chmielewski and Abken 2015, 2017; Pegram et al. 2014; Chmielewski et al. 2011; Pegram et al. 2012; Hu et al. 2017; Kunert et al. 2017); other cytokines or proteins are also feasible. CAR IL-12 T cells (IL-12 TRUCKs) recruited and activated an innate immune response in the targeted tumors (Chmielewski et al. 2011), resisted suppression by Treg cells (Pegram et al. 2012), and showed an increased cytokine release and expansion (Koneru et al. 2015a). CAR T cells targeting Muc16 and secreting IL-12 are currently tested in a clinical trial (NCT02498912) (Koneru et al. 2015b); other transgenic cytokines are also evaluated. For instance, IL-15 improved T cell amplification and anti-tumor activity (Xu et al. 2016), however, is potentially leukemogenic (Hsu et al. 2007) which demands a suicide gene to eliminate the CAR T cells in the case of uncontrolled amplification (Hoyos et al. 2010). Other applications can likewise be envisaged like protecting the attacking T cells from oxidative stress through the release of catalase (Ligtenberg et al. 2016) or sustaining tumor penetration by delivering the soluble HVEM ectodomain which targets the tumor vasculature (Boice et al. 2016).

(b) *CAR T cells with multiple specificities*

CD19 CAR T cell treatment of B cell leukemia/lymphoma is associated with a substantial risk of relapse by tumor cells lacking the targeted CD19 epitope or the entire CD19 protein. The situation is addressed by targeting two antigens which basically can be achieved by a mixture of CAR T cells with different specificities, by T cells with two co-expressed CARs or T cells with one CAR with two specificities. The latter is a bispecific or tandem CAR ("TanCAR") with two scFvs linked by a short linker; binding to either antigen is sufficient to induce CAR T cell activation (Grada et al. 2013). A TanCAR with anti-CD19 and anti-CD20 scFv is aimed at targeting even those leukemic cells which lost CD19 upon a primary CAR T cell attack (Zah et al. 2016). Pediatric acute lymphocytic leukemia with known high heterogeneity in CD19 and CD20 expression can be controlled by bispecific CD20-CD19 CAR T cells, while monospecific CD20 CAR T cells failed in a transplanted mouse model (Martyniszyn et al. 2017). Dual targeting CD19 and CD123 is aiming at eliminating CD123-positive blasts in the treatment of B-ALL (Ruella et al. 2016a); other antigens are also co-targeted like CD22 (Haso et al. 2013), ROR1 (Hudecek et al. 2010), and immunoglobulin kappa light chain (Igκ) (Vera et al. 2006). TanCAR T cells have an additional advantage in that they exhibit improved avidity to target cells with both antigens which helps to stabilize the CAR synapse.

T cells can also be equipped with two specificities by co-expressing two CARs, each recognizing a different antigen and each capable to initiate full T cell activation. In contrast, co-expressed CARs which provide complementary signals, e.g., through CD3ζ and CD28, require simultaneous recognition of the cognate antigens to initiate full T cell activation; engagement of only one antigen is insufficient. Such a combination of CARs integrates antigen recognition in a Boolean "AND" logic computation and aims at reducing off-tumor toxicities toward healthy tissues. Examples of combinatorial antigen recognition are CARs targeting ErbB2 by the CD3ζ CAR and Muc1 by the CD28 CAR (Wilkie et al. 2012), or CD3ζ CAR targeting mesothelin and CD28 CAR targeting folate receptor-α (Lanitis et al. 2013). In contrast, a bispecific CAR with both primary and costimulatory signaling initiates full T cell activating also upon engagement of one target antigen providing a Boolean "OR" computation of antigen recognition.

An alternative "AND" gate recognition is based on Notch which upon activation mediates the proteolysis of the internal domain and the release of a transcription regulator which finally controls the transcription of a CAR (synNotch CAR) for cancer cell recognition and T cell activation (Roybal et al. 2016a, b; Morsut et al. 2016).

(c) *CARs with exchangeable antigen recognition*

The prototype CAR has a defined specificity for the targeted antigen; targeting a new antigen requires engineering and expressing a new CAR with novel specificity. In order to make the strategy more flexible, a high-affinity CD16 variant CAR was used to capture a tumor-specific antibody through binding the Ig Fc region, while the variable region of the captured antibody recognizes the tumor-associated antigen (Kudo et al. 2014). CD16 CAR T cells in the presence of the Herceptin antibody can target Her2$^+$ cancer cells; the specificity can be changed by using different antibodies for targeting. T cells with such "universal" CARs can be equipped with various specificities by adding a labeled targeting antibody which is recognized by the CAR. Toxicity can be controlled by titrating the amount of targeting antibody. In alternative developments, the CAR has specificity for epitopes linked to the targeting antibody, like fluorescein isothiocyanate (FITC) (Tamada et al. 2012), avidin (Urbanska et al. 2012), or a protein epitope (Cartellieri et al. 2016; Kim et al. 2015). Adding antibodies of different specificities allows redirecting CAR T cells toward a plethora of antigens without the need of de novo CAR T cell engineering which becomes relevant when targeting tumor lesions with a heterogeneous pattern of antigens.

(d) *Conditional CARs*

In the case of CAR-related toxicity, a "switch-on/switch-off" mechanism will help to fine-tune the CAR T cell response. The aim is achieved by a titrated dimerization of two co-expressed CAR chains, one of which is the "first-generation" CAR and the second is a rudimentary chain with a costimulatory moiety and without extracellular domains. Both chains dimerize and co-signal upon adding a small dimerizer molecule ("switch-on"), while without dimerizer the CAR remains "switched-off" (Kim et al. 2015; Rodgers et al. 2016; Wu et al. 2015). Increasing concentrations of the dimerizer improves CAR signaling upon antigen engagement which allows a fine-tuned titration of T cell response.

(e) *Switch CARs: converting a suppressor into an activator*

Since many solid tumors express inhibitory ligands at high levels, an activating CAR targeting the inhibitory ligand will convert the inhibitory into an activating signal. A CAR recognizing PD-L1 through its extracellular PD-1 domain and providing CD28 costimulation converts the inhibitory into an activating signal (Kobold et al. 2015; Liu et al. 2016; Prosser et al. 2012). Such PD-1:CD28 switch CAR competes with available PD-L1 and overruns the inhibitory PD-1 signal through CD28 signaling. Other inhibitory ligands may likewise be targeted by a switch CAR.

(f) *CARs providing inhibitory signals: iCARs*

Most currently used CARs provide an activating signal; CARs with inhibitory signals are also useful in certain situations. Such an inhibitory CAR (iCAR) blocks T cell activation, for instance, when engaging antigens on healthy cells in order to suppress off-tumor toxicities (Fedorov et al. 2013).

(g) *Armored CAR T cells with cytokine receptors*

In order to increase T cell amplification in response to cytokines, CAR T cells were equipped with the transgenic IL-7 receptor-α chain to restore responsiveness to IL-7 and to promote a Th1 response without stimulating Treg cells (Vera et al. 2009; Perna et al. 2014). Similarly, in prostate cancer with increased IL-4 levels, co-expression of the IL-4 binding/IL-7 signaling receptor improved anti-tumor activity of T cells with anti-PSCA CAR (Mohammed et al. 2017). On the other hand, a dominant negative receptor on CAR T cells can compete with an inhibitory cytokine, for instance, co-expression of the dominant negative TGF-β DNRII improved T cell anti-tumor activity in the presence of TGF-β in a melanoma model (Zhang et al. 2013).

4 Exploring Allogeneic Effector Cells: "Universal" T Cells and NK Cells

"Universal" T cells

In most adoptive cell therapy trials, patients were treated with autologous CAR T cells. Such individualized treatment is labor- and cost-intensive and hampers in the current fashion the widespread delivery of CAR T cells. T cells without HLA barriers are potential "universal" T cells that can be manufactured in advance and applied "off-the-shelf" to a number of patients. In this line, cells were derived from a non-HLA matched donor, disrupted in the TCR α chain locus using transcription activator-like effector nucleases (TALENs), thereby producing TCR-negative T cells which were finally engineered with an anti-CD19 CAR for the treatment of pediatric B cell acute lymphoblastic leukemia (B-ALL) (Poirot et al. 2015; Qasim et al. 2017). Subsequent depleting of remaining TCRαβ T cells reduces the risk of graft versus host disease (GvHD) through contaminating allogeneic TCR+ cells (Poirot et al. 2015; Bertaina et al. 2014). In a first clinical application, TALEN-edited CAR T cells were administered to a pediatric patient with B-ALL for whom autologous T cells could not be produced in sufficient numbers; no substantial GvHD was induced (Qasim et al. 2017). However, genetic editing by TALENs produces translocations also between other target sites, although at low frequencies (Qasim et al. 2017), which basically also applies to other gene-editing procedures like virus-transmitted zinc-finger nucleases (Provasi et al. 2012) or non-virally transmitted megaTALs (Osborn et al. 2016). While CRISPR guide RNA and Cas9 were encoded by the viral vector for constitutive expression (Shalem et al. 2014), current research is aiming at providing both the CAR expression cassette and the gene-editing tools with one transducing vector. In the further development of gene editing, the endogenous TCR and β2-microglobulin locus were targeted by CRISPR RNA electroporation in order to disrupt TCR and MHC class I by transiently available tools in CAR T cells in order to minimize off-target editing (Ren et al. 2017a, b).

NK cells

Human NK cells can also be used to initiate a potent anti-tumor response in model systems and to secrete a panel of cytokines, like GM-CSF, IFN-γ and IL-3, required for a productive anti-tumor response (Kruschinski et al. 2008; Klingemann 2014; Huenecke et al. 2010). While the prototype CAR for T cells is also active in NK cells, a CAR with the NK cell signaling proteins 2DS and DAP12 produced higher levels of NK cell activation and anti-tumor activity (Wang et al. 2015a). However, NK cells have a limited life span and rapidly disappear from circulation. Instead of primary NK cells, cells of the established NK92 line were engineered with an anti-Her2 CAR which showed potent anti-tumor activity upon local installation in a glioblastoma xenograft (Zhang et al. 2016) and an orthotopic breast cancer model (Schönfeld et al. 2015). The advantage is the "off-the-shelf" manufacturing of the cell product for immediate use; however, the CAR NK92 cells need to be irradiated prior to infusion which results in short-term NK cell survival and requires repetitive administration.

5 CAR T Cell Production: Challenges in Translating Individualized CAR T Cell Therapy to the Clinic

Adoptive therapy with CAR-modified T cells requires the manufacturing of cell products in accordance with the good manufacturing practice (GMP) rules; the procedure includes collecting the cells by leukapheresis in most cases, genetic engineering by viral gene transfer or electroporation, T cell amplification, and quality control of the final cell product. T cells are stimulated ex vivo by incubation with beads coated with agonistic anti-CD3 and anti-CD28 antibodies. In the majority of trials, T cells are ex vivo modified by γ-retroviral or lentiviral gene transfer; some trials use RNA-modified T cells obtained by electroporation. Viral transduction is performed at moderate-to-low virus titers, aiming to obtain less than 5 integrates per cell. Transposon-based vectors like Sleeping Beauty and PiggyBac were recently applied for clinical applications as well (Singh et al. 2013, 2015; Manuri et al. 2010). With the currently used transfer systems and the use of mature T cells, the risk of insertional mutagenesis and subsequent oncogenic transformation seems to be low; no oncogenic event due to transformed T cells was reported so far. Unintended engineering of a single leukemic B cell with the anti-CD19 CAR during the manufacturing process resulted in relapse of leukemia and resistance to CD19 CAR therapy mainly due to masking of the CD19 epitope (Ruella et al. 2018).

Modified cells are furthermore amplified in the presence of cytokines to high cell numbers using shaking reactors or bags; gas-permeable rapid expansion cultureware is currently preferred. Stimulation in the presence of IL-2 triggers effector T cell differentiation (Pipkin et al. 2010), while T cells amplified in the presence of IL-7 or IL-15 display a central memory phenotype with robust cytokine release, clonotypic persistence, and clinical anti-tumor activity (Kaneko et al. 2009; Butler et al. 2007). IL-21 is alternatively used to amplify cells with a less differentiated phenotype (Li et al. 2005; Hinrichs et al. 2008). Used for ex vivo amplification of CAR T cells, γ-cytokines also impact the metabolism in a specific fashion. IL-15 improves the oxidative metabolism as well as carnitine palmitoyl transferase expression which is involved in the rate-limiting step in fatty acid oxidation (van der Windt et al. 2012). IL-7 increases Glut1 by STAT5 and Akt activation (Wofford et al. 2008) and induces glycerol transport and triglyceride synthesis (Cui et al. 2015), all improving T cell persistence and survival.

While most CAR T cell products are currently manufactured in a manual process, great efforts are made to translate the process into a fully automated and supervised system. The aim is to allow manufacturing with high reproducibility and quality and to produce cells from multiple patients in the same production facility in parallel. The latter is of practical relevance to deliver sufficient numbers of cell products when the CAR T cell strategy becomes standard of treatment for a number of cancer patients.

The maturation stage of amplified T cells substantially impacts the redirected anti-tumor activity and CAR T cell persistence; the most suitable T cell population for CAR therapy is thought to be a naïve or young central memory cell with an acute inflammatory signature. The rationale is based on the observation that non-responding patients in trials accumulated T cells with an early memory and exhaustion signature, while responder patients did not (O'Rourke et al. 2017). $CD45RO^+$ $CD62L^+$ memory CAR T cells provide a more durable anti-tumor response than effector T cells in more advanced stages of differentiation (Klebanoff et al. 2012; Gattinoni et al. 2011; Singh et al. 2016). Therefore, $CD62L^+$-enriched CAR T cells are currently explored in trials. However, it is still unresolved how to keep CAR T cells in the early stage of maturation, in particular after repetitive CAR activation.

6 The Second-Generation CAR T Cells Produced Lasting Remissions in Leukemia and Lymphoma

While adoptive therapy with the "first-generation" CAR T cells failed to show therapeutic efficacy, the "second-generation" CAR T cells achieved spectacular remissions in so far refractory leukemia and lymphoma, changing the overall therapeutic landscape in the long term. The standard treatment procedure is a sequence of events starting with leukapheresis of the patient for T cell donation, non-myeloablative lymphodepletion, and administration of the CAR T cells to the patient in one or more doses by i.v. infusion with or without IL-2 support. The vast majority of trials are designed for the treatment of hematologic malignancies (Holzinger et al. 2016); still a minority of trials is aiming at treating solid cancer (Abken 2017). Since CAR T cell persistence is crucial for clinical efficacy (Porter et al. 2015) and T cell persistence depends on appropriate costimulation, CARs with one or two costimulatory endodomains are used in trials, mostly providing CD28 or 4-1BB costimulation. CARs with alternative costimulatory domains are also clinically explored including CARs with OX40 (Hombach and Abken 2011), ICOS (Shen et al. 2013; Guedan et al. 2014), CD27 (Song et al. 2012), CD40-MyD88 (Foster et al. 2017), CD2 (Cheadle et al. 2012), and CD244 (Altvater et al. 2009).

One of the first successfully treated patients received anti-CD19 CAR T cells for the treatment of chronic lymphocytic leukemia (CLL) resulting in complete and maintained remission (Porter et al. 2011); other groups also successfully treated patients with CLL at the same time with CD19 CAR T cells (Porter et al. 2015; Grupp et al. 2013; Kochenderfer et al. 2013, 2015; Cruz et al. 2013; Brentjens et al. 2013; Maude et al. 2014a; Davila et al. 2014; Lee et al. 2015). CAR T cells with 4-1BB costimulation appear superior to CD28 CAR T cells (Porter et al. 2015) with prolonged persistence of 4-1BB CAR T cells for more than 4 years compared with 30 days of CD28 CAR T cells (Brentjens et al. 2011). All patients experienced lasting depletion of healthy B cells, at least as long as CD19 CAR T cells persisted. For the treatment of chronic lymphocytic leukemia (CLL), the Fcμ receptor is potentially a more tumor-selective target sparing healthy B cells from elimination by CAR T cells (Faitschuk et al. 2016b). Pediatric and adult patients with B cell acute lymphocytic leukemia (B-ALL) and follicular lymphoma were also successfully treated, even with higher frequencies of remissions. Remarkably, patients with multiple myeloma were also experienced remissions after CD19 CAR T cell therapy (Garfall et al. 2015) although multiple myeloma consists entirely of CD19-negative plasma cells. The observation led to the speculation that CD19 CAR T cells eliminated a $CD19^+$ cancer stem cell population responsible for tumor repopulation; alternatively, a suppressor B cell population may have been eliminated by CAR T cells. Apart from CD19, alternative antigens are also targeted, i.e., CD20, CD22, the Igκ light chain, ROR-1 for B-NHL and B-ALL, and CD30 for Hodgkin's lymphoma.

Currently, nearly 400 early-phase trials using the "second-generation" CAR T cells are in clinical exploration, mostly performed by academic centers or major pharmaceutical companies like Novartis, Juno Therapeutics, and Kite Pharma (now

Gilead). The anti-CD19 CAR for the treatment of pediatric B-ALL (Kymriah^{TM}, tisagenlecleucel, Novartis) and adult large B cell lymphoma (Yescarta^{TM}, axicabtagene ciloleucel, Gilead) have recently obtained FDA approval in 2017 and subsequently EMA approval in 2018. The CAR provides specificity by a murine anti-CD19 scFv and mediates T cell activation through CD28-CD3ζ signaling; fully humanized CARs are currently developed to avoid an anti-CAR immune response which potentially may deplete CAR T cells by the patient's immune system in the long term.

The success of CAR T cell therapy in various trials is difficult to compare due to a number of differences in the trial design, CAR composition, targeted antigen, preconditioning, and others. Apart thereof, CAR T cell dose and lymphodepletion were recently identified as key factors which impact CAR T cell amplification and persistence and finally therapeutic efficacy (Zhang et al. 2015). It is therefore reasonable that much effort is currently put into optimizing the "preconditioning" regimen in order to optimize the engraftment and initial amplification of CAR T cells. Only a small number of trials do not perform preconditioning.

During complete remission, most patients treated with 4-1BB CAR T cells did not receive further cancer-specific treatment; patients with CD28 CAR therapy frequently underwent allogeneic stem cell transplantation. Further exploration needs to identify a more successful strategy. However, the clinical observation that CD28 CAR T cells less persist than 4-1BB CAR T cells, i.e., few months compared with some years, underlines a potential benefit of transplantation after CD28 CAR T cell therapy.

Persistence of CAR T cells in the periphery is crucial for a lasting remission; repetitive re-stimulation of CAR T cells may improve persistence and finally anti-tumor activity. Therefore, virus-specific T cells, which are re-stimulated upon contact with viral antigens, are being used for a CAR-redirected anti-tumor response. In particular, T cells specific for Epstein–Barr virus (EBV) were engineered with a CAR with cancer specificity; EBV viral antigens are recognized by the endogenous TCR of the engineered T cells triggering their repetitive activation and amplification (Savoldo et al. 2007). EBV-specific CAR T cells persisted substantially longer after infusion to the patient than CAR T cells without virus specificity (Louis et al. 2011).

7 CAR T Cell Therapy of Solid Cancer Is Still Challenging

In the treatment of solid cancer lesions, some specific properties of T cells provide advantages over standard drug treatment regimens. Basically, CAR T cells have the capability to migrate through nearly all tissues, to amplify upon activation, and to execute their cytolytic and pro-inflammatory activity in a repetitive fashion. These properties make CAR T cells ideal for targeting widespread solid tumor lesions and metastases; however, the therapy of solid cancer is still challenging (Fig. 1, Table 1).

Fig. 1 Challenges and
modifications of CAR T cells
to overcome the barriers in
solid tumors

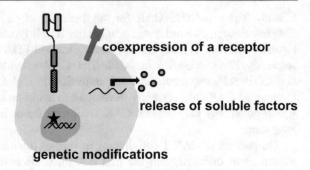

Trafficking of T cells to specific targets depends on sensing chemokines; however, the process is impaired since most tumors exhibit an altered chemokine milieu (Franciszkiewicz et al. 2012) and some adhesion factors are lost on tumor endothelia (Bouzin et al. 2007), making T cell penetration and migration less efficient. Locally deposited TNF-α increased vascular adhesion molecules, such as vascular cell adhesion protein-1 and intracellular adhesion molecule-2 on endothelial cells, resulting in enhanced T cell extravasation and tumor accumulation (Calcinotto et al. 2012). Endothelial cell adhesion and/or transmigration of T cells is improved by targeting vascular endothelial growth factor (VEGF) receptor-2 (Chinnasamy et al. 2010) or blocking migration inhibitory factors like the endothelin B receptor (Kandalaft et al. 2009). T cells can also accumulate in privileged tissues like testes and eyes (Brudno and Kochenderfer 2016), penetrate the blood–brain barrier, and infiltrate the brain (Pule et al. 2008), which is thought to be the cause of neurotoxicity (Mackall and Miklos 2017). On the other hand, several chemokine receptors are downregulated on the T cell surface upon extensive ex vivo propagation, making amplified T cell products less sensitive to chemokine-driven trafficking. Transgenic re-expression of chemokine receptors, like CXCR2 (CXCL1 receptor) for targeting melanoma (Kershaw et al. 2002) or CCR2b for targeting neuroblastoma (Craddock et al. 2010), is aiming at improving specific trafficking of CAR T cells toward the tumor lesion.

Infiltration into the tumor tissue is a major hurdle for CAR-modified T cells (Joyce and Fearon 2015). Local T cell installation circumvents this limitation and may improve therapeutic efficacy (Adusumilli et al. 2014). For instance, CAR T cells were applied intrapleurally and intraperitoneally for the treatment of mesothelioma and ovarian cancer, respectively (Koneru et al. 2015b). Anti-CEA CAR T cells were applied by endoscopy into hepatic metastases (Katz et al. 2015); anti-c-Met CAR T cells were applied by intratumoral injections into breast cancer metastases inducing necrosis of injected tumor lesions (Tchou et al. 2017) (NCT01837602). On the other hand, T cell penetration can be improved by transgenic expression of heparanase which degrades heparan sulfate proteoglycans in the stroma; moreover, endogenous heparanase expression is frequently downregulated during the manufacturing process (Caruana et al. 2015).

Table 1 Challenges and modifications of CAR T cells to overcome the barriers in solid tumors

Challenge	Barriers in the tumor environment	CAR T cell engineering	References
Co-expression of a receptor			
T cell activation	Lack of costimulation, e.g., 4-1BB-L, OX40-L, CD80/86	Expression of costimulatory receptors, e.g., CD28, 4-1BB, OX40	Curran et al. (2015)
T cell homing	Reduced release of chemokines by tumors	Expression of stimulatory ligands, e.g., CD40L	Craddock et al. (2010), Di Stasi et al. (2009), Peng et al. (2010)
		Expression of chemokine receptors, e.g., CCR4, CXCR2	
T cell suppression	Treg cells	Modified CD28 signaling deficient in IL-2 induction	Kofler et al. (2011)
Nutrient resources	Low glucose, glutamine, arginine, tryptophan	Expression of transporters, e.g., for glucose or amino acids	Cretenet et al. (2016)
Inhibitory pathways	Inhibitory ligands displayed by cancer cells, e.g., PD-L1/2	Expression of a switch receptor, e.g., PD-1:CD28, expression of dnPD-1	Kobold et al. (2015), Liu et al. (2016), Prosser et al. (2012)
	Inhibitory cytokines, e.g., TGF-β	Expression of dnTGF-β receptor; expression of synthetic receptor	Zhang et al. (2013); Golumba-Nagy et al. (2018)
Extravasation	Tumor-associated vasculature	Expression of anti-VEGF-R2 CAR	Chinnasamy et al. (2010)
Penetration	Stromal tissue	Expression of anti-FAP CAR	Kakarla et al. (2013)
Release of soluble factors			
Extravasation	Tumor-associated vasculature	Secretion of endothelin B receptor blocking Ab	Kandalaft et al. (2009)
Penetration	Stromal tissue	Release of degrading enzymes, e.g., heparanase	Caruana et al. (2015)
Immune suppression	Inhibitory ligands on cancer cells, e.g., PD-L1/L2, VISTA	Checkpoint blockade, e.g., expression of anti-PD-1 Ab, anti-PD-L1 Ab, anti-CTLA-4 Ab	
	Suppressor cells, e.g., Tregs, MDSCs	Release of IL-18	Chmielewski and Abken (2017)
	Deficient innate immune response, M2 macrophages	Release of IL-12	Chmielewski et al. (2011)

(continued)

Table 1 (continued)

Challenge	Barriers in the tumor environment	CAR T cell engineering	References
Metabolic situation	Metabolic exhaustion	Overexpression of intracellular proteins, e.g., transcription co-activator PGC1-α	
	Oxidative stress	Overexpression of catalase	Ligtenberg et al. (2016)
Genetic modifications			
Immune suppression	Inhibitory ligands, e.g., PD-L1	PD-1 suppression by siRNA, shRNA, Gene knockout by CRISPR/Cas9, e.g., PD-1, Cbl-b	Ren et al. (2017a)
	Low γ-cytokine levels	Enhanced sensitivity to γ-cytokines by miR-155 overexpression	Ji et al. (2015)

CAR T cells are facing a hostile environment after successful penetration into the tumor tissue. CAR T cells need to break the stroma and extracellular matrix barrier to get in near vicinity to the cancer cells; IFN-γ is required to eliminate the stromal cells (Textor et al. 2014). As a consequence, targeting tumor stroma by CAR T cells in addition to targeting the cancer cells likely improves the overall efficacy in eliminating solid tumor lesions. Fibroblast activation protein (FAP), a serine protease involved in extracellular matrix remodeling and expressed by stromal cells of a majority of epithelial cancers, is a candidate protein for targeting the stroma. Consequently, targeting FAP in addition to cancer cell targeting improved the overall anti-tumor activity (Kakarla et al. 2013).

Myeloid-derived suppressor cells (MDSCs) and tumor-associated macrophages deprive CAR T cells in the tumor tissue of essential amino acids through decreasing tryptophan levels (Ninomiya et al. 2015). Regulatory T (Treg) cells, MDSCs, and tumor-associated M2 macrophages release suppressive cytokines, like IL-4, IL-10, leukemia inhibitory factor, and TGF-β; MDSCs and Tregs can be suppressed by sunitinib, a multi-kinase inhibitor, which may be used in combination with CAR T cell treatment. The stromal cells are releasing IDO and deprive the tissue of glucose and other nutrients; profound acidosis moreover counteracts the anti-tumor activity of CAR T cells. IDO inhibits CAR T cells through accumulating kynurenine which blocks expansion, cytotoxicity, and cytokine secretion by CAR T cells (Ninomiya et al. 2015). On the other hand, fludarabine and cyclophosphamide, used for pre-conditioning in patients, decrease IDO levels through depletion from Treg cells. Low levels of arginine in the tumor tissue result in CD3ζ repression and inhibition of T cell amplification and cytokine release (Rodriguez et al. 2007). MDSCs moreover suppress T cell function in a direct fashion through arginase-mediated TCR CD3ζ chain repression (Rodriguez et al. 2002). Protein kinase A (PKA) is the effector molecule in the downstream cascade of prostaglandin E2 and adenosine, both produced in the tumor tissue and both inhibiting T cell function. Consequently, disruption of the PKA membrane anchoring increases CAR T cell infiltration, chemotaxis, persistence, and anti-tumor activity (Newick et al. 2016).

Inhibitory ligands suppress CAR T cell activity by binding to programmed cell death-1 (PD-1), cytotoxic T lymphocyte-associated antigen-4 (CTLA-4), or Fas, among others. Much effort is currently undertaken to make CAR T cells resistant to this type of suppression, e.g., by suppressing PD-1 expression (Cherkassky et al. 2016) or a PD-1 switch receptor which binds to PD-L1 and conveys the suppressing into an activating signal (Liu et al. 2016; Prosser et al. 2012). Alternatively, checkpoint inhibitors to block the PD-1/PD-L1, e.g., nivolumab, or CTLA-4 axis, e.g., ipilimumab, are currently explored as adjuvant in CAR T cell trials. Along this line, CAR T cell therapy combined with PD-1 blockade increased the anti-tumor efficacy (John et al. 2013). In a case report, a patient showed tumor reduction and increase in circulating CAR T cells upon PD-1 blockade by pembrolizumab (Chong et al. 2017); a trial is exploring PD-1 blockade in CD19 CAR T cell-resistant or relapsing leukemia patients (NCT02650999). A PD-L1 mini-body improved the anti-tumor activity of CAR T cells in a preclinical model (Tanoue et al. 2017).

Taken together, blocking inhibitory checkpoints can enhance the efficacy of CAR T cell therapy against tumors.

On the other hand, CAR T cell therapy is combined with agonistic activation of 4-1BB (Mardiana et al. 2017) or vaccination with viral antigen recognized by anti-tumor CAR and antivirus TCR-engineered T cells (Slaney et al. 2017). Other strategies including the use of EBV-specific T cells are in line with specifically re-stimulating CAR T cells by non-tumor antigens.

8 CAR T Cell Therapy-Associated Toxicities

CAR T cell therapy so far showed efficacy in the treatment of B cell leukemia, however, provokes side effects which need clinical intervention (Table 2). An updated review on grading and management of CRS was recently published by Riegler et al. (2019).

Table 2 Clinical management of toxicities associated with CAR T cell therapy

Toxicity	Potential prevention or treatment
Cytokine release syndrome (CRS)	Blocking the IL-6R/IL-6 axis by tocilizumab or siltuximab or sarilumab Depleting from CAR T cells Reducing or fractionating CAR T cell dose
Vascular leakage syndrome (VLS)	Plasma expansion Plasmapheresis to deplete serum factors
Tumor lysis syndrome (TLS)	Plasmapheresis Reducing tumor mass prior cell therapy Reducing or fractionating CAR T cell dose
Macrophage activation syndrome (MAS)	Blocking the IL-6R/IL-6 axis by tocilizumab or siltuximab
Neurotoxicity	Corticosteroids
"On-target off-tumor" toxicities	Targeting of tumor-selective antigens, e.g., neo-antigens Blocking the target antigen on healthy cells Co-expression of iCARs to protect healthy cells Combinatorial antigen recognition Transient CAR expression after RNA transfer Conditional CAR activation by a dimerizer Local CAR T cell application CAR T cell elimination by suicide gene activation, e.g., iCasp9, or by depleting antibodies
GvHD after allogeneic T cell therapy	TCR-negative CAR T cells
Tumor relapse by antigen escape of cancer cells	Targeting of co-expressed antigens
Poor in vivo expansion	Intensifying lymphodepletion Increasing cytokine substitution
B cell aplasia after CD19 CAR T cell therapy	Replacement of immunoglobulins Antibiotic and antifungal prophylaxis

(a) Most CAR-targeted antigens are not exclusively expressed by cancer cells but also by healthy cells. The lack of tumor selectivity becomes obvious, for instance, when targeting CD19 to treat B cell leukemia; also, healthy B cells are eliminated resulting in a lasting B cell depletion which requires immunoglobulin substitution and antibiotic and antifungal protection. Such "on-target off-tumor" toxicity in the treatment of leukemia is clinically manageable and, however, is more severe when the targeted antigen is expressed by vital tissues. For instance, targeting ErB2 by the third-generation CAR T cells resulted in a fatal cardiopulmonary failure likely due to the attack against healthy lung tissues (Morgan et al. 2010). The toxicity depends also on the particular binding domain and on CAR signaling since CAR T cells with another anti-Her2 binding domain and with one costimulatory domain produced no dose-limiting toxicity (Ahmed et al. 2015; Feng et al. 2017).

(b) Rapid destruction of a large tumor mass may induce a tumor lysis syndrome which is initiated by the release of tumor cell components and accompanied by electrolyte and metabolic disturbances with the risk of multi-organ failure.

(c) The CAR itself can induce "off-target off-tumor" toxicity through the IgG1 Fc spacer which binds to the Fc γ receptor (FcγR) (CD64) and can thereby activate innate cells like NK cells and macrophages. Deleting the IgG1 CH2 domain or mutating the Asn297 side (Hudecek et al. 2015; Hombach et al. 2010) reduces the risk; IgG4 or extracellular CD8 is used as an alternative spacer.

(d) The cytokine release syndrome (CRS) is an acute immune activation resulting in elevated serum levels of pro-inflammatory cytokines including IFN-γ and TNF-α, IL-10 and in particular IL-6 (Maude et al. 2014a, b; Davila et al. 2014; Lee et al. 2015). CRS is clinically characterized by high fever, malaise, fatigue, myalgia, nausea, anorexia, tachycardia, hypotension, capillary leak, cardiac dysfunction, renal impairment, hepatic failure, and disseminated intravascular coagulation (Lee et al. 2014). The severity of CRS may, but must not, correlate with tumor burden (Maude et al. 2014a; Teachey et al. 2016), often occurs together with the vascular leakage syndrome (VLS), and is closely associated with the systemic macrophage activation syndrome, clinically resembling hemophagocytic lymphohistiocytosis, which makes clinical diagnosis and management difficult. A score to identify CRS/VLS in early stages and clinical guidelines in management were recently proposed (Davila et al. 2014; Maude et al. 2014b; Teachey et al. 2016). Three markers were identified to predict CRS, i.e., in adults, soluble gp130 (sgp130), IFN-γ, and IL1Rα and in pediatric patients, IFN-γ, IL-13, and MIP1α. C-reactive protein, which is released by hepatocytes in response to IL-6, currently serves as a laboratory marker of CRS onset and severity (Davila et al. 2014).

Systemic corticosteroid treatment rapidly reversed CRS without compromising the initial anti-tumor response as long as steroids are applied short term, i.e., below 14 days (Davila et al. 2014; Lee et al. 2015). Current CRS therapy is based on blocking the IL-6/IL-6 receptor signaling axis by tocilizumab application which neutralizes the IL-6 receptor and does not interfere with CAR T cell efficacy (Grupp et al. 2013; Teachey et al. 2016; Chen et al. 2016);

the IL-6 blocking antibody siltuximab has also been used. The long-term impact of blocking IL-6 on the anti-tumor efficacy needs to be explored in detail.

(e) Neurotoxicity with aphasia, hallucinations, confusion, delirium, expressive aphasia, obtundation, myoclonus, and delirium occurs in about 40% of patients during CAR T cell therapy, is reversible, and is often observed after CD19 CAR T cell therapy (Maude et al. 2014a; Davila et al. 2014; Lee et al. 2015; Teachey et al. 2016). The mechanism is less understood; a diffuse encephalopathy caused by infiltrating CAR T cells is thought to be the cause.

(f) Anaphylaxis with elevated IgE levels was reported for one patient after repeated doses of CAR T cells; the patient developed antibodies against murine domains of the CAR (Maus et al. 2013).

9 Strategies to Improve Safety of CAR T Cell Therapy

(a) *CAR T cells recognizing more than one antigen*

The strategy is based on the rationale that a pattern of antigens is more indicative for cancer cells versus healthy cells than one antigen only; this is particularly the case since a truly cancer-specific antigen is rare. To drive T cell activation upon recognizing two antigens, two CARs are co-expressed, one CAR providing the primary activating signal and the other CAR, the costimulatory signal, thereby complementing the signals for full T cell activation only in the presence of both antigens (Wilkie et al. 2012; Lanitis et al. 2013; Kloss et al. 2012).

(b) *Inhibitory CARs*

The inhibitory CAR (iCAR) is co-expressed by T cells together with an activating CAR and aimed at providing an inhibitory signal when engaging an antigen on healthy cells which is absent on cancer cells. The iCAR signaling domain is derived from PD-1 or CTLA-4 which is dominant over the activating signals through CD3ζ and costimulation (Fedorov et al. 2013). The T cell is blocked by the inhibitory signal as long as the iCAR engages healthy cells; without iCAR signaling, the T cell can be activated through the co-expressed tumor-specific CAR.

(c) *Transient CAR expression*

In the case of potential toxicity, transient CAR expression by the T cell may limit the side effects. The CAR is transiently expressed upon RNA transfer due to the short RNA half-life and RNA dilution upon T cell division which is even more rapid after T cell activation. However, the CAR is present on the T cell surface in the order of several days and mediates efficient T cell activation upon target cell engagement (Birkholz et al. 2009). Such RNA-modified T cells were applied in trials with some, although transient efficacy (Maus et al. 2013; Beatty et al. 2014).

(d) *CAR T cell elimination*

In the case of uncontrolled toxicity, CAR T cells need to be rapidly and efficiently eliminated. High-dose steroid treatment was applied to stop autoimmunity after treatment with carboanhydrase IX-specific CAR T cells (Lamers et al. 2006). More selective elimination of CAR T cells is achieved by antibody targeting a specific domain in the extracellular CAR moiety (Philip et al. 2014) or by targeting a co-expressed marker, for instance, the truncated EGFR which can be targeted by cetuximab (Wang et al. 2011). The CAR binding domain can also be targeted by an anti-idiotypic antibody (Jena et al. 2013). Alternatively, a suicide gene is co-expressed with the CAR, for instance, the truncated caspase-9 and a mutated FK506 binding protein; the apoptotic cascade is initiated upon applying a synthetic drug for dimerizing caspase-9 (Straathof et al. 2005).

(e) Routes of T cell administration

Usually, CAR T cells are applied by i.v. injection to approach the target side through blood circulation. Local administration by endoscopy or by intrapleural or intraperitoneal application may avoid off-tumor T cell activation to some extent while providing high CAR T cell doses at the tumor side (Parente-Pereira et al. 2011; Katz et al. 2016). However, in most tumor patients, puncture of tumor lesions is technically not feasible and is not applicable in a disseminated tumor disease.

---

10   Future Developments in CAR T Cell Therapy: Challenges Remain

Current clinical trials in phase I and II are promising to establish CAR T cell therapy in the front-line treatment of leukemia and lymphoma within the next years. However, major hurdles remain, in particular in the CAR T cell therapy of solid cancer.

(a) *Which antigen serves best in targeting solid tumors while avoiding off-tumor toxicities?*

Extensive research is aiming at identifying new and more selective antigens suitable for safe targeting tumor lesions while sparing healthy tissues. Truly tumor-selective antigens are rare; however, more selective antigens are tumor-specific mutations of surface proteins or glycosylation variants like Muc1 or Muc16 which can be targeted by CAR T cells (Posey et al. 2016). Apart from tumor-specific antigens, CAR T cell treatment of solid tumors proved safe by targeting carcinoembryonic antigen (CEA) as an auto-antigen which is strictly luminal expressed by healthy epithelial cells while depolarized on cancer cells. Two trials provided some clinical efficacy in the treatment of gastrointestinal adenocarcinoma by systemic application of CEA-specific CAR T cells (NCT01212887, NCT02349724) (Thistlethwaite et al.

2017; Zhang et al. 2017); local administration of anti-CEA CAR T cells by hepatic artery infusion also declined tumor progression (NCT01373047) without the induction of treatment-related colitis (Katz et al. 2015).

(b) *How to prevent tumor relapse after CAR T cell therapy?*

CD19 CAR T cell therapy induces complete remissions in pediatric B-ALL patients with high frequencies; however, leukemia relapses in about 40% of patients despite persisting CAR T cells (Grupp et al. 2013; Maude et al. 2014a; Lee et al. 2015). A frequent cause of relapse is the expression of a functionally active CD19 isoform which is not recognized by the CAR due to the lack of exon-2 (Sotillo et al. 2015). Targeting a CD19 epitope which is not lost by splicing or co-targeting a second antigen, e.g., CD20 by a bispecific CAR, likely increases the therapeutic pressure on leukemic cells. Switching to a CD19-negative myeloid lineage was observed in the relapse of two cases of B-ALL after CD19 CAR treatment (Gardner et al. 2016), again pointing to the need to target leukemic cells by two independent antigens. Profound heterogeneity in the expression of the targeted antigen may also be the cause of early tumor relapse after initial tumor regression. A CAR T cell-initiated antigen-independent anti-tumor response through innate immune cells in the tumor lesion may improve the overall therapeutic efficacy. Designed for these purposes, IL-12 or IL-18 TRUCK cells, i.e., CAR T cells with the inducible release of transgenic cytokines, are capable to induce an innate response against antigen-negative cancer cells in an experimental model (Chmielewski et al. 2011; Chmielewski and Abken 2017).

(c) *What is the optimal CAR design?*

Research during the last two decades established the prototype design of a CAR; however, each CAR needs to be optimized with respect to the potential target antigen and the T cell subset. In particular, the binding affinity, the targeted antigen epitope, the extracellular spacer length, the transmembrane domain, and finally the primary and costimulatory signaling domains need to be individually evaluated with respect to the specific tumor situation. Early preclinical research established that CAR T cell activation depends on the affinity of antigen binding and the epitope of the targeted antigen (Chmielewski et al. 2004; Hombach et al. 2007). Recently confirmed by others (Liu et al. 2015; Caruso et al. 2015), there is an affinity window in which CAR T cells target tumor cells with high antigen load while sparing healthy cells with low antigen levels. Consequently, a trial targeting Her2 caused no toxicity (Ahmed et al. 2015), while a high-affinity CAR targeting a different epitope caused fatal adverse events (Morgan et al. 2010).

(d) *Which T cell subset performs best in the long term against solid tumors?*

The most suitable stage in T cell maturation for adoptive cell therapy seems to be a naïve or early central memory cell with an enhanced capacity for amplification and long-lived persistence. In some trials, T cells with a $CD62L^+$ phenotype are selected prior engineering with a CAR (Sabatino et al. 2016). Reducing T cell amplification during manufacturing improves the anti- tumor activity of CAR T cells (Ghassemi et al. 2018). On the other hand, the T cell maturation can be directed by costimulation and/or cytokine signals; 4-1BB costimulation initiates a central memory T cell response in young T cells, while CD28 mediates a more short-lived effector cell response (Kawalekar et al. 2016). In more matured stages of T cell development, other costimuli or combinations thereof are needed; for instance, $CCR7^-$ T cells require combined CD28-OX40 costimulation for lasting persistence, while young T cells respond upon CD28 costimulation (Hombach et al. 2013). The T cell phenotype and functional capacities can also be modulated by co-treatment with kinase inhibitors. Ibrutinib, a Bruton tyrosine kinase (BTK) inhibitor used for CLL treatment, reduces PD-1 and exhaustion of CAR T cells and thereby increases persistence and anti-tumor activity in the long term (Ruella et al. 2016b).

(e) *How can a high-quality T cell product be manufactured for an increasing number of patients in a standardized process?*

Currently, most CAR T cells are produced by a manual process in specialized GMP units, frozen, and shipped to the patient's hospital (Köhl et al. 2018). Manufacturing a growing number of cell products in this fashion will come to its limits, in particular, when thousands of patients require their own cell products in due time. A decentralized, in-hospital manufacturing by an automated, fully controlled and entirely closed system needs to be established. This will also require a high degree of standardization in the manufacturing process, will be less cost-intensive, and would avoid sophisticated logistics in transportation of blood and cell products.

(f) *Will "universal" CAR T cells outsmart patient's "individualized" CAR T cells?*

So far, patient's T cells are genetically engineered with the CAR for the individual patient and the individual tumor. A number of efforts are aiming at generating "universal" T cells which can be applied to a number of patients independently of their MHC which requires making the CAR T cell invisible to the patient's immune system. Moreover, the allogeneic CAR T cell needs to be deficient in alloreactivity against the patient's healthy tissues which is achieved by targeted disruption of the TCR α-chain locus (Qasim et al. 2017). In this line, CAR-modified virus-specific T cells and T cells with silenced endogenous TCR are explored toward a "universal" cell product (Poirot et al. 2015; Cruz et al. 2013; Wang et al. 2015b). While additional manipulations need to be performed to avoid immune destruction of such "universal" CAR T cells, a cell product "off-the-shelf" or a "third-party" cell bank would provide much more flexibility in the clinical application and would help to establish adoptive cell therapy for a higher number of patients.

(g) *Will major CAR T cell therapy-associated adverse events be controlled?*

CAR T cell treatment can cause severe side effects which need intensive care hospitalization; the cytokine release syndrome (CRS) is a frequently occurring; first, steps to standardize grading and treatment regimens are made (Davila et al. 2014; Maude et al. 2014b; Riegler et al. 2019; Teachey et al. 2016). However, as long as the CAR T cell protocols and treatment procedures differ and the various parameters were not clinically evaluated in a comparative clinical setting, more general conclusions cannot be drawn from individual trials and further optimization in mono- and combo-immune therapies is difficult to perform in a timely fashion. In the case of uncontrolled toxicity, CAR T cells need to be selectively and rapidly eliminated; co-expressed suicide genes or domains targeted by depleting antibodies may be mandatory. An example is the induced apoptosis by dimerization of the inducible caspase-9 (iCasp9) upon addition of the dimerizing agent AP1903 resulting in the elimination of >90% of T cells within 30 min (Thomis et al. 2001; Tey et al. 2007; Di Stasi et al. 2011; Zhou et al. 2014). However, spontaneous dimerization occurs in a substantial basal frequency producing a constant level of apoptotic cells. Alternatively, CAR T cells can be cleared by antibody-dependent cellular cytotoxicity (ADCC) using antibodies targeting a CAR domain, for instance, rituximab for a co-expressed CD20 epitope or cetuximab for EGFR targeting (Philip et al. 2014; Wang et al. 2011; Serafini et al. 2004). The caveat is that cancer patients with a dysfunctional immune system may have limited capacities to remove the CAR cells by ADCC, especially in the case of toxicity.

(h) *Will there be a specific preconditioning for each type of cancer?*

In order to sustain CAR T cell engraftment and amplification, patients are subjected to a non-myeloablative lymphodepletion prior to adoptive T cell transfer and IL-2 substitution in the following weeks. The pretreatment with fludarabine and cyclophosphamide also impacts the tumor tissue by depleting suppressor cells and mild cell destruction releasing tumor-associated antigens to the immune system. Although basically effective, the currently used preconditioning regimen still needs further optimization. A cancer-specific protocol may be required to meet the particular situation of solid or disseminated tumors. For instance, the non-myeloablative conditioning regimen used in the treatment of Her2$^+$ tumors (Morgan et al. 2010) was modified to nab-paclitaxel and cyclophosphamide pretreatment of biliary tract and pancreatic cancers in order to deplete from desmoplastic stroma and to increase T cell infiltration (Von Hoff et al. 2011). Depleting tumor stroma by nab-paclitaxel may promote HER2 antigen presentation; cyclophosphamide can deplete inhibitory cells like Tregs and MDSCs among others. These and other preconditioning regimens may create a more appropriate environment for CAR T cell activities. On the other hand, preconditioning can be highly toxic in the context of CAR T cell therapy. Cerebral edema and CAR T cells in cerebral spinal fluid are commonly observed in CD19 CAR T cell trials (Maude et al. 2014a; Davila et al. 2014; Hu et al. 2016). Following intensified lymphodepletion with fludarabine, neurologic toxicities caused fatal complications in a recent trial, reducing lymphodepletion still induced uncontrolled toxicities and deaths (NCT02535364). Further research is needed to elucidate the mechanism of toxicity and to establish more effective pretreatment regimens.

(i) *Can the immune network be manipulated in order to induce a broad inflammatory response?*

The host immune system is substantially involved in tumor rejection initiated by CAR T cell transfer. Evidences raised in experimental tumor models in which anti-EGFRvIII CAR T cells conferred resistance to EGFRvIII-negative tumors (Sampson et al. 2014). A secondary innate cell response can be induced by treatment with IL-12-releasing CAR T cells (IL-12 TRUCKs) which attract and activate M1 macrophages in the tumor tissue to eliminate those cancer cells which are invisible to CAR T cells (Chmielewski et al. 2011). IL-18 CAR T cells shape the immune cell environment of targeted tumors in a specific fashion by increasing the numbers of tumor-associated CD206$^-$ M1 macrophages and NKG2D$^+$ NK cells and reducing Treg cells, suppressive CD103$^+$ dendritic cells, and M2 macrophages (Chmielewski and Abken 2017). Other immune response modifiers deposited in the tumor tissue by CAR T cells will be explored in the near future in order to shape a broader anti-tumor immune response. Checkpoint blockade is the first step in this direction; targeting PD-1 in the context of CAR T cell therapy is currently explored in a trial (NCT02650999); other checkpoints or combinations thereof need likewise clinical exploration, in particular, since checkpoints are part of a regulatory network and specific checkpoints like TIM-3 are upregulated upon PD-1 blockade (Koyama et al. 2016).

11 CAR T Cell Therapy Beyond Cancer

Redirected T cell activation by a CAR is not limited to targets on cancer cells; moreover, it can be used to target other diseased tissues including infected cells. CARs were engineered to target viral antigens on the surface of cells infected by hepatitis B virus (Krebs et al. 2013), hepatitis C virus (Sautto et al. 2016), cytomegalovirus (Full et al. 2010), and HIV (Romeo and Seed 1991; Deeks et al. 2002). Carbohydrate epitopes on aspergillus can be targeted by using dectin-1, a pattern-recognition receptor from the innate immune system, as binder to disrupt germination of the fungus (Kumaresan et al. 2014). B cells can also be targeted by CAR T cells which are used to eliminate memory B cells expressing an anti-Dsg3 antibody, responsible for the pathology of pemphigus vulgaris (Ellebrecht et al. 2016). Auto-reactive T cells were targeted by CAR T cells recognizing MHC-presented auto-antigen (Jyothi et al. 2002; Margalit et al. 2003). Of broader clinical interest is the development of CAR Treg cells for use in the long-term control of autoimmune diseases like colitis (Elinav et al. 2008), allergic asthma (Skuljec et al. 2017), and graft versus host disease by targeting HLA (MacDonald et al. 2016; Boardman et al. 2017; Noyan et al. 2017). The experimental data sustain the concept that CAR Tregs can be used to promote immune tolerance in the therapy of autoimmune diseases.

Acknowledgements The work in the authors' laboratory was supported by grants from the Deutsche Forschungsgemeinschaft, Bonn; Deutsche Krebshilfe, Bonn; Bundesministerium für Bildung und Forschung, Berlin; Deutsche José Carreras-Leukämie Stiftung, München; Wilhelm Sander-Stiftung, München; Else Kröner-Fresenius Stiftung, Bad Homburg v.d.H.; the German-Israeli Foundation, Jerusalem; and the Fortune Program of the Medical Faculty of the University of Cologne.

References

Abken H (2017) Driving CARs on the highway to solid cancer: some considerations on the adoptive therapy with CAR T cells. Hum Gene Ther 28(11):1047–1060

Adusumilli PS, Cherkassky L, Villena-Vargas J, Colovos C, Servais E, Plotkin J et al (2014) Regional delivery of mesothelin-targeted CAR T cell therapy generates potent and long-lasting CD4-dependent tumor immunity. Sci Transl Med 6(261):261ra151

Ahmed N, Brawley VS, Hegde M, Robertson C, Ghazi A, Gerken C et al (2015) Human epidermal growth factor receptor 2 (HER2)—specific chimeric antigen receptor-modified T cells for the immunotherapy of HER2-positive sarcoma. J Clin Oncol Off J Am Soc Clin Oncol 33 (15):1688–1696

Altvater B, Landmeier S, Pscherer S, Temme J, Juergens H, Pule M et al (2009) 2B4 (CD244) signaling via chimeric receptors costimulates tumor-antigen specific proliferation and in vitro expansion of human T cells. Cancer Immunol Immunother CII 58(12):1991–2001

Alvarez-Vallina L, Hawkins RE (1996) Antigen-specific targeting of CD28-mediated T cell co-stimulation using chimeric single-chain antibody variable fragment-CD28 receptors. Eur J Immunol 26(10):2304–2309

Beatty GL, Haas AR, Maus MV, Torigian DA, Soulen MC, Plesa G et al (2014) Mesothelin-specific chimeric antigen receptor mRNA-engineered T cells induce anti-tumor activity in solid malignancies. Cancer Immunol Res 2(2):112–120

Bertaina A, Merli P, Rutella S, Pagliara D, Bernardo ME, Masetti R et al (2014) HLA-haploidentical stem cell transplantation after removal of αβ+ T and B cells in children with nonmalignant disorders. Blood 124(5):822–826

Birkholz K, Hombach A, Krug C, Reuter S, Kershaw M, Kämpgen E et al (2009) Transfer of mRNA encoding recombinant immunoreceptors reprograms CD4+ and CD8+ T cells for use in the adoptive immunotherapy of cancer. Gene Ther 16(5):596–604

Boardman DA, Philippeos C, Fruhwirth GO, Ibrahim MAA, Hannen RF, Cooper D et al (2017) Expression of a chimeric antigen receptor specific for donor HLA class I enhances the potency of human regulatory T cells in preventing human skin transplant rejection. Am J Transplant Off J Am Soc Transplant Am Soc Transpl Surg 17(4):931–943

Boice M, Salloum D, Mourcin F, Sanghvi V, Amin R, Oricchio E et al (2016) Loss of the HVEM tumor suppressor in lymphoma and restoration by modified CAR-T cells. Cell 167(2):405–418. e13

Bouzin C, Brouet A, De Vriese J, Dewever J, Feron O (2007) Effects of vascular endothelial growth factor on the lymphocyte-endothelium interactions: identification of caveolin-1 and nitric oxide as control points of endothelial cell anergy. J Immunol Baltim Md 1950 178 (3):1505–1511

Brentjens RJ, Rivière I, Park JH, Davila ML, Wang X, Stefanski J et al (2011) Safety and persistence of adoptively transferred autologous CD19-targeted T cells in patients with relapsed or chemotherapy refractory B-cell leukemias. Blood 118(18):4817–4828

Brentjens RJ, Davila ML, Riviere I, Park J, Wang X, Cowell LG et al (2013) CD19-targeted T cells rapidly induce molecular remissions in adults with chemotherapy-refractory acute lymphoblastic leukemia. Sci Transl Med 5(177):177ra38

Bridgeman JS, Hawkins RE, Bagley S, Blaylock M, Holland M, Gilham DE (2010) The optimal antigen response of chimeric antigen receptors harboring the CD3 transmembrane domain is dependent upon incorporation of the receptor into the endogenous TCR/CD3 complex. J Immunol 184(12):6938–6949

Brudno JN, Kochenderfer JN (2016) Toxicities of chimeric antigen receptor T cells: recognition and management. Blood 127(26):3321–3330

Butler MO, Lee J-S, Ansén S, Neuberg D, Hodi FS, Murray AP et al (2007) Long-lived antitumor CD8+ lymphocytes for adoptive therapy generated using an artificial antigen-presenting cell. Clin Cancer Res Off J Am Assoc Cancer Res 13(6):1857–1867

Calcinotto A, Grioni M, Jachetti E, Curnis F, Mondino A, Parmiani G et al (2012) Targeting TNF-α to neoangiogenic vessels enhances lymphocyte infiltration in tumors and increases the therapeutic potential of immunotherapy. J Immunol Baltim Md 1950 188(6):2687–2694

Cartellieri M, Feldmann A, Koristka S, Arndt C, Loff S, Ehninger A et al (2016) Switching CAR T cells on and off: a novel modular platform for retargeting of T cells to AML blasts. Blood Cancer J 6(8):e458

Caruana I, Savoldo B, Hoyos V, Weber G, Liu H, Kim ES et al (2015) Heparanase promotes tumor infiltration and antitumor activity of CAR-redirected T lymphocytes. Nat Med 21(5):524–529

Caruso HG, Hurton LV, Najjar A, Rushworth D, Ang S, Olivares S et al (2015) Tuning sensitivity of CAR to EGFR density limits recognition of normal tissue while maintaining potent antitumor activity. Cancer Res 75(17):3505–3518

Cheadle EJ, Rothwell DG, Bridgeman JS, Sheard VE, Hawkins RE, Gilham DE (2012) Ligation of the CD2 co-stimulatory receptor enhances IL-2 production from first-generation chimeric antigen receptor T cells. Gene Ther 19(11):1114–1120

Chen F, Teachey DT, Pequignot E, Frey N, Porter D, Maude SL et al (2016) Measuring IL-6 and sIL-6R in serum from patients treated with tocilizumab and/or siltuximab following CAR T cell therapy. J Immunol Methods

Cherkassky L, Morello A, Villena-Vargas J, Feng Y, Dimitrov DS, Jones DR et al (2016) Human CAR T cells with cell-intrinsic PD-1 checkpoint blockade resist tumor-mediated inhibition. J Clin Invest 126(8):3130–3144

Chinnasamy D, Yu Z, Theoret MR, Zhao Y, Shrimali RK, Morgan RA et al (2010) Gene therapy using genetically modified lymphocytes targeting VEGFR-2 inhibits the growth of vascularized syngenic tumors in mice. J Clin Invest 120(11):3953–3968

Chmielewski M, Abken H (2015) TRUCKs: the fourth generation of CARs. Expert Opin Biol Ther 15(8):1145–1154

Chmielewski M, Abken H (2017) CAR T cells releasing IL-18 convert to T-bet[high] FoxO1[low] effectors which exhibit augmented activity against advanced solid tumors. Cell Rep (in press)

Chmielewski M, Hombach A, Heuser C, Adams GP, Abken H (2004) T cell activation by antibody-like immunoreceptors: increase in affinity of the single-chain fragment domain above threshold does not increase T cell activation against antigen-positive target cells but decreases selectivity. J Immunol Baltim Md 1950 173(12):7647–7653

Chmielewski M, Kopecky C, Hombach AA, Abken H (2011) IL-12 release by engineered T cells expressing chimeric antigen receptors can effectively Muster an antigen-independent macrophage response on tumor cells that have shut down tumor antigen expression. Cancer Res 71(17):5697–5706

Chmielewski M, Hombach AA, Abken H (2014) Of CARs and TRUCKs: chimeric antigen receptor (CAR) T cells engineered with an inducible cytokine to modulate the tumor stroma. Immunol Rev 257(1):83–90

Chong EA, Melenhorst JJ, Lacey SF, Ambrose DE, Gonzalez V, Levine BL et al (2017) PD-1 blockade modulates chimeric antigen receptor (CAR)-modified T cells: refueling the CAR. Blood 129(8):1039–1041

Craddock JA, Lu A, Bear A, Pule M, Brenner MK, Rooney CM et al (2010) Enhanced tumor trafficking of GD2 chimeric antigen receptor T cells by expression of the chemokine receptor CCR2b. J Immunother Hagerstown Md 1997 33(8):780–788

Cretenet G, Clerc I, Matias M, Loisel S, Craveiro M, Oburoglu L et al (2016) Cell surface Glut1 levels distinguish human CD4 and CD8 T lymphocyte subsets with distinct effector functions. Sci Rep 12(6):24129

Cruz CRY, Micklethwaite KP, Savoldo B, Ramos CA, Lam S, Ku S et al (2013) Infusion of donor-derived CD19-redirected virus-specific T cells for B-cell malignancies relapsed after allogeneic stem cell transplant: a phase 1 study. Blood 122(17):2965–2973

Cui G, Staron MM, Gray SM, Ho P-C, Amezquita RA, Wu J et al (2015) IL-7-induced glycerol transport and TAG synthesis promotes memory CD8+ T cell longevity. Cell 161(4):750–761

Curran KJ, Seinstra BA, Nikhamin Y, Yeh R, Usachenko Y, van Leeuwen DG et al (2015) Enhancing antitumor efficacy of chimeric antigen receptor T cells through constitutive CD40L expression. Mol Ther J Am Soc Gene Ther 23(4):769–778

Davila ML, Riviere I, Wang X, Bartido S, Park J, Curran K et al (2014) Efficacy and toxicity management of 19-28z CAR T cell therapy in B cell acute lymphoblastic leukemia. Sci Transl Med 6(224):224ra25

Deeks SG, Wagner B, Anton PA, Mitsuyasu RT, Scadden DT, Huang C et al (2002) A phase II randomized study of HIV-specific T-cell gene therapy in subjects with undetectable plasma viremia on combination antiretroviral therapy. Mol Ther J Am Soc Gene Ther 5(6):788–797

Di Stasi A, De Angelis B, Rooney CM, Zhang L, Mahendravada A, Foster AE et al (2009) T lymphocytes coexpressing CCR207 and a chimeric antigen receptor targeting CD30 have improved homing and antitumor activity in a Hodgkin tumor model. Blood 113(25):6392–6402

Di Stasi A, Tey S-K, Dotti G, Fujita Y, Kennedy-Nasser A, Martinez C et al (2011) Inducible apoptosis as a safety switch for adoptive cell therapy. N Engl J Med 365(18):1673–1683

Dudley ME, Wunderlich JR, Robbins PF, Yang JC, Hwu P, Schwartzentruber DJ et al (2002) Cancer regression and autoimmunity in patients after clonal repopulation with antitumor lymphocytes. Science 298(5594):850–854

Elinav E, Waks T, Eshhar Z (2008) Redirection of regulatory T cells with predetermined specificity for the treatment of experimental colitis in mice. Gastroenterology 134(7):2014–2024

Ellebrecht CT, Bhoj VG, Nace A, Choi EJ, Mao X, Cho MJ et al (2016) Reengineering chimeric antigen receptor T cells for targeted therapy of autoimmune disease. Science 353(6295):179–184

Faitschuk E, Nagy V, Hombach AA, Abken H (2016a) A dual chain chimeric antigen receptor (CAR) in the native antibody format for targeting immune cells towards cancer cells without the need of an scFv. Gene Ther

Faitschuk E, Hombach AA, Frenzel LP, Wendtner C-M, Abken H (2016b) Chimeric antigen receptor T cells targeting Fc μ receptor selectively eliminate CLL cells while sparing healthy B cells. Blood

Fedorov VD, Themeli M, Sadelain M (2013) PD-1- and CTLA-4-based inhibitory chimeric antigen receptors (iCARs) divert off-target immunotherapy responses. Sci Transl Med 5 (215):215ra172

Feng K, Liu Y, Guo Y, Qiu J, Wu Z, Dai H et al (2017) Phase I study of chimeric antigen receptor modified T cells in treating HER2-positive advanced biliary tract cancers and pancreatic cancers. Protein Cell

Finney HM, Lawson AD, Bebbington CR, Weir AN (1998) Chimeric receptors providing both primary and costimulatory signaling in T cells from a single gene product. J Immunol Baltim Md 1950 161(6):2791–2797

Foster AE, Mahendravada A, Shinners NP, Chang W-C, Crisostomo J, Lu A et al (2017) Regulated expansion and survival of chimeric antigen receptor-modified T cells using small molecule-dependent inducible MyD88/CD40. Mol Ther J Am Soc Gene Ther 25(9):2176–2188

Franciszkiewicz K, Boissonnas A, Boutet M, Combadière C, Mami-Chouaib F (2012) Role of chemokines and chemokine receptors in shaping the effector phase of the antitumor immune response. Cancer Res 72(24):6325–6332

Frauwirth KA, Riley JL, Harris MH, Parry RV, Rathmell JC, Plas DR et al (2002) The CD28 signaling pathway regulates glucose metabolism. Immunity 16(6):769–777

Full F, Lehner M, Thonn V, Goetz G, Scholz B, Kaufmann KB et al (2010) T cells engineered with a cytomegalovirus-specific chimeric immunoreceptor. J Virol 84(8):4083–4088

Gardner R, Wu D, Cherian S, Fang M, Hanafi L-A, Finney O et al (2016) Acquisition of a CD19-negative myeloid phenotype allows immune escape of MLL-rearranged B-ALL from CD19 CAR-T-cell therapy. Blood 127(20):2406–2410

Garfall AL, Maus MV, Hwang W-T, Lacey SF, Mahnke YD, Melenhorst JJ et al (2015) Chimeric antigen receptor T cells against CD19 for multiple myeloma. N Engl J Med 373(11):1040–1047

Gattinoni L, Zhong X-S, Palmer DC, Ji Y, Hinrichs CS, Yu Z et al (2009) Wnt signaling arrests effector T cell differentiation and generates CD8+ memory stem cells. Nat Med 15(7):808–813

Gattinoni L, Lugli E, Ji Y, Pos Z, Paulos CM, Quigley MF et al (2011) A human memory T cell subset with stem cell-like properties. Nat Med 17(10):1290–1297

Ghassemi S, Nunez-Cruz S, O'Connor RS, Fraietta JA, Patel PR, Scholler J, Barrett DM, Lundh SM, Davis MM, Bedoya F, C Zhang, Leferovich J, Lacey SF, Levine BL, Grupp SA, June CH, Melenhorst JJ, Milone MC (2018) Reducing culture improves the antileukemic activity of chimeric antigen receptor (CAR) T cells. Cancer Immunol Res 6(9):1100–1109

Golumba-Nagy V, Kuehle J, Hombach AA, Abken H (2018) CD28-ζ CAR T cells resist TGF-β repression through IL-2 signaling, which can be mimicked by an engineered IL-7 autocrine loop. Mol Ther 26(9):2218–2230

Grada Z, Hegde M, Byrd T, Shaffer DR, Ghazi A, Brawley VS et al (2013) TanCAR: a novel bispecific chimeric antigen receptor for cancer immunotherapy. Mol Ther Nucleic Acids 2: e105

Grakoui A, Bromley SK, Sumen C, Davis MM, Shaw AS, Allen PM et al (1999) The immunological synapse: a molecular machine controlling T cell activation. Science 285 (5425):221–227

Gross G, Waks T, Eshhar Z (1989) Expression of immunoglobulin-T-cell receptor chimeric molecules as functional receptors with antibody-type specificity. Proc Natl Acad Sci U S A 86 (24):10024–10028

Grupp SA, Kalos M, Barrett D, Aplenc R, Porter DL, Rheingold SR et al (2013) Chimeric antigen receptor-modified T cells for acute lymphoid leukemia. N Engl J Med 368(16):1509–1518

Guedan S, Chen X, Madar A, Carpenito C, McGettigan SE, Frigault MJ et al (2014) ICOS-based chimeric antigen receptors program bipolar TH17/TH1 cells. Blood 124(7):1070–1080

Hammill JA, VanSeggelen H, Helsen CW, Denisova GF, Evelegh C, Tantalo DGM et al (2015) Designed ankyrin repeat proteins are effective targeting elements for chimeric antigen receptors. J Immunother Cancer 3:55

Han X, Cinay GE, Zhao Y, Guo Y, Zhang X, Wang P (2017) Adnectin-based design of chimeric antigen receptor for T cell engineering. Mol Ther J Am Soc Gene Ther 25(11):2466–2476

Haso W, Lee DW, Shah NN, Stetler-Stevenson M, Yuan CM, Pastan IH et al (2013) Anti-CD22-chimeric antigen receptors targeting B-cell precursor acute lymphoblastic leukemia. Blood 121(7):1165–1174

Hinrichs CS, Spolski R, Paulos CM, Gattinoni L, Kerstann KW, Palmer DC et al (2008) IL-2 and IL-21 confer opposing differentiation programs to CD8+ T cells for adoptive immunotherapy. Blood 111(11):5326–5333

Holzinger A, Barden M, Abken H (2016) The growing world of CAR T cell trials: a systematic review. Cancer Immunol Immunother CII

Hombach A, Abken H (2007) Costimulation tunes tumor-specific activation of redirected T cells in adoptive immunotherapy. Cancer Immunol Immunother CII. 56(5):731–737

Hombach AA, Abken H (2011) Costimulation by chimeric antigen receptors revisited the T cell antitumor response benefits from combined CD28-OX40 signalling. Int J Cancer 129 (12):2935–2944

Hombach A, Sent D, Schneider C, Heuser C, Koch D, Pohl C et al (2001) T-cell activation by recombinant receptors CD28 costimulation is required for interleukin 2 secretion and receptor-mediated T-cell proliferation but does not affect receptor-mediated target cell lysis. Cancer Res 61(5):1976–1982

Hombach AA, Schildgen V, Heuser C, Finnern R, Gilham DE, Abken H (2007) T cell activation by antibody-like immunoreceptors: the position of the binding epitope within the target molecule determines the efficiency of activation of redirected T cells. J Immunol Baltim Md 1950 178(7):4650–4657

Hombach A, Hombach AA, Abken H (2010) Adoptive immunotherapy with genetically engineered T cells: modification of the IgG1 Fc "spacer" domain in the extracellular moiety of chimeric antigen receptors avoids "off-target" activation and unintended initiation of an innate immune response. Gene Ther 17(10):1206–1213

Hombach AA, Chmielewski M, Rappl G, Abken H (2013) Adoptive immunotherapy with redirected T cells produces CCR6− cells that are trapped in the periphery and benefit from combined CD28-OX40 costimulation. Hum Gene Ther 24(3):259–269

Hoyos V, Savoldo B, Quintarelli C, Mahendravada A, Zhang M, Vera J et al (2010) Engineering CD19-specific T lymphocytes with interleukin-15 and a suicide gene to enhance their anti-lymphoma/leukemia effects and safety. Leukemia 24(6):1160–1170

Hsu C, Jones SA, Cohen CJ, Zheng Z, Kerstann K, Zhou J et al (2007) Cytokine-independent growth and clonal expansion of a primary human CD8+ T-cell clone following retroviral transduction with the IL-15 gene. Blood 109(12):5168–5177

Hu Y, Sun J, Wu Z, Yu J, Cui Q, Pu C et al (2016) Predominant cerebral cytokine release syndrome in CD19-directed chimeric antigen receptor-modified T cell therapy. J Hematol Oncol 9(1):70

Hu B, Ren J, Luo Y, Keith B, Young RM, Scholler J et al (2017) Augmentation of antitumor immunity by human and mouse CAR T cells secreting IL-18. Cell Rep 20(13):3025–3033

Hudecek M, Schmitt TM, Baskar S, Lupo-Stanghellini MT, Nishida T, Yamamoto TN et al (2010) The B-cell tumor-associated antigen ROR1 can be targeted with T cells modified to express a ROR1-specific chimeric antigen receptor. Blood 116(22):4532–4541

Hudecek M, Sommermeyer D, Kosasih PL, Silva-Benedict A, Liu L, Rader C et al (2015) The nonsignaling extracellular spacer domain of chimeric antigen receptors is decisive for in vivo antitumor activity. Cancer Immunol Res 3(2):125–135

Huenecke S, Zimmermann SY, Kloess S, Esser R, Brinkmann A, Tramsen L et al (2010) IL-2-driven regulation of NK cell receptors with regard to the distribution of CD16+ and CD16 − subpopulations and in vivo influence after haploidentical NK cell infusion. J Immunother Hagerstown Md 1997 33(2):200–210

Jena B, Maiti S, Huls H, Singh H, Lee DA, Champlin RE et al (2013) Chimeric antigen receptor (CAR)-specific monoclonal antibody to detect CD19-specific T cells in clinical trials. PLoS ONE 8(3):e57838

Ji Y, Wrzesinski C, Yu Z, Hu J, Gautam S, Hawk NV et al (2015) miR-155 augments CD8+ T-cell antitumor activity in lymphoreplete hosts by enhancing responsiveness to homeostatic γc cytokines. Proc Natl Acad Sci U S A 112(2):476–481

John LB, Devaud C, Duong CPM, Yong CS, Beavis PA, Haynes NM et al (2013) Anti-PD-1 antibody therapy potently enhances the eradication of established tumors by gene-modified T cells. Clin Cancer Res Off J Am Assoc Cancer Res 19(20):5636–5646

Joyce JA, Fearon DT (2015) T cell exclusion, immune privilege, and the tumor microenvironment. Science 348(6230):74–80

Jyothi MD, Flavell RA, Geiger TL (2002) Targeting autoantigen-specific T cells and suppression of autoimmune encephalomyelitis with receptor-modified T lymphocytes. Nat Biotechnol 20 (12):1215–1220

Kahlon KS, Brown C, Cooper LJN, Raubitschek A, Forman SJ, Jensen MC (2004) Specific recognition and killing of glioblastoma multiforme by interleukin 13-zetakine redirected cytolytic T cells. Cancer Res 64(24):9160–9166

Kakarla S, Chow KKH, Mata M, Shaffer DR, Song X-T, Wu M-F et al (2013) Antitumor effects of chimeric receptor engineered human T cells directed to tumor stroma. Mol Ther J Am Soc Gene Ther 21(8):1611–1620

Kandalaft LE, Facciabene A, Buckanovich RJ, Coukos G (2009) Endothelin B receptor, a new target in cancer immune therapy. Clin Cancer Res Off J Am Assoc Cancer Res 15(14):4521–4528

Kaneko S, Mastaglio S, Bondanza A, Ponzoni M, Sanvito F, Aldrighetti L et al (2009) IL-7 and IL-15 allow the generation of suicide gene-modified alloreactive self-renewing central memory human T lymphocytes. Blood 113(5):1006–1015

Katz SC, Burga RA, McCormack E, Wang LJ, Mooring W, Point GR et al (2015) Phase I hepatic immunotherapy for metastases study of intra-arterial chimeric antigen receptor-modified T-cell therapy for CEA+ liver metastases. Clin Cancer Res Off J Am Assoc Cancer Res 21(14):3149–3159

Katz SC, Point GR, Cunetta M, Thorn M, Guha P, Espat NJ et al (2016) Regional CAR T cell infusions for peritoneal carcinomatosis are superior to systemic delivery. Cancer Gene Ther

Kawalekar OU, O'Connor RS, Fraietta JA, Guo L, McGettigan SE, Posey AD et al (2016) Distinct signaling of coreceptors regulates specific metabolism pathways and impacts memory development in CAR T Cells. Immunity 44(2):380–390

Kershaw MH, Wang G, Westwood JA, Pachynski RK, Tiffany HL, Marincola FM et al (2002) Redirecting migration of T cells to chemokine secreted from tumors by genetic modification with CXCR2. Hum Gene Ther 13(16):1971–1980

Kim MS, Ma JSY, Yun H, Cao Y, Kim JY, Chi V et al (2015) Redirection of genetically engineered CAR-T cells using bifunctional small molecules. J Am Chem Soc 137(8):2832–2835

Klebanoff CA, Gattinoni L, Restifo NP (2012) Sorting through subsets: which T-cell populations mediate highly effective adoptive immunotherapy? J Immunother Hagerstown Md 1997 35 (9):651–660

Klingemann H (2014) Are natural killer cells superior CAR drivers? Oncoimmunology 3:e28147

Kloss CC, Condomines M, Cartellieri M, Bachmann M, Sadelain M (2012) Combinatorial antigen recognition with balanced signaling promotes selective tumor eradication by engineered T cells. Nat Biotechnol 31(1):71–75

Kobold S, Grassmann S, Chaloupka M, Lampert C, Wenk S, Kraus F et al (2015) Impact of a new fusion receptor on PD-1-mediated immunosuppression in adoptive T cell therapy. J Natl Cancer Inst 107(8)

Kochenderfer JN, Dudley ME, Carpenter RO, Kassim SH, Rose JJ, Telford WG et al (2013) Donor-derived CD19-targeted T cells cause regression of malignancy persisting after allogeneic hematopoietic stem cell transplantation. Blood 122(25):4129–4139

Kochenderfer JN, Dudley ME, Kassim SH, Somerville RPT, Carpenter RO, Stetler-Stevenson M et al (2015) Chemotherapy-refractory diffuse large B-cell lymphoma and indolent B-cell malignancies can be effectively treated with autologous T cells expressing an anti-CD19 chimeric antigen receptor. J Clin Oncol 33(6):540–549

Kofler DM, Chmielewski M, Rappl G, Hombach A, Riet T, Schmidt A et al (2011) CD28 costimulation Impairs the efficacy of a redirected t-cell antitumor attack in the presence of regulatory t cells which can be overcome by preventing Lck activation. Mol Ther J Am Soc Gene Ther 19(4):760–767

Köhl U, Arsenieva S, Holzinger A, Abken H (2018) CAR T cells in Trials: recent achievements and challenges that remain in the production of modified T cells for clinical applications. Hum Gene Ther 29(5):559–568

Koneru M, Purdon TJ, Spriggs D, Koneru S, Brentjens RJ (2015a) IL-12 secreting tumor-targeted chimeric antigen receptor T cells eradicate ovarian tumors in vivo. Oncoimmunology 4(3): e994446

Koneru M, O'Cearbhaill R, Pendharkar S, Spriggs DR, Brentjens RJ (2015b) A phase I clinical trial of adoptive T cell therapy using IL-12 secreting MUC-16(ecto) directed chimeric antigen receptors for recurrent ovarian cancer. J Transl Med 28(13):102

Kong S, Sengupta S, Tyler B, Bais AJ, Ma Q, Doucette S et al (2012) Suppression of human glioma xenografts with second-generation IL13R-specific chimeric antigen receptor-modified T cells. Clin Cancer Res Off J Am Assoc Cancer Res 18(21):5949–5960

Koyama S, Akbay EA, Li YY, Herter-Sprie GS, Buczkowski KA, Richards WG et al (2016) Adaptive resistance to therapeutic PD-1 blockade is associated with upregulation of alternative immune checkpoints. Nat Commun 17(7):10501

Krebs K, Böttinger N, Huang L-R, Chmielewski M, Arzberger S, Gasteiger G et al (2013) T cells expressing a chimeric antigen receptor that binds hepatitis B virus envelope proteins control virus replication in mice. Gastroenterology 145(2):456–465

Krebs S, Chow KKH, Yi Z, Rodriguez-Cruz T, Hegde M, Gerken C et al (2014) T cells redirected to interleukin-13Rα2 with interleukin-13 mutein–chimeric antigen receptors have anti-glioma activity but also recognize interleukin-13Rα1. Cytotherapy 16(8):1121–1131

Kruschinski A, Moosmann A, Poschke I, Norell H, Chmielewski M, Seliger B et al (2008) Engineering antigen-specific primary human NK cells against HER-2 positive carcinomas. Proc Natl Acad Sci U S A 105(45):17481–17486

Kudo K, Imai C, Lorenzini P, Kamiya T, Kono K, Davidoff AM et al (2014) T lymphocytes expressing a CD16 signaling receptor exert antibody-dependent cancer cell killing. Cancer Res 74(1):93–103

Kumaresan PR, Manuri PR, Albert ND, Maiti S, Singh H, Mi T et al (2014) Bioengineering T cells to target carbohydrate to treat opportunistic fungal infection. Proc Natl Acad Sci U S A 111 (29):10660–10665

Kunert A, Chmielewski M, Wijers R, Berrevoets C, Abken H, Debets R (2017) Intra-tumoral production of IL18, but not IL12, by TCR-engineered T cells is non-toxic and counteracts immune evasion of solid tumors. Oncoimmunology (in press)

Lamers CHJ, Sleijfer S, Vulto AG, Kruit WHJ, Kliffen M, Debets R et al (2006) Treatment of metastatic renal cell carcinoma with autologous T-lymphocytes genetically retargeted against carbonic anhydrase IX: first clinical experience. J Clin Oncol Off J Am Soc Clin Oncol 24(13): e20–e22

Lanitis E, Poussin M, Klattenhoff AW, Song D, Sandaltzopoulos R, June CH et al (2013) Chimeric antigen receptor T Cells with dissociated signaling domains exhibit focused antitumor activity with reduced potential for toxicity in vivo. Cancer Immunol Res 1(1):43–53

Lee DW, Gardner R, Porter DL, Louis CU, Ahmed N, Jensen M et al (2014) Current concepts in the diagnosis and management of cytokine release syndrome. Blood 124(2):188–195

Lee DW, Kochenderfer JN, Stetler-Stevenson M, Cui YK, Delbrook C, Feldman SA et al (2015) T cells expressing CD19 chimeric antigen receptors for acute lymphoblastic leukaemia in children and young adults: a phase 1 dose-escalation trial. Lancet Lond Engl 385(9967):517–528

Li Y, Bleakley M, Yee C (2005) IL-21 influences the frequency, phenotype, and affinity of the antigen-specific CD8 T cell response. J Immunol Baltim Md 1950 175(4):2261–2269

Ligtenberg MA, Mougiakakos D, Mukhopadhyay M, Witt K, Lladser A, Chmielewski M et al (2016) Coexpressed catalase protects chimeric antigen receptor-redirected T cells as well as bystander cells from oxidative stress-induced loss of antitumor activity. J Immunol Baltim Md 1950 196(2):759–766

Liu X, Jiang S, Fang C, Yang S, Olalere D, Pequignot EC et al (2015) Affinity-tuned ErbB2 or EGFR chimeric antigen receptor T cells exhibit an increased therapeutic index against tumors in mice. Cancer Res 75(17):3596–3607

Liu X, Ranganathan R, Jiang S, Fang C, Sun J, Kim S et al (2016) A chimeric switch-receptor targeting PD1 augments the efficacy of second-generation CAR T cells in advanced solid tumors. Cancer Res 76(6):1578–1590

Louis CU, Savoldo B, Dotti G, Pule M, Yvon E, Myers GD et al (2011) Antitumor activity and long-term fate of chimeric antigen receptor-positive T cells in patients with neuroblastoma. Blood 118(23):6050–6056

Ma Q, Garber HR, Lu S, He H, Tallis E, Ding X et al (2016) A novel TCR-like CAR with specificity for PR1/HLA-A2 effectively targets myeloid leukemia in vitro when expressed in human adult peripheral blood and cord blood T cells. Cytotherapy 18(8):985–994

MacDonald KG, Hoeppli RE, Huang Q, Gillies J, Luciani DS, Orban PC et al (2016) Alloantigen-specific regulatory T cells generated with a chimeric antigen receptor. J Clin Invest 126(4):1413–1424

Mackall CL, Miklos DB (2017) CNS endothelial cell activation emerges as a driver of CAR T cell-associated neurotoxicity. Cancer Discov 7(12):1371–1373

Manuri PVR, Wilson MH, Maiti SN, Mi T, Singh H, Olivares S et al (2010) piggyBac transposon/transposase system to generate CD19-specific T cells for the treatment of B-lineage malignancies. Hum Gene Ther 21(4):427–437

Mardiana S, John LB, Henderson MA, Slaney CY, von Scheidt B, Giuffrida L et al (2017) A multifunctional role for adjuvant anti-4-1BB therapy in augmenting antitumor response by chimeric antigen receptor T cells. Cancer Res 77(6):1296–1309

Margalit A, Fishman S, Berko D, Engberg J, Gross G (2003) Chimeric beta2 microglobulin/CD3zeta polypeptides expressed in T cells convert MHC class I peptide ligands into T cell activation receptors: a potential tool for specific targeting of pathogenic CD8 (+) T cells. Int Immunol 15(11):1379–1387

Martyniszyn A, Krahl A-C, André MC, Hombach AA, Abken H (2017) CD20-CD19 bispecific CAR T cells for the treatment of B cell malignancies. Hum Gene Ther

Maude SL, Frey N, Shaw PA, Aplenc R, Barrett DM, Bunin NJ et al (2014a) Chimeric antigen receptor T cells for sustained remissions in leukemia. N Engl J Med 371(16):1507–1517

Maude SL, Barrett D, Teachey DT, Grupp SA (2014b) Managing cytokine release syndrome associated with novel T cell-engaging therapies. Cancer J Sudbury Mass 20(2):119–122

Maus MV, Haas AR, Beatty GL, Albelda SM, Levine BL, Liu X et al (2013) T cells expressing chimeric antigen receptors can cause anaphylaxis in humans. Cancer Immunol Res 1(1):26–31

Mohammed S, Sukumaran S, Bajgain P, Watanabe N, Heslop HE, Rooney CM et al (2017) Improving chimeric antigen receptor-modified T cell function by reversing the immunosuppressive tumor microenvironment of pancreatic cancer. Mol Ther J Am Soc Gene Ther 25 (1):249–258

Morgan RA, Yang JC, Kitano M, Dudley ME, Laurencot CM, Rosenberg SA (2010) Case report of a serious adverse event following the administration of T cells transduced with a chimeric antigen receptor recognizing ERBB2. Mol Ther J Am Soc Gene Ther 18(4):843–851

Morsut L, Roybal KT, Xiong X, Gordley RM, Coyle SM, Thomson M et al (2016) Engineering customized cell sensing and response behaviors using synthetic notch receptors. Cell 164 (4):780–791

Newick K, O'Brien S, Sun J, Kapoor V, Maceyko S, Lo A et al (2016) Augmentation of CAR T cell trafficking and antitumor efficacy by blocking protein kinase A (PKA) localization. Cancer Immunol Res

Ninomiya S, Narala N, Huye L, Yagyu S, Savoldo B, Dotti G et al (2015) Tumor indoleamine 2,3-dioxygenase (IDO) inhibits CD19-CAR T cells and is downregulated by lymphodepleting drugs. Blood 125(25):3905–3916

Noyan F, Zimmermann K, Hardtke-Wolenski M, Knoefel A, Schulde E, Geffers R et al (2017) Prevention of Allograft rejection by use of regulatory T cells with an MHC-specific chimeric antigen receptor. Am J Transplant Off J Am Soc Transplant Am Soc Transpl Surg 17(4):917–930

O'Rourke DM, Nasrallah MP, Desai A, Melenhorst JJ, Mansfield K, Morrissette JJD et al (2017) A single dose of peripherally infused EGFRvIII-directed CAR T cells mediates antigen loss and induces adaptive resistance in patients with recurrent glioblastoma. Sci Transl Med 9(399)

Osborn MJ, Webber BR, Knipping F, Lonetree C, Tennis N, DeFeo AP et al (2016) Evaluation of TCR gene editing achieved by TALENs, CRISPR/Cas9, and megaTAL nucleases. Mol Ther J Am Soc Gene Ther 24(3):570–581

Parente-Pereira AC, Burnet J, Ellison D, Foster J, Davies DM, van der Stegen S et al (2011) Trafficking of CAR-engineered human T cells following regional or systemic adoptive transfer in SCID beige mice. J Clin Immunol 31(4):710–718

Pearce EL, Walsh MC, Cejas PJ, Harms GM, Shen H, Wang L-S et al (2009) Enhancing CD8 T-cell memory by modulating fatty acid metabolism. Nature 460(7251):103–107

Pegram HJ, Lee JC, Hayman EG, Imperato GH, Tedder TF, Sadelain M et al (2012) Tumor-targeted T cells modified to secrete IL-12 eradicate systemic tumors without need for prior conditioning. Blood 119(18):4133–4141

Pegram HJ, Park JH, Brentjens RJ (2014) CD28z CARs and armored CARs. Cancer J Sudbury Mass 20(2):127–133

Peng W, Ye Y, Rabinovich BA, Liu C, Lou Y, Zhang M et al (2010) Transduction of tumor-specific T cells with CXCR208 chemokine receptor improves migration to tumor and antitumor immune responses. Clin Cancer Res Off J Am Assoc Cancer Res 16(22):5458–5468

Perna SK, Pagliara D, Mahendravada A, Liu H, Brenner MK, Savoldo B et al (2014) Interleukin-7 mediates selective expansion of tumor-redirected cytotoxic T lymphocytes (CTLs) without enhancement of regulatory T-cell inhibition. Clin Cancer Res Off J Am Assoc Cancer Res 20 (1):131–139

Philip B, Kokalaki E, Mekkaoui L, Thomas S, Straathof K, Flutter B et al (2014) A highly compact epitope-based marker/suicide gene for easier and safer T-cell therapy. Blood 124 (8):1277–1287

Pipkin ME, Sacks JA, Cruz-Guilloty F, Lichtenheld MG, Bevan MJ, Rao A (2010) Interleukin-2 and inflammation induce distinct transcriptional programs that promote the differentiation of effector cytolytic T cells. Immunity 32(1):79–90

Poirot L, Philip B, Schiffer-Mannioui C, Le Clerre D, Chion-Sotinel I, Derniame S et al (2015) Multiplex genome-edited T-cell manufacturing platform for "off-the-shelf" adoptive T-cell immunotherapies. Cancer Res 75(18):3853–3864

Porter DL, Levine BL, Kalos M, Bagg A, June CH (2011) Chimeric antigen receptor-modified T cells in chronic lymphoid leukemia. N Engl J Med 365(8):725–733

Porter DL, Hwang W-T, Frey NV, Lacey SF, Shaw PA, Loren AW et al (2015) Chimeric antigen receptor T cells persist and induce sustained remissions in relapsed refractory chronic lymphocytic leukemia. Sci Transl Med 7(303):303ra139

Posey AD, Schwab RD, Boesteanu AC, Steentoft C, Mandel U, Engels B et al (2016) Engineered CAR T cells targeting the cancer-associated Tn-glycoform of the membrane mucin MUC1 control adenocarcinoma. Immunity 44(6):1444–1454

Prosser ME, Brown CE, Shami AF, Forman SJ, Jensen MC (2012) Tumor PD-L1 co-stimulates primary human CD8(+) cytotoxic T cells modified to express a PD1:CD28 chimeric receptor. Mol Immunol 51(3–4):263–272

Provasi E, Genovese P, Lombardo A, Magnani Z, Liu P-Q, Reik A et al (2012) Editing T cell specificity towards leukemia by zinc finger nucleases and lentiviral gene transfer. Nat Med 18 (5):807–815

Pule MA, Savoldo B, Myers GD, Rossig C, Russell HV, Dotti G et al (2008) Virus-specific T cells engineered to coexpress tumor-specific receptors: persistence and antitumor activity in individuals with neuroblastoma. Nat Med 14(11):1264–1270

Qasim W, Zhan H, Samarasinghe S, Adams S, Amrolia P, Stafford S et al (2017) Molecular remission of infant B-ALL after infusion of universal TALEN gene-edited CAR T cells. Sci Transl Med 9(374)

Ren J, Zhang X, Liu X, Fang C, Jiang S, June CH et al (2017a) A versatile system for rapid multiplex genome-edited CAR T cell generation. Oncotarget 8(10):17002–17011

Ren J, Liu X, Fang C, Jiang S, June CH, Zhao Y (2017b) Multiplex genome editing to generate universal CAR T cells resistant to PD1 inhibition. Clin Cancer Res Off J Am Assoc Cancer Res 23(9):2255–2266

Riegler LL, Jones GP, Lee DW (2019) Current approaches in the grading and management of cytokine release syndrome after chimeric antigen receptor T-cell therapy. Ther Clin Risk Manag 15:323–335

Rodgers DT, Mazagova M, Hampton EN, Cao Y, Ramadoss NS, Hardy IR et al (2016) Switch-mediated activation and retargeting of CAR-T cells for B-cell malignancies. Proc Natl Acad Sci U S A 113(4):E459–E468

Rodriguez PC, Zea AH, Culotta KS, Zabaleta J, Ochoa JB, Ochoa AC (2002) Regulation of T cell receptor CD3zeta chain expression by L-arginine. J Biol Chem 277(24):21123–21129

Rodriguez PC, Quiceno DG, Ochoa AC (2007) l-arginine availability regulates T-lymphocyte cell-cycle progression. Blood 109(4):1568–1573

Romeo C, Seed B (1991) Cellular immunity to HIV activated by CD4 fused to T cell or Fc receptor polypeptides. Cell 64(5):1037 1046

Roybal KT, Rupp LJ, Morsut L, Walker WJ, McNally KA, Park JS et al (2016a) Precision tumor recognition by T cells with combinatorial antigen-sensing circuits. Cell 164(4):770–779

Roybal KT, Williams JZ, Morsut L, Rupp LJ, Kolinko I, Choe JH et al (2016b) Engineering T cells with customized therapeutic response programs using synthetic notch receptors. Cell 167 (2):419–432.e16

Ruella M, Barrett DM, Kenderian SS, Shestova O, Hofmann TJ, Perazzelli J et al (2016a) Dual CD19 and CD123 targeting prevents antigen-loss relapses after CD19-directed immunother-apies. J Clin Invest 126(10):3814–3826

Ruella M, Kenderian SS, Shestova O, Fraietta JA, Qayyum S, Zhang Q et al (2016b) The addition of the btk inhibitor ibrutinib to anti-CD19 chimeric antigen receptor T cells (CART19) improves responses against mantle cell lymphoma. Clin Cancer Res Off J Am Assoc Cancer Res 22(11):2684–2696

Ruella M, Xu J, Barrett DM, Fraietta JA, Reich TJ, Ambrose DE, Klichinsky M, Shestova O, Patel PR, Kulikovskaya I, Nazimuddin F, Bhoj VG, Orlando EJ, Fry TJ, Bitter H, Maude SL, Levine BL, Nobles CL, Bushman FD, Young RM, Scholler J, Gill SL, June CH, Grupp SA, Lacey SF, Melenhorst JJ (2018) Induction of resistance to chimeric antigen receptor T cell therapy by transduction of a single leukemic B cell. Nat Med 24(10):1499–1503

Sabatino M, Hu J, Sommariva M, Gautam S, Fellowes V, Hocker JD et al (2016) Generation of clinical-grade CD19-specific CAR-modified CD8+ memory stem cells for the treatment of human B-cell malignancies. Blood 128(4):519–528

Sampson JH, Choi BD, Sanchez-Perez L, Suryadevara CM, Snyder DJ, Flores CT et al (2014) EGFRvIII mCAR-modified T-cell therapy cures mice with established intracerebral glioma and generates host immunity against tumor-antigen loss. Clin Cancer Res Off J Am Assoc Cancer Res 20(4):972–984

Sautto GA, Wisskirchen K, Clementi N, Castelli M, Diotti RA, Graf J et al (2016) Chimeric antigen receptor (CAR)-engineered T cells redirected against hepatitis C virus (HCV) E2 glycoprotein. Gut 65(3):512–523

Savoldo B, Rooney CM, Di Stasi A, Abken H, Hombach A, Foster AE et al (2007) Epstein Barr virus specific cytotoxic T lymphocytes expressing the anti-CD30zeta artificial chimeric T-cell receptor for immunotherapy of Hodgkin disease. Blood 110(7):2620–2630

Schönfeld K, Sahm C, Zhang C, Naundorf S, Brendel C, Odendahl M et al (2015) Selective inhibition of tumor growth by clonal NK cells expressing an ErbB2/HER2-specific chimeric antigen receptor. Mol Ther J Am Soc Gene Ther 23(2):330–338

Serafini M, Manganini M, Borleri G, Bonamino M, Imberti L, Biondi A et al (2004) Characterization of CD20-transduced T lymphocytes as an alternative suicide gene therapy approach for the treatment of graft-versus-host disease. Hum Gene Ther 15(1):63–76

Shalem O, Sanjana NE, Hartenian E, Shi X, Scott DA, Mikkelson T et al (2014) Genome-scale CRISPR-Cas9 knockout screening in human cells. Science 343(6166):84–87

Shen C-J, Yang Y-X, Han EQ, Cao N, Wang Y-F, Wang Y et al (2013) Chimeric antigen receptor containing ICOS signaling domain mediates specific and efficient antitumor effect of T cells against EGFRvIII expressing glioma. J Hematol Oncol 6:33

Singh H, Figliola MJ, Dawson MJ, Olivares S, Zhang L, Yang G et al (2013) Manufacture of clinical-grade CD19-specific T cells stably expressing chimeric antigen receptor using Sleeping Beauty system and artificial antigen presenting cells. PLoS ONE 8(5):e64138

Singh H, Moyes JSE, Huls MH, Cooper LJN (2015) Manufacture of T cells using the Sleeping Beauty system to enforce expression of a CD19-specific chimeric antigen receptor. Cancer Gene Ther 22(2):95–100

Singh N, Perazzelli J, Grupp SA, Barrett DM (2016) Early memory phenotypes drive T cell proliferation in patients with pediatric malignancies. Sci Transl Med 8(320):320ra3

Skuljec J, Chmielewski M, Happle C, Habener A, Busse M, Abken H et al (2017) Chimeric antigen receptor-redirected regulatory T cells suppress experimental allergic airway inflammation, a model of asthma. Front Immunol 8:1125

Slaney CY, von Scheidt B, Davenport AJ, Beavis PA, Westwood JA, Mardiana S et al (2017) Dual-specific chimeric antigen receptor T cells and an indirect vaccine eradicate a variety of large solid tumors in an immunocompetent, self-antigen setting. Clin Cancer Res Off J Am Assoc Cancer Res 23(10):2478–2490

Song D-G, Ye Q, Poussin M, Harms GM, Figini M, Powell DJ (2012) CD27 costimulation augments the survival and antitumor activity of redirected human T cells in vivo. Blood 119 (3):696–706

Sotillo E, Barrett DM, Black KL, Bagashev A, Oldridge D, Wu G et al (2015) Convergence of acquired mutations and alternative splicing of CD19 enables resistance to CART-19 immunotherapy. Cancer Discov 5(12):1282–1295

Srivastava S, Riddell SR (2015) Engineering CAR-T cells: design concepts. Trends Immunol 36 (8):494–502

Stewart-Jones G, Wadle A, Hombach A, Shenderov E, Held G, Fischer E et al (2009) Rational development of high-affinity T-cell receptor-like antibodies. Proc Natl Acad Sci U S A 106 (14):5784–5788

Straathof KC, Pulè MA, Yotnda P, Dotti G, Vanin EF, Brenner MK et al (2005) An inducible caspase 9 safety switch for T-cell therapy. Blood 105(11):4247–4254

Sukumar M, Liu J, Ji Y, Subramanian M, Crompton JG, Yu Z et al (2013) Inhibiting glycolytic metabolism enhances CD8+ T cell memory and antitumor function. J Clin Invest 123 (10):4479–4488

Tamada K, Geng D, Sakoda Y, Bansal N, Srivastava R, Li Z et al (2012) Redirecting gene-modified T cells toward various cancer types using tagged antibodies. Clin Cancer Res Off J Am Assoc Cancer Res 18(23):6436–6445

Tanoue K, Rosewell Shaw A, Watanabe N, Porter C, Rana B, Gottschalk S et al (2017) Armed oncolytic adenovirus-expressing PD-L1 mini-body enhances antitumor effects of chimeric antigen receptor T cells in solid tumors. Cancer Res 77(8):2040–2051

Tchou J, Zhao Y, Levine BL, Zhang PJ, Davis MM, Melenhorst JJ et al (2017) Safety and efficacy of intratumoral injections of chimeric antigen receptor (CAR) T cells in metastatic breast cancer. Cancer Immunol Res 5(12):1152–1161

Teachey DT, Lacey SF, Shaw PA, Melenhorst JJ, Maude SL, Frey N et al (2016) Identification of predictive biomarkers for cytokine release syndrome after chimeric antigen receptor T-cell therapy for acute lymphoblastic leukemia. Cancer Discov 6(6):664–679

Textor A, Listopad JJ, Wührmann LL, Perez C, Kruschinski A, Chmielewski M et al (2014) Efficacy of CAR T-cell therapy in large tumors relies upon stromal targeting by IFNγ. Cancer Res 74(23):6796–6805

Tey S-K, Dotti G, Rooney CM, Heslop HE, Brenner MK (2007) Inducible caspase 9 suicide gene to improve the safety of allodepleted T cells after haploidentical stem cell transplantation. Biol Blood Marrow Transplant J Am Soc Blood Marrow Transplant 13(8):913–924

Thistlethwaite FC, Gilham DE, Guest RD, Rothwell DG, Pillai M, Burt DJ et al (2017) The clinical efficacy of first-generation carcinoembryonic antigen (CEACAM5)-specific CAR T cells is limited by poor persistence and transient pre-conditioning-dependent respiratory toxicity. Cancer Immunol Immunother CII

Thomis DC, Marktel S, Bonini C, Traversari C, Gilman M, Bordignon C et al (2001) A Fas-based suicide switch in human T cells for the treatment of graft-versus-host disease. Blood 97 (5):1249–1257

Torikai H, Reik A, Liu P-Q, Zhou Y, Zhang L, Maiti S et al (2012) A foundation for universal T-cell based immunotherapy: T cells engineered to express a CD19-specific chimeric-antigen-receptor and eliminate expression of endogenous TCR. Blood 119 (24):5697–5705

Urbanska K, Lanitis E, Poussin M, Lynn RC, Gavin BP, Kelderman S et al (2012) A universal strategy for adoptive immunotherapy of cancer through use of a novel T-cell antigen receptor. Cancer Res 72(7):1844–1852

van der Waart AB, van de Weem NMP, Maas F, Kramer CSM, Kester MGD, Falkenburg JHF et al (2014) Inhibition of Akt signaling promotes the generation of superior tumor-reactive T cells for adoptive immunotherapy. Blood 124(23):3490–3500

van der Windt GJW, Pearce EL (2012) Metabolic switching and fuel choice during T-cell differentiation and memory development. Immunol Rev 249(1):27–42

van der Windt GJW, Everts B, Chang C-H, Curtis JD, Freitas TC, Amiel E et al (2012) Mitochondrial respiratory capacity is a critical regulator of CD8+ T cell memory development. Immunity 36(1):68–78

Vera J, Savoldo B, Vigouroux S, Biagi E, Pule M, Rossig C et al (2006) T lymphocytes redirected against the kappa light chain of human immunoglobulin efficiently kill mature B lymphocyte derived malignant cells. Blood 108(12):3890–3897

Vera JF, Hoyos V, Savoldo B, Quintarelli C, Giordano Attianese GMP, Leen AM et al (2009) Genetic manipulation of tumor-specific cytotoxic T lymphocytes to restore responsiveness to IL-7. Mol Ther J Am Soc Gene Ther 17(5):880–888

Von Hoff DD, Ramanathan RK, Borad MJ, Laheru DA, Smith LS, Wood TE et al (2011) Gemcitabine plus nab-paclitaxel is an active regimen in patients with advanced pancreatic cancer: a phase I/II trial. J Clin Oncol Off J Am Soc Clin Oncol 29(34):4548–4554

Wang X, Chang W-C, Wong CW, Colcher D, Sherman M, Ostberg JR et al (2011) A transgene-encoded cell surface polypeptide for selection, in vivo tracking, and ablation of engineered cells. Blood 118(5):1255–1263

Wang E, Wang L-C, Tsai C-Y, Bhoj V, Gershenson Z, Moon E et al (2015a) Generation of potent T-cell immunotherapy for cancer using DAP12-based, multichain, chimeric immunoreceptors. Cancer Immunol Res 3(7):815–826

Wang X, Wong CW, Urak R, Mardiros A, Budde LE, Chang W-C et al (2015b) CMVpp65 vaccine enhances the antitumor efficacy of adoptively transferred CD19-redirected CMV-specific T cells. Clin Cancer Res Off J Am Assoc Cancer Res 21(13):2993–3002

Wang X, Popplewell LL, Wagner JR, Naranjo A, Blanchard MS, Mott MR et al (2016) Phase 1 studies of central memory-derived CD19 CAR T-cell therapy following autologous HSCT in patients with B-cell NHL. Blood 127(24):2980–2990

Wilkie S, van Schalkwyk MCI, Hobbs S, Davies DM, van der Stegen SJC, Pereira ACP et al (2012) Dual targeting of ErbB2 and MUC1 in breast cancer using chimeric antigen receptors engineered to provide complementary signaling. J Clin Immunol 32(5):1059–1070

Wofford JA, Wieman HL, Jacobs SR, Zhao Y, Rathmell JC (2008) IL-7 promotes Glut1 trafficking and glucose uptake via STAT5-mediated activation of Akt to support T-cell survival. Blood 111(4):2101–2111

Wu C-Y, Roybal KT, Puchner EM, Onuffer J, Lim WA (2015) Remote control of therapeutic T cells through a small molecule-gated chimeric receptor. Science

Xu A, Bhanumathy KK, Wu J, Ye Z, Freywald A, Leary SC et al (2016) IL-15 signaling promotes adoptive effector T-cell survival and memory formation in irradiation-induced lymphopenia. Cell Biosci 6:30

Zah E, Lin M-Y, Silva-Benedict A, Jensen MC, Chen YY (2016) T cells expressing CD19/CD20 bispecific chimeric antigen receptors prevent antigen escape by malignant B cells. Cancer Immunol Res 4(6):498–508

Zhang L, Yu Z, Muranski P, Palmer DC, Restifo NP, Rosenberg SA et al (2013) Inhibition of TGF-β signaling in genetically engineered tumor antigen-reactive T cells significantly enhances tumor treatment efficacy. Gene Ther 20(5):575–580

Zhang T, Cao L, Xie J, Shi N, Zhang Z, Luo Z et al (2015) Efficiency of CD19 chimeric antigen receptor-modified T cells for treatment of B cell malignancies in phase I clinical trials: a meta-analysis. Oncotarget 6(32):33961–33971

Zhang C, Burger MC, Jennewein L, Genßler S, Schönfeld K, Zeiner P et al (2016) ErbB2/HER2-specific NK cells for targeted therapy of glioblastoma. J Natl Cancer Inst 108(5)

Zhang C, Wang Z, Yang Z, Wang M, Li S, Li Y et al (2017) Phase I escalating-dose trial of CAR-T therapy targeting CEA(+) metastatic colorectal cancers. Mol Ther J Am Soc Gene Ther

Zhou X, Di Stasi A, Tey S-K, Krance RA, Martinez C, Leung KS et al (2014) Long-term outcome after haploidentical stem cell transplant and infusion of T cells expressing the inducible caspase 9 safety transgene. Blood 123(25):3895–3905

Targeting Cancer with Genetically Engineered TCR T Cells

Thomas W. Smith Jr. and Michael I. Nishimura

1 Historical Perspective

Although adoptive cell transfer (ACT) of genetically engineered T cell receptor (TCR) T cells is a trending topic within the field of immunotherapy, its origins can be traced back to the late 1960s. In 1969, Alexander Fefer showed 30–40% complete regression in Moloney sarcoma virus (MSV) induced tumor mice when treated with splenocytes or serum from syngeneic mice that had previous tumor regression (Fefer 1969). The next major breakthrough in the field came when lymphocytes could be isolated and cultured ex vivo for extended periods of time. Human and murine cytotoxic T cells were cultured and grown with T cell growth factor (TCGF) which was obtained from antigen-stimulated lymphocytes (Gillis and Smith 1977; Morgan et al. 1976). It was not known what in TCGF drove T-lymphocyte development, and subsequent advancements in ACT focused on the isolation of the specific growth factor in TCGF, which led to the discovery of IL-2 (Morgan et al. 1976; Liao et al. 2013). Studies initially began with IL-2 activating isolated murine splenocytes, thus transferring lymphokine-activated killer (LAK) cells to treat pulmonary metastases in mice (Mule et al. 1984). Subsequent clinical trials using LAK cells showed promising results, with 11 out of 25 patients with metastatic melanoma having objective responses (greater than 50% volume reduction) and one patient having a complete response (Rosenberg et al. 1985). However, it was subsequently shown that the administration of IL-2 alone provided the anti-tumor response calling into question the role of LAK cells in anti-tumor immunity (Rosenberg et al. 1987, 1993). LAK cells were deficient in tumor specificity and were compromised of aggregates of lymphoid cells with differential antigen targeting. Further studies showed that 26% of metastatic melanoma patients

T. W. Smith Jr. (✉) · M. I. Nishimura
Loyola University Medical Center, Maywood, IL, USA
e-mail: thomas.w.smith@lumc.edu

© Springer Nature Switzerland AG 2020
M. Theobald (ed.), *Current Immunotherapeutic Strategies in Cancer*,
Recent Results in Cancer Research 214,
https://doi.org/10.1007/978-3-030-23765-3_4

who responded to systemic IL-2 mono-therapy treatment reported vitiligo; however, none of the IL-2 non-responders (27 patients) reported vitiligo (Rosenberg and White 1996). Vitiligo being autoimmune destruction of melanocytes suggested that the mechanism behind IL-2-mediated cancer regression was antigen-specific, thus likely requiring T cells.

The next major development in ACT was the isolating and expansion of T lymphocytes from tumor explants (Yron et al. 1980). Improved isolation of T cells from tumor samples led to a subpopulation of reactive T cells, named tumor-infiltrating lymphocytes (TIL) (Rosenberg et al. 1986). Expanded TIL populations consisted of CD3$^+$ T cells and were found to produce interferon-γ (IFNγ) and tumor necrosis factor-α (TNFα) when presented with autologous tumors and led to tumor regression in vivo in both human and murine models (Barth et al. 1991; Yannelli et al. 1996). TIL were more effective than LAK cells, with murine studies showing TIL to be 50–100 times more effective than LAK at eliminating pulmonary micrometastases (Rosenberg et al. 1986). TIL were able to be isolated from multiple cancer models in humans and mice and could be expanded large-scale ex vivo (Yannelli et al. 1996; Topalian et al. 1987). In humans, TIL were reported to be isolated from melanoma, renal cell cancer, lung cancer, hepatocellular carcinoma, colorectal cancer, breast, and ovarian cancer lesions (Yoong and Adams 1996). However, clinical response rates varied significantly for TIL clinical trials, with overall response rates from 60 to 0% of the patients treated (Rosenberg et al. 1986, 1988; Yoong and Adams 1996). Moreover, TIL isolation was difficult and had poor yields, with isolates often contaminated with tumor cells. With varying clinical responses and difficulties standardizing TIL isolation and expansion across multiple cancer models continued research expanded into the mechanism behind TIL tumor identification and killing.

1.1 Target Antigen Identification

Further development with ACT involved the identification of the antigens recognized by TIL. T cell activation and function is restricted by the major histocompatibility (MHC) allele presenting antigen to the T cell. CD8$^+$ and CD4$^+$ T cells recognize peptide antigens presented by MHC class I or II molecules, respectively (Spear et al. 2016a). MHC class I molecules are present in all nucleated cells and are encoded by the human leukocyte antigen (HLA)—A, B, or C genes in humans and the H-2 K, D, and L genes in mice. MHC class molecules generally present peptides derived from intracellularly encoded antigens to CD8$^+$ T cells. MHC class II molecules are present in professional antigen-presenting cells (APC) and are encoded by HLA—DP, DR, and DQ genes in humans and I-A and I-E genes in mice. MHC class II molecules generally present peptides derived from extracellularly encoded antigens to CD4$^+$ T cells. CD8$^+$ T cells are generally considered cytotoxic T lymphocytes (CTL) secreting cytokines and cytotoxic granules leading to target cell destruction, while CD4$^+$ T cells are generally considered T helper cells secreting cytokines that augment the CTL function. Understanding of the mechanisms behind T cell target antigen selection by TCRs led to specific research into cancer antigens isolated to tumor cells, so-called tumor-associated antigens (TAA) (Townsend and Bodmer 1989). The first TAA discovered in humans was identified in melanoma tumor cells, named melanoma-associated antigen 1 (MAGE-1) (van der Bruggen et al. 1991). Ensuing melanoma differentiation antigens identified are numerous and included MAGE-3, tyrosinase, gp100 (PMEL), MART-1 (Melan-A), and gp75 (Yoong and Adams 1996). A clinical trial involving metastatic melanoma patients showed patients who received TIL having specificity for MART-1 peptide had a median survival time 15 times longer than patients who received TIL lacking specificity for MART-1 peptide, and this highlights the importance of tumor antigen specificity in the success of ACT (Benlalam et al. 2007).

TAA have been discovered beyond melanoma across multiple human cancer types. T cell antigens have been identified in melanoma, colon cancer, lung cancer, breast cancer, prostate cancer, pancreatic cancer, thyroid cancer, cervical cancer, anal cancer, oropharyngeal cancer, mesothelioma, and multiple B cell malignancies (Yarchoan et al. 2017) (Table 1). TAA are numerous, and many antigens are specific to not only a single cancer type but to an individual patient due to specific isolated mutations. Much interest surrounded finding tumor antigen targets that were shared across multiple cancer histologies and were present in all patients with the disease of interest. MAGE-1, the melanoma TAA, was subsequently further classified as a cancer-testis antigen (CTA) found to be associated with multiple malignancies (including breast, lung, bladder, ovary, and melanoma), but only expressed on a minimal amount of endogenous tissue (Sang et al. 2011). CTA antigens are naturally reserved primarily for fetal development being isolated on germ-line tissue, trophoblasts, and placenta (Sang et al. 2011). CTA antigens are numerous and include MAGE-1, MAGE-3/9/12, and NY-ESO (Hinrichs and Restifo 2013). Although CTAs linked multiple malignancies, significant interest surrounded the discovery of a TAA linked with all malignancies, a so-called universal TAA.

Research into universal TAA has led to targets that are aberrantly produced in tumor cells, including p53, Her-2, and hTERT (Nishimura et al. 2005). A tumor suppressor gene, p53, is commonly mutated in many cancers, Her-2 is a receptor tyrosine kinase overexpressed in multiple cancer models, and hTERT is human telomerase reverse transcriptase commonly mutated for telomerase activation (Theobald and Offringa 2003; Kuball et al. 2002; Theobald et al. 1995; Vogelstein et al. 2000; Kyte et al. 2016; Lustgarten et al. 1997; Weiss et al. 2012). Although these are attractive tumor targets shared with many cancers, there is considerable concern of cross-reactivity due to the protein presence in all endogenous tissues.

With concern for cross-reactivity toward endogenous tissue, antigens isolated to tumor cells alone are an attractive T cell target. All cancer histologies share a common transformation pathway, and cancer cell growth is driven by mutagenesis leading to mutations affecting cell regulation and growth (Garraway and Lander 2013). These genetic mutations lead to mutated proteins, which are specific to the cancer cells compared to endogenous proteins, thus termed neoantigens (Yarchoan

Table 1 Tumor Associated Antigens (TAA)

Target	Malignancy	Tumor-associated antigen (TAA) type	References
Tyrosinase	Melanoma	Melanoma/melanocyte differentiation antigen (MDA)	Yoong and Adams (1996), Roszkowski et al. (2003), Nishimura et al. (1999), Moore et al. (2017)
gp100 (PMEL)	Melanoma	Melanoma/melanocyte differentiation antigen (MDA)	Yoong and Adams (1996), Johnson et al. (2009), Moore et al. (2009), Voelkl et al. (2009)
gp75	Melanoma	Melanoma/melanocyte differentiation antigen (MDA)	Yoong and Adams (1996)
TRP-1	Melanoma	Melanoma/melanocyte differentiation antigen (MDA)	Yoong and Adams (1996)
MART-1 (MELAN-A)	Melanoma	Melanoma/melanocyte differentiation antigen (MDA)	Yoong and Adams (1996), Benlalam et al. (2007), Johnson et al. (2009)
MAGE-1	Melanoma	Cancer–testis antigen (CTA)	van der Bruggen et al. (1991), Sang et al. (2011), Hinrichs and Restifo (2013)
MAGE-3/9/12	Melanoma, multiple myeloma, esophageal, and synovial cell sarcoma	Cancer–testis antigen (CTA)	Yoong and Adams (1996), Sang et al. (2011), Hinrichs and Restifo (2013), Morgan et al. (2013)
NY-ESO-1	Melanoma, synovial cell sarcoma	Cancer–testis antigen (CTA)	Hinrichs and Restifo (2013), Robbins et al. (2011), Rapoport et al. (2015)
p53	Numerous	Aberrantly regulated/expressed	Vogelstein et al. (2000), Theobald and Offringa (2003), Theobald et al. (1995), Kuball et al. (2002, 2005)
Her2/Neu	Numerous (colon, breast)	Aberrantly regulated/expressed	Lustgarten et al. (1997), Weiss et al. (2012)
KRAS	Numerous (pancreatic, colon, lung)	Aberrantly regulated/expressed	Wang et al. (2016)
hTERT	Numerous	Aberrantly regulated/expressed	Hiyama et al. (2001)
MUC1	Numerous (pancreatic, colon, and lung)	Aberrantly regulated/expressed	Mukherjee et al. (2004)
WT1	Myelodysplastic syndrome, non-small cell lung cancer, and mesothelioma	Aberrantly regulated/expressed	Ochi et al. (2011), Call et al. (1990)
CD19	B cell malignancies	Aberrantly regulated/expressed	Uckun et al. (1988)

(continued)

Table 1 (continued)

Target	Malignancy	Tumor-associated antigen (TAA) type	References
CAIX	Renal cell cancer	Aberrantly regulated/expressed	Lamers et al. (2006)
HERV-E	Renal cell cancer	Aberrantly regulated/expressed	Cherkasova et al. (2013)
PSMA	Prostate cancer	Aberrantly regulated/expressed	Ma et al. (2014)
PSA	Prostate cancer	Aberrantly regulated/expressed	Xue et al. (1997), Harada et al. (2003)
PSCA	Prostate cancer	Aberrantly regulated/expressed	Morgenroth et al. (2007)
PAP	Prostate cancer	Aberrantly regulated/expressed	Machlenkin et al. (2005)
CEA	Colon cancer	Aberrantly regulated/expressed	Parkhurst et al. (2009, 2011)
Thyroglobulin	Thyroid	Aberrantly regulated/expressed	Verginis et al. (2002), Papewalis et al. (2010)
Gag	HIV	Viral antigens	Ueno et al. (2004)
HCV	HCV	Viral antigens	Pasetto et al. (2012), Spear et al. (2016b)
HPV E6/7	HPV	Viral antigens	Scholten et al. (2011)
LMP 2	EBV	Viral antigens	Zheng et al. (2015)

et al. 2017). Melanoma has a high rate of mutagenicity, compared to other cancers, thus has an increased mutational load making neoantigens plentiful (Kamta et al. 2017). An example of an initial neoantigen discovered was a mutated β-catenin protein differing by one amino acid for the endogenous protein, discovered while screening TIL T cell reactivity (Robbins et al. 1996). Furthermore, a separate TAA group target viral induced malignancies and have immediate tumor target antigens linked to viral proteins, including malignancies related to HPV, HCV, HIV, EBV, and CMV infections (Scholten et al. 2011; Pasetto et al. 2012; Spear et al. 2016b; Ueno et al. 2004; Zheng et al. 2015).

Ideal targets for ACT would target specific peptides presented by tumor cells and not normal tissues or cells. MAGE-1, being a CTA antigen, is tumor-specific (endogenously only present on non-MHC bearing human testes), however, other TAA, including MART-1, gp100, and tyrosinase, are present on both normal melanocytes and melanoma tumor cells (Sang et al. 2011). There have been reports of adoptively transferred cells targeting tyrosinase, gp100, and MART-1 leading to the destruction of not only melanoma cells but healthy melanocytes, leading to vitiligo (Rosenberg and White 1996; Yee et al. 2000). Furthermore, gp100 reactive adoptively transferred cells have been shown to cause ocular toxicity in patients, due to the destruction of melanocytes present in the eye (Palmer et al. 2008). This "on-target, off-tumor" reaction to the TCRs targeting the gp100 peptide is an example of adverse reaction and illustrates the importance of proper TAA selection (Spear et al. 2016a).

There are numerous TAA for multiple cancer types, and studies have shown that melanoma patients have endogenous T cells reactive to TAA in approximately 60–75% of patients; however, cancer does not regress (Cohen et al. 2015; Gros et al. 2016). Moreover, reactive TIL can only be isolated from approximately 50% of melanoma tumor explants, and for other tumor histologies, this number is significantly lower (Dudley et al. 2003). Even with endogenous T cell populations specific for cancer, TIL processing is a challenging and long process; this is the setting for which genetically engineered TCR T cells are being developed.

2   TCR Engineered T Cells

T cells are antigen-specific, and their specificity is mediated by the TCR. TCRs are heterodimers, consisting of α and β membrane-bound subunits which couple with CD3 complexes leading to intracellular signal transduction when presented with MHC bound antigens (Spear et al. 2016a). Initial characterization of TCR α and β chains used individual clones of tumor-reactive TCRs, these clones were identified in numerous manners including screening individual TIL clones and testing for reactivity to peptide-loaded antigen-presenting cells and by immunizing transgenic mice with specific TAA and identifying reactive murine TCRs (Johnson et al. 2009; Hughes et al. 2005; Gao et al. 2000; Clay et al. 1999a, b; Cole et al. 1995).

Once individual tumor-reactive TCR α and β chains were identified, the next hurdle was to safely and efficiently transfer α and β genes to cells and see if the pair reconstitute as a functional TCR. This was initially accomplished by transfecting α and β chain genes from a MART-1-specific T cell clone (TIL 5) into Jurkat cells (immortalized T cell lymphoma line) (Cole et al. 1995). In vitro functional assays of Jurkat cells transfected with the α and β chain genes from the MART-1-specific T cell clone (TIL 5) showed reactivity to peptide-loaded cells with reactive tumor peptide; however, there was no reactivity toward HLA-matched melanoma tumor lines (Cole et al. 1995). The Jurkat studies led to the next major advance in TCR gene transfer which was the transduction of human PBL-derived T cells (Cole et al. 1995; Clay et al. 1999b). These transduced human T cells derived from PBL showed reactivity to not only peptide-loaded cells with reactive tumor peptide but also HLA-matched tumor cell lines (Clay et al. 1999b). This tumor recognition by transduced PBL-derived T cells and not Jurkat-derived T cells would later be discovered to be caused by Jurkat cells' lack of CD8 co-stimulatory effect and led a discussion into different affinity levels of newly discovered TCRs and their associated functional avidity.

2.1 Affinity Enhancements

Naturally occurring high-affinity TCRs are in the minority and difficult to find naturally due to central and peripheral tolerance leading to negative selection, and thus, groups have moved to increase the affinity of receptors with genetic modification (Schmitt et al. 2015). It was hypothesized that CD8 independence of reactive TCRs designates the receptor as high affinity (Roszkowski et al. 2003, 2005). The majority of TCRs used in ACT trials are MHC class I restricted, thus interacting with and requiring CD8 (Spear et al. 2016a). However, multiple groups have identified CD8 independent TCRs, including CD4$^+$ T cells MHC class I restricted with tumor reactivity (Nishimura et al. 1999; Callender et al. 2006). In other words, CD4 and CD8 interaction with MHC is required for low-affinity TCRs, when MHC/TCR binding affinity is weak (Cole et al. 1995; Clay et al. 1999b; Roszkowski et al. 2005; de Vries et al. 1989; Lyons et al. 2006). Using an HLA-A2 transgenic mouse model, high-affinity receptors could be screened for because murine CD8 cannot bind to human HLA-A2 α3 domain, and thus, all reactive TCRs were CD8 independent in this model (Theobald et al. 1995; Kuball et al. 2005). This led to a large effort to identify high-affinity TCRs, with the theory that the highest affinity receptors would have the highest functional avidity (Zhu et al. 2015). However, the relationship between affinity and functional avidity was found to not always be positively correlated (Roszkowski et al. 2005; Zeh et al. 1999; Moore et al. 2009). High-affinity receptors were difficult to identify and few in number compared to low-affinity receptors (Alexander-Miller et al. 1996).

Instead of relying on finding naturally occurring TCRs with high affinity and avidity, there was a movement toward genetically enhancing T cell affinity. Genetic modifications leading to changes in the TCR complementarity-determining region (CDR), site of the α and β chains involved in TCR surface interaction with peptide/MHC complex, have led to variations in the affinity and avidity of modified TCRs. CDR mutations initially discovered via bacteriophage and yeast display created increased affinity receptors, compared to wild type (Li et al. 2005; Richman et al. 2006). Murine studies showed that the transduction of affinity-enhanced TCRs, including WT1 and MSLN TCRs, did not lead to autoimmune reactivity in the mouse and had increased avidity in response to antigen stimulation (Li et al. 2005; Richman et al. 2006; Schmitt et al. 2013; Tan et al. 2017). It was shown that even single amino acid substitutions in the TCR CDR regions can lead to increased affinity and tumor recognition, across multiple receptors reacting to various peptides including NY-ESO-1 and MART-1 (Robbins et al. 2008).

A clinical trial performed using a genetically modified TCR targeting NY-ESO-1 with a two amino acid substitution in the CDR region, treated patients with metastatic melanoma and metastatic synovial cell sarcoma at National Cancer Institute (NCI) with objective responses seen in 5 of 11 patients with melanoma and 4 of 6 patients with synovial cell carcinoma (Robbins et al. 2011). Another clinical trial involving advanced disease multiple myeloma patients using affinity enhanced genetically modified TCRs targeting NY-ESO-1 and LAGE-1, after autologous stem cell transplant, showed 16 out of 20 patients with median survival greater than

19 months (Rapoport et al. 2015). Not only did this study show increased survival but it tracked the genetically modified T cells post ACT in the patients and showed trafficking to the bone marrow by day 7 and persistence beyond 6 months (Rapoport et al. 2015). Not all affinity-enhanced TCRs led to such positive results, a clinical trial reported of metastatic melanoma patients using an affinity-enhanced TCR targeting MAGE-A3 with specific alterations made via site-directed mutagenesis to the CDR3 region, which led to clinical regression in 5 out of 9 patients but also had significant neurological toxicities causing lethal adverse events in 2 out of 9 patients (Morgan et al. 2013). The cause of death of the patients was due to necrotizing leukoencephalopathy caused by cross-reactivity of the gene-modified TCR targeting MAGE-A3 with MAGE-A12 located on the human brain. The gene-modified TCR was known to have reactivity to MAGE-A3/A9/A12, so this adverse reaction is an example of "on-target, off-tumor" specificity leading to the neurologic toxicity. Another example of "on-target, off-tumor" adverse reaction was with a clinical trial involving metastatic colorectal patients with ACT of a transgenic murine TCR reactive against carcinoembryonic antigen (CEA) with a single amino acid affinity enhancement in the CDR region which led to objective regression of lung and liver metastasis in 1 out of 3 patients, however, also led to transient inflammatory colitis (Parkhurst et al. 2009, 2011). Not all toxicities are caused by "on-target" peptide recognition, a gene-modified TCR again targeting MAGE-A3 melanoma peptide, was affinity enhanced via screening bacteriophage display mutants, which led to acute cardiac failure and death in the first 2 patients enrolled in the cohort (Linette et al. 2013). It was discovered that the genetically modified TCR targeting MAGE-A3 was also reactive against the titin protein present in cardiac tissue leading to "off-target, off-tumor" autoimmune reaction that led to the death of the 2 patients enrolled (Cameron et al. 2013).

The goal of affinity-enhanced TCRs is to increase the T cell specificity and functionality; however, the evidence of multiple studies with adverse reactions due to cross-reactivity with endogenous tissue has led to concern. Beyond selecting for high-affinity receptors or affinity enhancing receptors, multiple strategies have been explored to improve TCR α and β vector delivery.

2.2 Vector Design and Pairing

There are multiple vector systems that have been used to transduce the α and β chain genes to human PBL-derived T cells, and a majority of vector delivery from multiple groups have focused on integrating viral vectors (including retroviral and lentiviral systems); however, different groups have experimented with multiple systems, including naked DNA/RNA transfection, adenovirus vectors, and poxvirus vectors (Clay et al. 1999a; Kessler et al. 1996; Fisher et al. 1997). The benefit of integrating viruses, specifically retroviral systems, includes stable transgene expression over an extended period of time and the ability to create stable cell packaging lines to produce replication competent virus (Clay et al. 1999a). The first gene transfer study performed on humans transferred neomycin resistance via a retroviral vector to TIL reactive against melanoma, thus transfusing genetically engineered TIL (Clay et al. 1999a; Rosenberg et al. 1990). Retroviral transduction allows for stable integration of the α and β chain genes into the genome leading to the transduced cells then having multiple copies of α and β TCR chains, the transduced and endogenous copies. Beyond vector delivery and integration, vector construction relied on facilitated translation and expression of the α and β chains of interest. Multiple mechanisms have been used to aid in the coordinated translation of the transduced α and β chains, including internal ribosome entry sites (IRES) and viral 2A self-cleaving protein sequences (Rosenberg et al. 2008). Viral 2A self-cleaving protein sequences and IRES components are designed between the α and β chains so that the α and β subunits would be translated in a 1:1 stoichiometric ratio (Leisegang et al. 2008).

The α and β subunits of transduced TCRs can dimerize with the T cell's endogenous TCR subunits leading to mispairing. Mispairing of the transduced and endogenous α and β subunits leads to decreased cell surface expression of the heterodimer of interest, which decreases reactivity toward tumor peptide antigen (Cole et al. 1995). Even more important is that mispairing of endogenous and transduced TCR subunits has the potential to create novel and unintended antigen specificity, including autoimmune reactivity (van Loenen et al. 2010; Sommermeyer et al. 2006). Murine models showed evidence of autoimmune graft-versus-host disease post ACT with transduced T cells with ovalbumin specific OT-1 TCR (Bendle et al. 2010). It was shown that mixed dimerization consisting of endogenous and transduced TCR subunits led to lethal graft-versus-host disease in these mice. However, this lethal autoimmune graft-versus-host disease has not been shown to date in humans, and the Rosenberg Group published a large cohort of 106 patients treated with multiple retroviral transduced TCR groups, including human and murine TCRs against melanoma antigens, and showed no evidence of graft-versus-host disease (Rosenberg 2010). The concern for "off-target, off-tumor" reactivity from the novel pairing of transduced and endogenous TCR subunits led to some investigators to reduce mispairing via genetic modifications of transduced TCRs (Spear et al. 2016a).

The goal of initial genetic modifications was to increase pairing of transduced TCR subunits post-translation by increasing the pairing the α subunit for the specific β subunit of interest. Codon optimization changed the genetic sequence, by increasing translational efficiency, without changing the protein sequence which led to increased production and surface dimerization of transduced α and β subunits (Scholten et al. 2006). Not only does codon optimization increase surface pairing between α and β subunits, it has been shown to increase in vitro tumor peptide recognition compared to wild-type receptors (Jorritsma et al. 2007; Leisegang et al. 2010). Beyond codon optimization, the addition of cysteine residues in the extracellular domains of the TCR leads to the creation of disulfide bonds across the α and β heterodimer leading to the increased potential pairing of the introduced chains (Cohen et al. 2007; Kuball et al. 2007). In a similar fashion, the addition of leucine zippers to the α and β chains leads to a coiled-coil formation lending increased binding between the subunits (Chang et al. 1994). Addition of murine constant regions in human TCRs led to an overexpression of the murine–human hybrid TCRs on the cell surface and increased T cell function when compared to pure human counterparts, and moreover, the murine–human hybrid showed increased CD3 binding stability (Cohen et al. 2006). Both of these factors led to increased in vitro function, evidenced by increased cytokine production (Cohen et al. 2006; Sommermeyer and Uckert 2010). To completely bypass the issue of mispairing, single-chain TCRs have been created fusing the α and β chain variable and constant regions only allowing for specific pairing (Voss et al. 2010; Knies et al. 2016). Although genetic modifications showed increased surface pairing of α and β chains and increased cytokine function, there is minimal comparison across the different genetic modifications. We compared codon optimization, leucine zipper, murine–human hybrid, and α and β single with a hepatitis C virus (HCV) reactive TCR transduced into human PBL and showed that the murine–human hybrid and leucine zipper significantly increased receptor cell surface expression and increased cytokine production when compared to wild-type and other modifications (Foley et al. 2017). Another approach to increased pairing of transduced α and β subunits is to knock out endogenous chains with either zinc finger nucleases, small interfering RNA (siRNA), transcription activator-like effector nucleases (TALENs), or clustered regularly interspaced short palindromic repeats (CRISPR) (Okamoto et al. 2009; Provasi et al. 2012; Knipping et al. 2017).

Although the increased pairing of the transduced α and β subunits increases the specificity of genetically engineered TCR T cells for tumor targets of interest in vitro, no trials have compared the pairing modifications clinically. To help mitigate the potential for cross-reactivity leading to adverse reactions, some groups have developed safety check mechanisms.

2.3 Suicide Switches

The development of suicide switches, which can lead to inducible cell death of the transduced cells, was created to help minimize potential toxicities of genetically modified TCRs. Multiple suicide switches have been developed with the overriding goal of reversing adverse events when observed in patients by activating death pathways of the genetically modified transduced T cells. One group co-transduced inducible caspase 9 (iCasp9) along with their TCR of interest, allowing activation of the intrinsic cellular apoptosis pathway via administration of a bio-inert drug, AP1903, which showed 90% elimination of gene-modified TCRs within 30 min (Di Stasi et al. 2011). Other groups have co-transduced herpes simplex virus thymidine kinase (HSV-TK) with the gene-modified T cells, leading to ganciclovir sensitivity of the transduced cells (Bonini et al. 1997). These genetic modifications allow for a controllable means to regulate adoptively transferred T cells in the instance of an adverse reaction.

2.4 Cytokines and Tumor Microenvironment

With multiple examples of adverse reactions with affinity-enhanced-gene-modified TCRs, there has been a focus on the survival and persistence of adoptively transferred cells in the tumor microenvironment. Many clinical protocols call for non-myeloablative chemotherapy for lymphodepletion prior to administration of adoptively transferred gene-modified T cells (Dudley et al. 2005). The purpose of this lymphodepletion is to decrease endogenous T cells, thereby decreasing competition for limited cytokines and decreasing populations of immunosuppressive cells, including T regulatory cells (Gattinoni et al. 2005). Furthermore, lymphodepletion removed antigenic competition by depleting endogenous T cells, thereby increasing the percentage of free peptide/MHC complexes for binding and activation of transduced T cell population (Kedl et al. 2000). A clinical trial involving refractory metastatic melanoma patients treated 35 patients with non-myeloablative chemotherapy, consisting of cyclophosphamide and fludarabine, followed by ACT of TIL and demonstrated over 50% objective response (Dudley et al. 2005). Beyond chemotherapy to provide lymphodepletion, multiple studies have involved total body irradiation (TBI) to reduce endogenous T cell populations prior to ACT. One such study compared the objective response rates of metastatic melanoma patients infused with autologous TIL with different preparative lymphodepletion regimens, including myeloablative chemotherapy and either 2 or 12 Gy of TBI (Dudley et al. 2008). The 2 Gy group had an objective response rate of 52%, and the 12 Gy group had an objective response rate of 72% (Dudley et al. 2008).

Beyond lymphodepletion many ACT protocols, including the clinical trial just referenced, called for systemic administration of exogenous IL-2 to augment the adoptively transferred cells function and persistence. A phase I clinical trial compared ACT post non-myeloablative chemotherapy with either no IL-2, low-dose (72,000 IU/kg 3× daily) IL-2, and high-dose (720,000 IU/kg 3× daily) IL-2 (Dudley et al. 2002). The study had no objective responses in disease progression; however, all toxicities with different dosages were transient and tolerated by the patients (Dudley et al. 2002). Both lymphodepletion and systemic IL-2 therapy are toxic and morbid to the patient. IL-2 treatment is extremely toxic to patients, leading to multiple morbidities including hypovolemic shock due to capillary leak syndrome so much so that multiple centers require an ICU admission for administration (Rosenberg et al. 1994). For these reasons, there has been a push to genetically engineer modified T cells to increase their survival and persistence in vivo, thereby potentially reducing the need for lymphodepletion and systemic IL-2 therapy, and the discussion has involved IL-15 in vivo stimulation of adoptively transferred T cell anti-tumor function with positive results in murine models but clinical trials still pending (Klebanoff et al. 2004).

There has been development into modifying adoptively transferred cells to express their own cytokines, obviating the need for exogenous administration and further giving the transduced cells survival and persistence advantage over endogenous lymphocytes. One group engineered a tumor-reactive TCR toward melanoma peptide gp100 to express single-chain IL-12, and in vivo murine models showed significant tumor regression with without the need for exogenous IL-2 administration (Kerkar et al. 2010). They found that the co-transduced cells expressing the gene-modified TCR and IL-12 produced supra-physiologic levels of IL-12 and required fewer transduced cells to be administered to cause tumor regression (Kerkar et al. 2010, 2011). Genetic modifications with cytokine development have not been limited to IL-12, much interest has surround IL-2 and its receptor complex (a heterotrimeric protein consisting of α, β, and γ chains) (Rubinstein et al. 2012). It was shown in a murine model that cell expressing higher levels of IL2Rα had increased proliferation and anti-tumor ability, and when IL2Rα was blocked by an antibody, this increase in function was lost (Su et al. 2015). It was subsequently shown in human T cells that transduction of IL-2 along with TCR of interest led to increased cell proliferation with low levels of IL-2, with continued anti-tumor ability (Liu and Rosenberg 2001). These and other studies have led to increased interest in genetically modifying TCRs to co-express cytokines and cytokines receptors of interest, allowing autocrine advancement of the gene-modified T cells.

Beyond T cell persistence and function, genetic modifications have also focused on T cell trafficking and migration to the tumor. A criticism of ACT has been inefficient trafficking of adoptively transferred cells to solid tumor sites, and this has been cited as one of the reason for minimal success in solid tumors (beyond melanoma) including breast, ovarian, and colon cancer (Galon et al. 2006). The tumor microenvironment has been studied and shown that high infiltrates of tumor-infiltrating lymphocytes lead to positive prognostic indications across multiple cancer models (Baier et al. 1998; Clemente et al. 1996). To increase trafficking to the site of tumor, a group transduced T cells with a chemokine receptor, CXCR2, which targeted tumor expressed chemokine CXCL1. They subsequently showed the increased chemotactic ability of transduced T cells toward CXCL1, both recombinant and tumor-derived; moreover, they showed increased functional avidity by increased IFNγ secretion (Kershaw et al. 2002). Beyond chemotaxis, to invade the tumor microenvironment cells need to roll, arrest, and extravasate through the vascular endothelium and this is mediated through selectins and integrins (Butcher and Picker 1996). To increase this process, a group increased the T cell surface expression of integrin α vβ 3 ligand, integrin α vβ 3 is expressed on tumor neoangiogenesis endothelial sites (Legler et al. 2004). In an in vivo murine model, they showed five times increased T cell trafficking to the tumor with integrin α vβ 3 ligand group compared to control (Legler et al. 2004).

2.5 T Cell Metabolic Profile

Beyond testing the external functional profile of T cells involved in ACT, including testing for cytokine patterns with IFNγ, IL-2, and TNFα, new attention has been brought to metabolic profiling of the T cells themselves to determine cellular features involved in T cell function and survival (Wilde et al. 2012). For example, much interest has surrounded research into T helper 17 (T_H17) cells, which are a subset of T helper cells which appear to be resistant to apoptosis and have long persistence in vivo while still maintaining anti-tumor function (Murphy and Stockinger 2010). This phenotype if transferred to genetically modified T cells of ACT could provide a significant anti-tumor functional advantage in the hostile tumor microenvironment. The persistence and survival of T_H17 cells are mediated by the hypoxia-inducible factor 1α (HIF-1 α), Notch, and Bcl-2 signaling cascades (Kryczek et al. 2011). There is thought that T cells could be metabolically programmed or driven to a phenotype of interest, including a T_H17 cell-like lineage to increase survival (Chatterjee et al. 2017). A group showed that by culturing T cells in conditions with IL6, IL1β, IL23, and TGFβlo, they could metabolically reprogram the cell to express a T_H17-like phenotype with increased anti-tumor activity compared to wild-type T_H1 cells and control T_H17 cells (Chatterjee et al. 2017). This is just one example of multiple studies involved in reprogramming the metabolic activity and downstream signaling of T cells to express a phenotype of interest, to augment T cell survival and functional anti-tumor activity.

3   Future Directions—Combined Approaches with ACT

Future directions with ACT of genetically modified TCR T cells will develop with combined treatment approaches adding additional immunotherapies to treatment approaches augmenting anti-tumor functionality (Dietrich and Theobald 2015). Clinical trials involving combined ACT with peptide tumor vaccination have shown initial promise, one such study involved metastatic melanoma patients and provided not only ACT of genetically engineered TCR T cells targeting the MART-1 TAA but also concurrent vaccination with MART-1 peptide-pulsed dendritic cell (DC) vaccination. This study showed that 69% of treated patients showed evidence of tumor regression determined by PET CT (Chodon et al. 2014). Beyond combined vaccination approaches, much development has been made with treatments involving immune checkpoint blockade. Tumors evade immune responses, specifically T cell recognition of tumor antigen, in multiple manners, including upregulation of inhibitory immune checkpoints. Immune checkpoint receptors, cytotoxic T-lymphocyte-associated protein 4 (CTLA-4) and programmed cell death 1 (PD-1), downregulate T cell activation and can decrease T cell response to tumor antigen allowing for immune tolerance and resistance (Pardoll 2012). Moreover, it has been shown that cancer cell lines, including melanoma and renal cell cancer, express and upregulate checkpoint inhibitor ligands upon cytokine stimulation (Blank et al. 2006). Ipilimumab, an anti-CTLA-4 antibody, was FDA approved for the treatment of metastatic melanoma in 2011 after a clinical trial showed increased survival of patients receiving the treatment compared to control of gp100 peptide vaccination (Hodi et al. 2010). There have been indirect comparisons of patients receiving ACT of genetically modified TCR T cells and subsequently receiving checkpoint blockade later in their treatment course, a clinical trial treated three patients with metastatic melanoma with autologous T cells transduced with a tyrosinase reactive TIL 1838I TCR (Moore et al. 2017). In this clinical trial, 2 out of 3 patients responded, the two patients who responded subsequently underwent checkpoint blockade with pembrolizumab (Moore et al. 2017). In one of the patients receiving pembrolizumab, there was a dramatic increase in the number of transduced cells evident in the patient post-checkpoint blockade treatment (Moore et al. 2017). Great future promise holds for combining ACT of genetically enhanced TCR T cells with checkpoint blockade inhibitors (Page et al. 2014). In vitro data has shown increased expression of PD-1 on TIL when compared to PBL, and moreover by blocking PD-L1, it has been shown to increase T cell function measured by IFNγ secretion (Blank et al. 2006).

4 Conclusions

Since Alexander Fefer's initial success treating murine MSV tumors with adoptively transferred serum and splenocytes, the field of immunotherapy and specifically ACT has been constantly evolving and progressing. Initial accomplishments in the field were continually mired by cancer's innate ability to escape immune monitoring and elimination, by creating immunosuppressive environments and blocking antigenic identification. Genetically engineered TCR T cells allow limitless modification potential to combat cancer's immune evasion. This potential is real and evidenced by the drastic amount of current clinical trials underway involving ACT. Future development surrounds continued studies involving combined approaches using multiple genetic modifications aimed at homing tumor specificity, increasing T cell persistence, and tumor elimination with sustained remission. This will be made possible with improvement in the engineering of genetically modified T cell (with vector design), growing cells in vitro (with cytokines and metabolic reprogramming), and supporting cells in vivo after adoptive cell transfer.

References

Alexander-Miller MA, Leggatt GR, Berzofsky JA (1996) Selective expansion of high- or low-avidity cytotoxic T lymphocytes and efficacy for adoptive immunotherapy. Proc Natl Acad Sci U S A 93(9):4102–4107. PubMed PMID: 8633023. Pubmed Central PMCID: 39494

Baier PK, Wimmenauer S, Hirsch T, von Specht BU, von Kleist S, Keller H et al (1998) Analysis of the T cell receptor variability of tumor-infiltrating lymphocytes in colorectal carcinomas. Tumour Biol 19(3):205-212. PubMed PMID: 9591047

Barth RJ Jr, Mule JJ, Spiess PJ, Rosenberg SA (1991) Interferon gamma and tumor necrosis factor have a role in tumor regressions mediated by murine CD8+ tumor-infiltrating lymphocytes. J Exp Med 173(3):647–658. PubMed PMID: 1900079. Pubmed Central PMCID: 2118834

Bendle GM, Linnemann C, Hooijkaas AI, Bies L, de Witte MA, Jorritsma A et al (2010) Lethal graft-versus-host disease in mouse models of T cell receptor gene therapy. Nat Med 16(5):565–570

Benlalam H, Vignard V, Khammari A, Bonnin A, Godet Y, Pandolfino MC et al (2007) Infusion of Melan-A/Mart-1 specific tumor-infiltrating lymphocytes enhanced relapse-free survival of melanoma patients. Cancer Immunol Immunother 56(4):515–526. PubMed PMID: 16874485

Blank C, Kuball J, Voelkl S, Wiendl H, Becker B, Walter B et al (2006) Blockade of PD-L1 (B7-H1) augments human tumor-specific T cell responses in vitro. Int J Cancer 119(2):317–327. PubMed PMID: 16482562

Bonini C, Ferrari G, Verzeletti S, Servida P, Zappone E, Ruggieri L et al (1997) HSV-TK gene transfer into donor lymphocytes for control of allogeneic graft-versus-leukemia. Science 276 (5319):1719–1724

Butcher EC, Picker LJ (1996) Lymphocyte homing and homeostasis. Science 272(5258):60–66. PubMed PMID: 8600538

Call KM, Glaser T, Ito CY, Buckler AJ, Pelletier J, Haber DA et al (1990) Isolation and characterization of a zinc finger polypeptide gene at the human chromosome 11 Wilms' tumor locus. Cell 60(3):509–520. PubMed PMID: 2154335

Callender GG, Rosen HR, Roszkowski JJ, Lyons GE, Li M, Moore T et al (2006) Identification of a hepatitis C virus-reactive T cell receptor that does not require CD8 for target cell recognition. Hepatology 43(5):973–981. PubMed PMID: 16628627

Cameron BJ, Gerry AB, Dukes J, Harper JV, Kannan V, Bianchi FC et al (2013) Identification of a Titin-derived HLA-A1–presented peptide as a cross-reactive target for engineered MAGE A3–directed T cells. Sci Transl Med 5(197):197ra03

Chang HC, Bao Z, Yao Y, Tse AG, Goyarts EC, Madsen M et al (1994) A general method for facilitating heterodimeric pairing between two proteins: application to expression of alpha and beta T-cell receptor extracellular segments. Proc Natl Acad Sci U S A 91(24):11408–11412. PubMed PMID: 7972074. Pubmed Central PMCID: 45240

Chatterjee S, Daenthanasanmak A, Chakraborty P, Wyatt MW, Dhar P, Selvam SP et al (2017) CD38-NAD(+) axis regulates immunotherapeutic anti-tumor T cell response. Cell Metab. PubMed PMID: 29129787

Cherkasova E, Weisman Q, Childs RW (2013) Endogenous retroviruses as targets for antitumor immunity in renal cell cancer and other tumors. Front Oncol

Chodon T, Comin-Anduix B, Chmielowski B, Koya RC, Wu Z, Auerbach M et al (2014) Adoptive transfer of MART-1 T-cell receptor transgenic lymphocytes and dendritic cell vaccination in patients with metastatic melanoma. Clin Cancer Res: An Official Journal of the American Association for Cancer Research 20(9):2457–2465. PubMed PMID: 24634374. Pubmed Central PMCID: 4070853

Clay TM, Custer MC, Spiess PJ, Nishimura MI (1999a) Potential use of T cell receptor genes to modify hematopoietic stem cells for the gene therapy of cancer. Pathol Oncol Res 5(1):3–15. PubMed PMID: 10079371

Clay TM, Custer MC, Sachs J, Hwu P, Rosenberg SA, Nishimura MI (1999b) Efficient transfer of a tumor antigen-reactive TCR to human peripheral blood lymphocytes confers anti-tumor reactivity. J Immunol 163(1):507–513

Clemente CG, Mihm MC, Jr., Bufalino R, Zurrida S, Collini P, Cascinelli N (1996) Prognostic value of tumor infiltrating lymphocytes in the vertical growth phase of primary cutaneous melanoma. Cancer 77(7):1303–1310. PubMed PMID: 8608507

Cohen CJ, Zhao Y, Zheng Z, Rosenberg SA, Morgan RA (2006) Enhanced antitumor activity of murine-human hybrid T-cell receptor (TCR) in human lymphocytes is associated with improved pairing and TCR/CD3 stability. Cancer Res 66(17):8878–8886. PubMed PMID: 16951205. Pubmed Central PMCID: 2147082

Cohen CJ, Li YF, El-Gamil M, Robbins PF, Rosenberg SA, Morgan RA (2007) Enhanced antitumor activity of T cells engineered to express T-cell receptors with a second disulfide bond. Cancer Res 67(8):3898–3903. PubMed PMID: 17440104. Pubmed Central PMCID: 2147081

Cohen CJ, Gartner JJ, Horovitz-Fried M, Shamalov K, Trebska-McGowan K, Bliskovsky VV et al (2015) Isolation of neoantigen-specific T cells from tumor and peripheral lymphocytes. J Clin Invest 125(10):3981–3991. PubMed PMID: 26389673. Pubmed Central PMCID: 4607110

Cole DJ, Weil DP, Shilyansky J, Custer M, Kawakami Y, Rosenberg SA et al (1995) Characterization of the functional specificity of a cloned T-cell receptor heterodimer recognizing the MART-1 melanoma antigen. Cancer Res 55(4):748–752. PubMed PMID: 7531614

de Vries JE, Yssel H, Spits H (1989) Interplay between the TCR/CD3 complex and CD4 or CD8 in the activation of cytotoxic T lymphocytes. Immunol Rev 109:119–141. PubMed PMID: 2527803

Di Stasi A, Tey SK, Dotti G, Fujita Y, Kennedy-Nasser A, Martinez C et al (2011) Inducible apoptosis as a safety switch for adoptive cell therapy. N Engl J Med 365(18):1673–1683. PubMed PMID: 22047558. Pubmed Central PMCID: 3236370

Dietrich K, Theobald M (2015) [Immunological tumor therapy]. Internist (Berl) 56(8):907–916; quiz 17. PubMed PMID: 26187335. Immunologische Tumortherapie

Dudley ME, Wunderlich JR, Yang JC, Hwu P, Schwartzentruber DJ, Topalian SL et al (2002) A phase I study of nonmyeloablative chemotherapy and adoptive transfer of autologous tumor antigen-specific T lymphocytes in patients with metastatic melanoma. J Immunother 25 (3):243–251. PubMed PMID: 12000866. Pubmed Central PMCID: 2413438

Dudley ME, Wunderlich JR, Shelton TE, Even J, Rosenberg SA (2003) Generation of tumor-infiltrating lymphocyte cultures for use in adoptive transfer therapy for melanoma patients. J Immunother 26(4):332–342. PubMed PMID: 12843795. Pubmed Central PMCID: 2305721

Dudley ME, Wunderlich JR, Yang JC, Sherry RM, Topalian SL, Restifo NP et al (2005) Adoptive cell transfer therapy following non-myeloablative but lymphodepleting chemotherapy for the treatment of patients with refractory metastatic melanoma. J Clin Oncol: Official Journal of the American Society of Clinical Oncology 23(10):2346–2357. PubMed PMID: 15800326. Pubmed Central PMCID: 1475951

Dudley ME, Yang JC, Sherry R, Hughes MS, Royal R, Kammula U et al (2008) Adoptive cell therapy for patients with metastatic melanoma: evaluation of intensive myeloablative chemoradiation preparative regimens. J Clin Oncol: Official Journal of the American Society of Clinical Oncology 26(32):5233–5239. PubMed PMID: 18809613. Pubmed Central PMCID: 2652090

Fefer A (1969) Immunotherapy and chemotherapy of Moloney sarcoma virus-induced tumors in mice. Cancer Res 29(12):2177–2183. PubMed PMID: 5369675

Fisher KJ, Jooss K, Alston J, Yang Y, Haecker SE, High K et al (1997) Recombinant adeno-associated virus for muscle directed gene therapy. Nat Med 3(3):306–312. PubMed PMID: 9055858

Foley KC, Spear TT, Murray DC, Nagato K, Garrett-Mayer E, Nishimura MI (2017) HCV T cell receptor chain modifications to enhance expression, pairing, and antigen recognition in T cells for adoptive transfer. Mol Ther Oncolytics 5:105–115. PubMed PMID: 28573185. Pubmed Central PMCID: 5447397

Galon J, Costes A, Sanchez-Cabo F, Kirilovsky A, Mlecnik B, Lagorce-Pagès C et al (2006) Type, density, and location of immune cells within human colorectal tumors predict clinical outcome. Science 313(5795):1960–1964

Gao L, Bellantuono I, Elsasser A, Marley SB, Gordon MY, Goldman JM et al (2000) Selective elimination of leukemic CD34(+) progenitor cells by cytotoxic T lymphocytes specific for WT1. Blood 95(7):2198–2203. PubMed PMID: 10733485

Garraway LA, Lander ES (2013) Lessons from the cancer genome. Cell 153(1):17–37. PubMed PMID: 23540688

Gattinoni L, Finkelstein SE, Klebanoff CA, Antony PA, Palmer DC, Spiess PJ et al (2005) Removal of homeostatic cytokine sinks by lymphodepletion enhances the efficacy of adoptively transferred tumor-specific CD8+ T cells. J Exp Med 202(7):907–912. PubMed PMID: 16203864. Pubmed Central PMCID: 1397916

Gillis S, Smith KA (1977) Long term culture of tumour-specific cytotoxic T cells. Nature 268 (5616):154–156. PubMed PMID: 145543

Gros A, Parkhurst MR, Tran E, Pasetto A, Robbins PF, Ilyas S et al (2016) Prospective identification of neoantigen-specific lymphocytes in the peripheral blood of melanoma patients. Nat Med 22(4):433–438. PubMed PMID: 26901407

Harada M, Kobayashi K, Matsueda S, Nakagawa M, Noguchi M, Itoh K (2003) Prostate-specific antigen-derived epitopes capable of inducing cellular and humoral responses in HLA-A24+ prostate cancer patients. Prostate 57(2):152–159. PubMed PMID: 12949939

Hinrichs CS, Restifo NP (2013) Reassessing target antigens for adoptive T-cell therapy. Nature Biotechnol 31(11):999–1008. PubMed PMID: 24142051. Pubmed Central PMCID: 4280065

Hiyama E, Hiyama K, Yokoyama T, Shay JW (2001) Immunohistochemical detection of telomerase (hTERT) protein in human cancer tissues and a subset of cells in normal tissues. Neoplasia 3(1):17–26. PubMed PMID: 11326312. Pubmed Central PMCID: 1505023

Hodi FS, O'Day SJ, McDermott DF, Weber RW, Sosman JA, Haanen JB et al (2010) Improved survival with ipilimumab in patients with metastatic melanoma. N Engl J Med 363(8):711–723. PubMed PMID: 20525992

Hughes MS, Yu YY, Dudley ME, Zheng Z, Robbins PF, Li Y et al (2005) Transfer of a TCR gene derived from a patient with a marked antitumor response conveys highly active T-cell effector functions. Hum Gene Ther 16(4):457–472. PubMed PMID: PMC1476695

Johnson LA, Morgan RA, Dudley ME, Cassard L, Yang JC, Hughes MS et al (2009) Gene therapy with human and mouse T-cell receptors mediates cancer regression and targets normal tissues expressing cognate antigen. Blood 114(3):535–546. PubMed PMID: 19451549. Pubmed Central PMCID: 2929689

Jorritsma A, Gomez-Eerland R, Dokter M, van de Kasteele W, Zoet YM, Doxiadis II et al (2007) Selecting highly affine and well-expressed TCRs for gene therapy of melanoma. Blood 110 (10):3564–3572. PubMed PMID: 17660381

Kamta J, Chaar M, Ande A, Altomare DA, Ait-Oudhia S (2017) Advancing cancer therapy with present and emerging immuno-oncology approaches. Front Oncol 7:64. 01/13/received 03/20/accepted. PubMed PMID: PMC5394116

Kedl RM, Rees WA, Hildeman DA, Schaefer B, Mitchell T, Kappler J et al (2000) T cells compete for access to antigen-bearing antigen-presenting cells. J Exp Med 192(8):1105–1113. PubMed PMID: 11034600. Pubmed Central PMCID: 2195874

Kerkar SP, Muranski P, Kaiser A, Boni A, Sanchez-Perez L, Yu Z et al (2010) Tumor-specific CD8+ T cells expressing IL-12 eradicate established cancers in lymphodepleted hosts. Cancer Res 70(17):6725–6734. PubMed PMID: PMC2935308

Kerkar SP, Goldszmid RS, Muranski P, Chinnasamy D, Yu Z, Reger RN et al (2011) IL-12 triggers a programmatic change in dysfunctional myeloid-derived cells within mouse tumors. J Clin Investig 121(12):4746–4757. 05/02/received 09/28/accepted. PubMed PMID: PMC3226001

Kershaw MH, Wang G, Westwood JA, Pachynski RK, Tiffany HL, Marincola FM et al (2002) Redirecting migration of T cells to chemokine secreted from tumors by genetic modification with CXCR2. Hum Gene Ther 13(16):1971–1980. PubMed PMID: 12427307

Kessler PD, Podsakoff GM, Chen X, McQuiston SA, Colosi PC, Matelis LA et al (1996) Gene delivery to skeletal muscle results in sustained expression and systemic delivery of a therapeutic protein. Proc Natl Acad Sci U S A 93(24):14082–14087. PubMed PMID: 8943064. Pubmed Central PMCID: 19498

Klebanoff CA, Finkelstein SE, Surman DR, Lichtman MK, Gattinoni L, Theoret MR et al (2004) IL-15 enhances the in vivo antitumor activity of tumor-reactive CD8(+) T cells. Proc Natl Acad Sci U S A 101(7):1969–1974. PubMed PMID: PMC357036

Knies D, Klobuch S, Xue SA, Birtel M, Echchannaoui H, Yildiz O et al (2016) An optimized single chain TCR scaffold relying on the assembly with the native CD3-complex prevents residual mispairing with endogenous TCRs in human T-cells. Oncotarget 7(16):21199–21221. PubMed PMID: 27028870. Pubmed Central PMCID: 5008279

Knipping F, Osborn MJ, Petri K, Tolar J, Glimm H, von Kalle C et al (2017) Genome-wide specificity of highly efficient TALENs and CRISPR/Cas9 for T cell receptor modification. Mol Ther Methods Clin Dev 4:213–224. PubMed PMID: 28345006. Pubmed Central PMCID: 5363317

Kryczek I, Zhao E, Liu Y, Wang Y, Vatan L, Szeliga W et al (2011) Human T_H17 cells are long-lived effector memory cells. Sci Transl Med 3(104):104ra0

Kuball J, Schuler M, Antunes Ferreira E, Herr W, Neumann M, Obenauer-Kutner L et al (2002) Generating p 53-specific cytotoxic T lymphocytes by recombinant adenoviral vector-based vaccination in mice, but not man. Gene Therapy 9:833

Kuball J, Schmitz FW, Voss RH, Ferreira EA, Engel R, Guillaume P et al (2005) Cooperation of human tumor-reactive CD4+ and CD8+ T cells after redirection of their specificity by a high-affinity p 53A2.1-specific TCR. Immunity 22(1):117–129. PubMed PMID: 15664164

Kuball J, Dossett ML, Wolfl M, Ho WY, Voss RH, Fowler C et al (2007) Facilitating matched pairing and expression of TCR chains introduced into human T cells. Blood 109(6):2331–2338. PubMed PMID: 17082316. Pubmed Central PMCID: 1852191

Kyte JA, Gaudernack G, Faane A, Lislerud K, Inderberg EM, Brunsvig P et al (2016) T-helper cell receptors from long-term survivors after telomerase cancer vaccination for use in adoptive cell therapy. Oncoimmunology 5(12):e1249090. 06/27/received 09/28/revised 10/12/accepted. PubMed PMID: PMC5214348

Lamers CH, Sleijfer S, Vulto AG, Kruit WH, Kliffen M, Debets R et al (2006) Treatment of metastatic renal cell carcinoma with autologous T-lymphocytes genetically retargeted against carbonic anhydrase IX: first clinical experience. J Clin Oncol: Official Journal of the American Society of Clinical Oncology 24(13):e20–e22. PubMed PMID: 16648493

Legler DF, Johnson-Leger C, Wiedle G, Bron C, Imhof BA (2004) The alpha v beta 3 integrin as a tumor homing ligand for lymphocytes. Eur J Immunol 34(6):1608–1616. PubMed PMID: 15162430

Leisegang M, Engels B, Meyerhuber P, Kieback E, Sommermeyer D, Xue SA et al (2008) Enhanced functionality of T cell receptor-redirected T cells is defined by the transgene cassette. J Mol Med (Berl) 86(5):573–583. PubMed PMID: 18335188

Leisegang M, Turqueti-Neves A, Engels B, Blankenstein T, Schendel DJ, Uckert W et al (2010) T-cell receptor gene-modified T cells with shared renal cell carcinoma specificity for adoptive T-cell therapy. Clin Cancer Res: An Official Journal of the American Association for Cancer Research 16(8):2333–2343. PubMed PMID: 20371691

Li Y, Moysey R, Molloy PE, Vuidepot AL, Mahon T, Baston E et al (2005) Directed evolution of human T-cell receptors with picomolar affinities by phage display. Nat Biotechnol 23(3):349–354. PubMed PMID: 15723046

Liao W, Lin J-X, Leonard WJ (2013) Interleukin-2 at the crossroads of effector responses, tolerance, and immunotherapy. Immunity 38(1):13–25. PubMed PMID: PMC3610532

Linette GP, Stadtmauer EA, Maus MV, Rapoport AP, Levine BL, Emery L et al (2013) Cardiovascular toxicity and titin cross-reactivity of affinity-enhanced T cells in myeloma and melanoma. Blood 122(6):863–871

Liu K, Rosenberg SA (2001) Transduction of an IL-2 gene into human melanoma-reactive lymphocytes results in their continued growth in the absence of exogenous IL-2 and maintenance of specific antitumor activity. J Immunol (Baltimore, Md: 1950) 167(11):6356–6365. PubMed PMID: PMC2430884

Lustgarten J, Theobald M, Labadie C, LaFace D, Peterson P, Disis ML et al (1997) Identification of Her-2/Neu CTL epitopes using double transgenic mice expressing HLA-A2.1 and human CD.8. Hum Immunol 52(2):109–118. PubMed PMID: 9077559

Lyons GE, Moore T, Brasic N, Li M, Roszkowski JJ, Nishimura MI (2006) Influence of human CD8 on antigen recognition by T-cell receptor-transduced cells. Cancer Res 66(23):11455–11461. PubMed PMID: 17145893

Ma Q, Gomes EM, Lo AS, Junghans RP (2014) Advanced generation anti-prostate specific membrane antigen designer T cells for prostate cancer immunotherapy. Prostate 74(3):286–296. PubMed PMID: 24174378

Machlenkin A, Paz A, Bar Haim E, Goldberger O, Finkel E, Tirosh B et al (2005) Human CTL epitopes prostatic acid phosphatase-3 and six-transmembrane epithelial antigen of prostate-3 as candidates for prostate cancer immunotherapy. Cancer Res 65(14):6435–6442. PubMed PMID: 16024648

Moore TV, Lyons GE, Brasic N, Roszkowski JJ, Voelkl S, Mackensen A et al (2009) Relationship between CD8-dependent antigen recognition, T cell functional avidity, and tumor cell recognition. Cancer Immunol Immunother 58(5):719–728. PubMed PMID: 18836717. Pubmed Central PMCID: 2773431

Moore T, Wagner CR, Scurti GM, Hutchens KA, Godellas C, Clark AL et al (2017) Clinical and immunologic evaluation of three metastatic melanoma patients treated with autologous melanoma-reactive TCR-transduced T cells. Cancer Immunol Immunother. PubMed PMID: 29052782

Morgan DA, Ruscetti FW, Gallo R (1976) Selective in vitro growth of T lymphocytes from normal human bone marrows. Science 193(4257):1007–1008. PubMed PMID: 181845

Morgan RA, Chinnasamy N, Abate-Daga DD, Gros A, Robbins PF, Zheng Z et al (2013) Cancer regression and neurologic toxicity following anti-MAGE-A3 TCR gene therapy. J Immunother (Hagerstown, Md: 1997) 36(2):133–151. PubMed PMID: PMC3581823

Morgenroth A, Cartellieri M, Schmitz M, Gunes S, Weigle B, Bachmann M et al (2007) Targeting of tumor cells expressing the prostate stem cell antigen (PSCA) using genetically engineered T-cells. Prostate 67(10):1121–1131. PubMed PMID: 17492652

Mukherjee P, Tinder TL, Basu GD, Pathangey LB, Chen L, Gendler SJ (2004) Therapeutic efficacy of MUC1-specific cytotoxic T lymphocytes and CD137 co-stimulation in a spontaneous breast cancer model. Breast Dis 20:53–63. PubMed PMID: 15687707

Mule JJ, Shu S, Schwarz SL, Rosenberg SA (1984) Adoptive immunotherapy of established pulmonary metastases with LAK cells and recombinant interleukin-2. Science 225 (4669):1487–1489. PubMed PMID: 6332379

Murphy KM, Stockinger B (2010) Effector T cell plasticity: flexibility in the face of changing circumstances. Nat Immunol 11(8):674–680. PubMed PMID: PMC3249647

Nishimura MI, Avichezer D, Custer MC, Lee CS, Chen C, Parkhurst MR et al (1999) MHC class I-restricted recognition of a melanoma antigen by a human CD4+ tumor infiltrating lymphocyte. Cancer Res 59(24):6230–6238. PubMed PMID: 10626817

Nishimura MI, Roszkowski JJ, Moore TV, Brasic N, McKee MD, Clay TM (2005) Antigen recognition and T-cell biology. Cancer Treat Res 123:37–59. PubMed PMID: 16211865

Ochi T, Fujiwara H, Okamoto S, An J, Nagai K, Shirakata T et al (2011) Novel adoptive T-cell immunotherapy using a WT1-specific TCR vector encoding silencers for endogenous TCRs shows marked antileukemia reactivity and safety. Blood 118(6):1495–1503. PubMed PMID: 21673345

Okamoto S, Mineno J, Ikeda H, Fujiwara H, Yasukawa M, Shiku H et al (2009) Improved expression and reactivity of transduced tumor-specific TCRs in human lymphocytes by specific silencing of endogenous TCR. Cancer Res 69(23):9003–9011. PubMed PMID: 19903853

Page DB, Postow MA, Callahan MK, Allison JP, Wolchok JD (2014) Immune modulation in cancer with antibodies. Annu Rev Med 65:185–202. PubMed PMID: 24188664

Palmer DC, Chan C-C, Gattinoni L, Wrzesinski C, Paulos CM, Hinrichs CS et al (2008) Effective tumor treatment targeting a melanoma/melanocyte-associated antigen triggers severe ocular autoimmunity. Proc Natl Acad Sci 105(23):8061–8066

Papewalis C, Ehlers M, Schott M (2010) Advances in cellular therapy for the treatment of thyroid cancer. J Oncol. 09/02/received

Pardoll DM (2012) The blockade of immune checkpoints in cancer immunotherapy. Nat Rev
    Cancer 12(4):252–264. PubMed PMID: 22437870. Pubmed Central PMCID: 4856023
Parkhurst MR, Joo J, Riley JP, Yu Z, Li Y, Robbins PF et al (2009) Characterization of genetically
    modified T-cell receptors that recognize the CEA:691–699 peptide in the context of HLA-A2.1
    on human colorectal cancer cells. Clin Cancer Res: An Official Journal of the American
    Association for Cancer Research 15(1):169–180. PubMed PMID: 19118044. Pubmed Central
    PMCID: 3474199
Parkhurst MR, Yang JC, Langan RC, Dudley ME, Nathan D-AN, Feldman SA et al (2011) T cells
    targeting carcinoembryonic antigen can mediate regression of metastatic colorectal cancer but
    induce severe transient colitis. Mol Ther 19(3):620–626. 10/14/received 11/08/accepted.
    PubMed PMID: PMC3048186
Pasetto A, Frelin L, Aleman S, Holmstrom F, Brass A, Ahlen G et al (2012) TCR-redirected
    human T cells inhibit hepatitis C virus replication: hepatotoxic potential is linked to antigen
    specificity and functional avidity. J Immunol 189(9):4510–4519. PubMed PMID: 23024278
Provasi E, Genovese P, Lombardo A, Magnani Z, Liu PQ, Reik A et al (2012) Editing T cell
    specificity towards leukemia by zinc finger nucleases and lentiviral gene transfer. Nat Med 18
    (5):807–815. PubMed PMID: 22466705. Pubmed Central PMCID: 5019824
Rapoport AP, Stadtmauer EA, Binder-Scholl GK, Goloubeva O, Vogl DT, Lacey SF et al (2015)
    NY-ESO-1 specific TCR engineered T-cells mediate sustained antigen-specific antitumor
    effects in myeloma. Nat Med 21(8):914–921. PubMed PMID: PMC4529359
Richman SA, Healan SJ, Weber KS, Donermeyer DL, Dossett ML, Greenberg PD et al (2006)
    Development of a novel strategy for engineering high-affinity proteins by yeast display. Protein
    Eng Des Sel 19(6):255–264. PubMed PMID: 16549400
Robbins PF, El-Gamil M, Li YF, Kawakami Y, Loftus D, Appella E et al (1996) A mutated
    beta-catenin gene encodes a melanoma-specific antigen recognized by tumor infiltrating
    lymphocytes. J Exp Med 183(3):1185–1192
Robbins PF, Li YF, El-Gamil M, Zhao Y, Wargo JA, Zheng Z et al (2008) Single and dual amino
    acid substitutions in TCR CDRs can enhance antigen-specific T cell functions. J Immunol 180
    (9):6116–6131
Robbins PF, Morgan RA, Feldman SA, Yang JC, Sherry RM, Dudley ME et al (2011) Tumor
    regression in patients with metastatic synovial cell sarcoma and melanoma using genetically
    engineered lymphocytes reactive with NY-ESO-1. J Clin Oncol: Official Journal of the
    American Society of Clinical Oncology 29(7):917–924. PubMed PMID: 21282551. Pubmed
    Central PMCID: 3068063
Rosenberg SA (2010) Of mice, not men: no evidence for graft-versus-host disease in humans
    receiving T-cell receptor–transduced autologous T cells. Mol Ther 18(10):1744–1745. PubMed
    PMID: PMC2951571
Rosenberg SA, White DE (1996) Vitiligo in patients with melanoma: normal tissue antigens can
    be targets for cancer immunotherapy. J Immunother Emphasis Tumor Immunol 19(1):81–84.
    PubMed PMID: 8859727
Rosenberg SA, Lotze MT, Muul LM, Leitman S, Chang AE, Ettinghausen SE et al (1985)
    Observations on the systemic administration of autologous lymphokine-activated killer cells
    and recombinant interleukin-2 to patients with metastatic cancer. New Engl J Med 313
    (23):1485–1492. PubMed PMID: 3903508
Rosenberg SA, Spiess P, Lafreniere R (1986) A new approach to the adoptive immunotherapy of
    cancer with tumor-infiltrating lymphocytes. Science 233(4770):1318–1321. PubMed PMID:
    3489291
Rosenberg SA, Lotze MT, Muul LM, Chang AE, Avis FP, Leitman S et al (1987) A progress
    report on the treatment of 157 patients with advanced cancer using lymphokine-activated killer
    cells and interleukin-2 or high-dose interleukin-2 alone. N Engl J Med. 316(15):889–897.
    PubMed PMID: 3493432

Rosenberg SA, Packard BS, Aebersold PM, Solomon D, Topalian SL, Toy ST et al (1988) Use of tumor-infiltrating lymphocytes and interleukin-2 in the immunotherapy of patients with metastatic melanoma. A preliminary report. N Engl J Med 319(25):1676–1680. PubMed PMID: 3264384

Rosenberg SA, Aebersold P, Cornetta K, Kasid A, Morgan RA, Moen R et al (1990) Gene transfer into humans–immunotherapy of patients with advanced melanoma, using tumor-infiltrating lymphocytes modified by retroviral gene transduction. N Engl J Med 323(9):570–578. PubMed PMID: 2381442

Rosenberg SA, Lotze MT, Yang JC, Topalian SL, Chang AE, Schwartzentruber DJ et al (1993) Prospective randomized trial of high-dose interleukin-2 alone or in conjunction with lymphokine-activated killer cells for the treatment of patients with advanced cancer. JNCI: J Natl Cancer Inst 85(8):622–632

Rosenberg SA, Yang JC, Topalian SL, Schwartzentruber DJ, Weber JS, Parkinson DR et al (1994) Treatment of 283 consecutive patients with metastatic melanoma or renal cell cancer using high-dose bolus interleukin 2. JAMA 271(12):907–913. PubMed PMID: 8120958

Rosenberg SA, Restifo NP, Yang JC, Morgan RA, Dudley ME (2008) Adoptive cell transfer: a clinical path to effective cancer immunotherapy. Nat Rev Cancer 8:299

Roszkowski JJ, Yu DC, Rubinstein MP, McKee MD, Cole DJ, Nishimura MI (2003) CD8-independent tumor cell recognition is a property of the T cell receptor and not the T cell. J Immunol 170(5):2582–2589. PubMed PMID: 12594285

Roszkowski JJ, Lyons GE, Kast WM, Yee C, Van Besien K, Nishimura MI (2005) Simultaneous generation of CD8+ and CD4+ melanoma-reactive T cells by retroviral-mediated transfer of a single T-cell receptor. Cancer Res 65(4):1570–1576. PubMed PMID: 15735047

Rubinstein MP, Cloud CA, Garrett TE, Moore CJ, Schwartz KM, Johnson CB et al (2012) Ex vivo interleukin-12-priming during CD8(+) T cell activation dramatically improves adoptive T cell transfer antitumor efficacy in a lymphodepleted host. J Am Coll Surg 214(4):700–707; discussion 7–8. PubMed PMID: 22360982. Pubmed Central PMCID: 3429131

Sang M, Lian Y, Zhou X, Shan B (2011) MAGE-A family: attractive targets for cancer immunotherapy. Vaccine 29(47):8496–8500. PubMed PMID: 21933694

Schmitt TM, Aggen DH, Stromnes IM, Dossett ML, Richman SA, Kranz DM et al (2013) Enhanced-affinity murine T-cell receptors for tumor/self-antigens can be safe in gene therapy despite surpassing the threshold for thymic selection. Blood 122(3):348–356. 01/11/received 05/03/accepted. PubMed PMID: PMC3716200

Schmitt TM, Stromnes IM, Chapuis AG, Greenberg PD (2015) New strategies in engineering T-cell receptor gene-modified T cells to more effectively target malignancies. Clin Cancer Res: An Official Journal of the American Association for Cancer Research 21(23):5191–5197. PubMed PMID: 26463711. Pubmed Central PMCID: 4746077

Scholten KBJ, Kramer D, Kueter EWM, Graf M, Schoedl T, Meijer CJLM et al (2006) Codon modification of T cell receptors allows enhanced functional expression in transgenic human T cells. Clin Immunol 119(2):135–145

Scholten KB, Turksma AW, Ruizendaal JJ, van den Hende M, van der Burg SH, Heemskerk MH et al (2011) Generating HPV specific T helper cells for the treatment of HPV induced malignancies using TCR gene transfer. J Transl Med 9:147. PubMed PMID: 21892941. Pubmed Central PMCID: 3176193

Sommermeyer D, Uckert W (2010) Minimal amino acid exchange in human TCR constant regions fosters improved function of TCR gene-modified T cells. J Immunol 184(11):6223–6231

Sommermeyer D, Neudorfer J, Weinhold M, Leisegang M, Engels B, Noessner E et al (2006) Designer T cells by T cell receptor replacement. Eur J Immunol 36(11):3052–3059. PubMed PMID: 17051621

Spear TT, Nagato K, Nishimura MI (2016a) Strategies to genetically engineer T cells for cancer immunotherapy. Cancer Immunol Immunother 65(6):631–649. PubMed PMID: 27138532. Pubmed Central PMCID: 5424608

Spear TT, Riley TP, Lyons GE, Callender GG, Roszkowski JJ, Wang Y et al (2016b) Hepatitis C virus-cross-reactive TCR gene-modified T cells: a model for immunotherapy against diseases with genomic instability. J Leukoc Biol 100(3):545–557. PubMed PMID: 26921345. Pubmed Central PMCID: 4982612

Su EW, Moore CJ, Suriano S, Johnson CB, Songalia N, Patterson A et al (2015) IL-2Rα mediates temporal regulation of IL-2 signaling and enhances immunotherapy. Sci Transl Med 7 (311):311ra170

Tan MP, Dolton GM, Gerry AB, Brewer JE, Bennett AD, Pumphrey NJ et al (2017) Human leucocyte antigen class I-redirected anti-tumour CD4(+) T cells require a higher T cell receptor binding affinity for optimal activity than CD8(+) T cells. Clin Exp Immunol 187(1):124–137. PubMed PMID: 27324616. Pubmed Central PMCID: 5167017

Theobald M, Offringa R (2003) Anti-p53-directed immunotherapy of malignant disease. Expert Rev Mol Med 5(11):1–13. PubMed PMID: 14987396

Theobald M, Biggs J, Dittmer D, Levine AJ, Sherman LA (1995) Targeting p 53 as a general tumor antigen. Proc Natl Acad Sci U S A 92(26):11993–11997. PubMed PMID: 8618830. Pubmed Central PMCID: 40282

Topalian SL, Muul LM, Solomon D, Rosenberg SA (1987) Expansion of human tumor infiltrating lymphocytes for use in immunotherapy trials. J Immunol Methods 102(1):127–141. PubMed PMID: 3305708

Townsend A, Bodmer H (1989) Antigen recognition by class I-restricted T lymphocytes. Annu Rev Immunol 7(1):601–624. PubMed PMID: 2469442

Uckun FM, Jaszcz W, Ambrus JL, Fauci AS, Gajl-Peczalska K, Song CW et al (1988) Detailed studies on expression and function of CD19 surface determinant by using B43 monoclonal antibody and the clinical potential of anti-CD19 immunotoxins. Blood 71(1):13–29. PubMed PMID: 3257143

Ueno T, Fujiwara M, Tomiyama H, Onodera M, Takiguchi M (2004) Reconstitution of anti-HIV effector functions of primary human CD8 T lymphocytes by transfer of HIV-specific alphabeta TCR genes. Eur J Immunol 34(12):3379–3388. PubMed PMID: 15517606

van der Bruggen P, Traversari C, Chomez P, Lurquin C, De Plaen E, Van den Eynde B et al (1991) A gene encoding an antigen recognized by cytolytic T lymphocytes on a human melanoma. Science 254(5038):1643–1647. PubMed PMID: 1840703

van Loenen MM, de Boer R, Amir AL, Hagedoorn RS, Volbeda GL, Willemze R et al (2010) Mixed T cell receptor dimers harbor potentially harmful neoreactivity. Proc Natl Acad Sci U S A 107(24):10972–10977. PubMed PMID: 20534461. Pubmed Central PMCID: 2890759

Verginis P, Stanford MM, Carayanniotis G (2002) Delineation of five thyroglobulin T cell epitopes with pathogenic potential in experimental autoimmune thyroiditis. J Immunol 169(9): 5332–5337

Voelkl S, Moore TV, Rehli M, Nishimura MI, Mackensen A, Fischer K (2009) Characterization of MHC class-I restricted TCRalphabeta+ CD4− CD8− double negative T cells recognizing the gp100 antigen from a melanoma patient after gp100 vaccination. Cancer Immunol Immunother 58(5):709–718. PubMed PMID: 18836718. Pubmed Central PMCID: 2832593

Vogelstein B, Lane D, Levine AJ (2000) Surfing the p53 network. Nature 408(6810):307–310. PubMed PMID: 11099028

Voss RH, Thomas S, Pfirschke C, Hauptrock B, Klobuch S, Kuball J et al (2010) Coexpression of the T-cell receptor constant alpha domain triggers tumor reactivity of single-chain TCR-transduced human T cells. Blood 115(25):5154–5163. PubMed PMID: 20378753

Wang QJ, Yu Z, Griffith K, Hanada K, Restifo NP, Yang JC (2016) Identification of T-cell receptors targeting KRAS-mutated human tumors. Cancer Immunol Res 4(3):204–214. PubMed PMID: 26701267. Pubmed Central PMCID: 4775432

Weiss VL, Lee TH, Song H, Kouo TS, Black CM, Sgouros G et al (2012) Trafficking of high avidity HER-2/neu-specific T cells into HER-2/neu-expressing tumors after depletion of effector/memory-like regulatory T cells. PloS one 7(2):e31962. PubMed PMID: 22359647. Pubmed Central PMCID: 3281086

Wilde S, Sommermeyer D, Leisegang M, Frankenberger B, Mosetter B, Uckert W et al (2012) Human antitumor CD8$^+$ T cells producing Th1 polycytokines show superior antigen sensitivity and tumor recognition. J Immunol 189(2):598–605

Xue BH, Zhang Y, Sosman JA, Peace DJ (1997) Induction of human cytotoxic T lymphocytes specific for prostate-specific antigen. Prostate 30(2):73–78. PubMed PMID: 9051144

Yannelli JR, Hyatt C, McConnell S, Hines K, Jacknin L, Parker L et al (1996) Growth of tumor-infiltrating lymphocytes from human solid cancers: summary of a 5-year experience. Int J Cancer 65(4):413–421. PubMed PMID: 8621219

Yarchoan M, Johnson BA, 3rd, Lutz ER, Laheru DA, Jaffee EM (2017) Targeting neoantigens to augment antitumour immunity. Nat Rev Cancer 17(9):569. PubMed PMID: 28835723

Yee C, Thompson JA, Roche P, Byrd DR, Lee PP, Piepkorn M et al (2000) Melanocyte destruction after antigen-specific immunotherapy of melanoma. Direct evidence of T cell-mediated vitiligo. J Exp Med 192(11):1637–1644

Yoong KF, Adams DH (1996) Tumour infiltrating lymphocytes: insights into tumour immunology and potential therapeutic implications. Clin Mol Pathol 49(5):M256–M67. PubMed PMID: 16696086. Pubmed Central PMCID: 408070

Yron I, Wood TA, Spiess PJ, Rosenberg SA (1980) In vitro growth of murine T cells. V. The isolation and growth of lymphoid cells infiltrating syngeneic solid tumors. J Immunol 125 (1):238–245

Zeh HJ, Perry-Lalley D, Dudley ME, Rosenberg SA, Yang JC (1999) High avidity CTLs for two self-antigens demonstrate superior in vitro and in vivo antitumor efficacy. J Immunol 162 (2):989–994

Zheng Y, Parsonage G, Zhuang X, Machado LR, James CH, Salman A et al (2015) Human leukocyte antigen (HLA) A*1101-restricted Epstein-Barr virus-specific T-cell receptor gene transfer to target nasopharyngeal carcinoma. Cancer Immunol Res 3(10):1138–1147. PubMed PMID: 25711537. Pubmed Central PMCID: 4456157

Zhu Z, Cuss SM, Singh V, Gurusamy D, Shoe JL, Leighty R et al (2015) CD4+ T cell help selectively enhances high-avidity tumor antigen-specific CD8+ T cells. J Immunol 195 (7):3482–3489. PubMed PMID: 26320256

Personalized Neo-Epitope Vaccines for Cancer Treatment

Mathias Vormehr, Mustafa Diken, Özlem Türeci, Ugur Sahin and Sebastian Kreiter

1 Introduction

After more than a century of efforts to establish cancer immunotherapy in clinical practice, the advent of checkpoint inhibition (CPI) therapy was a critical breakthrough toward this direction (Hodi et al. 2010; Wolchok et al. 2013; Herbst et al. 2014; Tumeh et al. 2014). Further, CPIs shifted the focus from long studied shared tumor-associated antigens to mutated ones. As cancer is caused by mutations in somatic cells, the concept to utilize these correlates of 'foreignness' to enable recognition and lysis of the cancer cell by T cell immunity seems an obvious thing to do. In this regard, a key scientific observation was that after surgical removal of methylcholanthrene-induced tumors, mice were protected against a second challenge with the same tumor cells (Foley 1953; Prehn and Main 1957; Klein et al. 1960). Based on observations in such transplantable mouse model systems from the 1950s and 1960s, the concept of a systemic anti-tumor immunity was developed. It was only in the late 1980s and early 1990s that Boon and co-workers generated first data in mice and humans demonstrating that non-synonymous point mutations can become immunogenic tumor antigens (Lurquin et al. 1989; Coulie et al. 1995).

M. Vormehr · M. Diken · Ö. Türeci · U. Sahin · S. Kreiter
BioNTech RNA Pharmaceuticals GmbH, Mainz, Germany

M. Vormehr · U. Sahin
University Medical Center of the Johannes Gutenberg University, Mainz, Germany

M. Diken · U. Sahin · S. Kreiter (✉)
TRON—Translational Oncology at the University Medical Center, Johannes Gutenberg University gGmbH, Mainz, Germany
e-mail: sebastian.kreiter@tron-mainz.de

Ö. Türeci
CI3 Cluster for Individualized Immunointervention e.V, Hölderlinstr 8, 55131 Mainz, Germany

© Springer Nature Switzerland AG 2020
M. Theobald (ed.), *Current Immunotherapeutic Strategies in Cancer*,
Recent Results in Cancer Research 214,
https://doi.org/10.1007/978-3-030-23765-3_5

Various mutated neo-epitopes were identified as targets of tumor-reactive CD4$^+$ or CD8$^+$ T cell clones isolated from cancer patients (Sibille et al. 1990; Wölfel et al. 1995; Wang et al. 1999). In 2005, a study by Lennerz et al. indicated that neo-epitopes rather than non-mutated tumor-associated proteins are the dominant T cell antigens recognized by the native immune response in melanoma patients. Altogether, these data supported the notion that expanding preexisting and priming new neo-epitope specific T cells could provide a rational therapeutic approach (Lennerz et al. 2005). It was only after the recent advent of next-generation sequencing technologies, however, that an important technological prerequisite for the concept of actively individualized neo-epitope vaccination was laid out, enabling the realization of this innovative treatment approach.

In this chapter, we describe the basic concepts and recent developments in neo-epitope vaccination and we define the challenges to be overcome in order to make neo-epitope vaccination a standard of care therapy.

2   Mutations as Sources of Neo-Epitopes

Cancer formation is accompanied by the accumulation of genetic and epigenetic changes that introduce malignant properties in tumor cells (Hanahan and Weinberg 2011). Mutations that foster tumor growth and survival are called 'drivers.' The vast majority of mutations are considered functionally neutral 'passengers.' Irrespective of their functional impact, mutations that alter the amino acid sequence of a protein can be recognized by the immune system. A mutated protein which can be recognized by lymphocytes is called a 'neo-antigen' and the sequence bound to the lymphocyte receptor is termed 'neo-epitope.' Neo-antigens are not expressed in healthy tissues, including the thymus. As a result, mutation-specific T cells are unlikely to be affected by central immune tolerance and to cause autoimmune toxicities.

Single-nucleotide variations (SNVs) are the most abundant type of tumor mutations (Alexandrov et al. 2013). They can be categorized into silent, missense, and nonsense. Silent SNVs do not alter the amino acid sequence of a protein. They occur in non-coding regions of the genome or in exons (in case of the latter called 'synonymous') and do not constitute neo-antigens. Nonsense mutations form a premature stop codon resulting in translation of a truncated protein. A fraction of SNVs (between about ten to a couple of thousands depending on the tumor type (Vormehr et al. 2016) alters the protein sequence and therefore can give rise to neo-epitopes recognized by T cells. Such mutations are called missense or non-synonymous.

Besides SNVs, small insertions and deletions (indels) and large chromosomal aberrations, like gene fusions or duplications, occur in tumors. In rare cases, indels and fusions are in frame and do not alter the reading frame of the gene. In-frame indels may result in neo-epitopes by insertion or deletion of amino acids. In-frame gene fusions can cause breakpoint-spanning (the intersection between two formerly distinct genetic regions) neo-epitopes, as shown for the BCR-ABL fusion protein

(Bosch et al. 1996). The majority of indels and fusions cause a frameshift, which may result in new amino acids.

Furthermore, gene fusions may additionally lead to the translation of intronic sequences. Of note, due to nonsense-mediated mRNA decay, posttranscriptional quality control mechanisms, not all mutations, manifest themselves on the protein level (Popp and Maquat 2013). For example, a premature termination codon about 24 nucleotides upstream of a splicing-generated exon–exon junction may trigger the decay of aberrant mRNA.

Neo-epitope specific immunotherapies currently focus on SNVs and indels. More complex mutation events are known to occur in cancer, e.g., mutations at an exon–intron splice site can cause an altered open reading frame leading to amino acid substitutions that could give rise to neo-epitopes. Technologies to detect such genetic aberrations, however, are not mature yet.

3 Preclinical Proof of Concept for Individualized Mutanome Vaccination

Until recently, cancer vaccination focused on tumor antigens shared across patients. These included only a few mutated targets such as Ras, BRAF, and p53 (Houbiers et al. 1993; Gjertsen et al. 1995; Somasundaram et al. 2006), as the vast majority of tumor mutations are private to the individual patient, and personalized treatment settings were considered as not feasible.

In 2005 with the advent of next-generation sequencing (NGS), a critical step toward enabling personalized treatment approaches was made (Margulies et al. 2005; Shendure et al. 2005). NGS was first used for systematic identification of mutated neo-epitopes in 2012 by the groups of Sahin and Schreiber (Castle et al. 2012; Matsushita et al. 2012). Castle et al. suggested the use of NGS for identification of mutated neo-epitopes for cancer vaccination. In the first proof of concept, they identified neo-antigens derived from point mutations in the B16F10 melanoma mouse model. Peptide vaccination addressing predicted neo-epitopes frequently gave rise to mutation specific T cells and conferred potent tumor control in vivo. Matsushita et al. determined neo-antigens in tumor cell lines and proofed immune editing by neo-epitope specific CD8$^+$ T cells. These two landmark publications were succeeded by several studies. The group of Schreiber followed up on its 2012 paper by showing that neo-epitope specific T cells are induced upon anti-PD-1/anti-CTLA-4 antibody treatment. They demonstrated that vaccination against neo-antigens was equally efficient as checkpoint blockade (Gubin et al. 2014). Experiments in two syngeneic mouse tumor models, CMS5 and Meth A, indicated that a strong disparity in the binding affinity to MHC class I between the mutant and the wild-type variant of the gene is a good predictor for its immunogenicity (Duan et al. 2014). An advancement of NGS-based neo-epitope prediction was suggested by Yadav and colleagues. By using mass spectrometry analysis of MHC ligands on tumor cells, they were able to narrow down the NGS predicted neo-antigens to factually expressed MHC ligands.

Vaccination against three identified neo-epitopes resulted in potent control of sub-cutaneous MC38 tumors (Yadav et al. 2014). Nevertheless, as the author's state in their discussion, this process is not yet suitable for clinical application due to technical and practical reasons. They rather suggested using 'a purely computational approach' as initially performed by Sahin and Schreiber. In 2015, Sahin's group showed that such a purely in silico guided approach can indeed be successful. Screening almost 200 mutations across three different mouse tumors, they found that neo-epitopes are more frequent than previously anticipated (Kreiter et al. 2015). Between 21 and 45% of mutations were immunogenic, and the majority of neo-epitopes were recognized by CD4$^+$ T cells. Depending on the mouse model, neo-antigen-specific CD4$^+$ T cells conferred tumor control by inducing tumor-specific CD8$^+$ T cell responses or by direct IFNγ-mediated tumor growth inhibition. Importantly, several candidate epitopes selected via MHC class II binding prediction and encoded as RNA vaccine-mediated potent tumor control without prior selection of immunogenic variants. Of note, the experimental determination of immunogenic epitopes in tumor patients' prior vaccination is not trivial and restricted to preexisting T cell responses. Thus, by indicating that immunogenic mutations can be enriched in silico without wet-bench validation, these data contributed substantially to the translation of individualized cancer vaccines into the clinics.

4 Prediction of Neo-Epitopes

Tumors of patients display dozens to thousands of expressed mutations with the majority of them being point mutations (Vormehr et al. 2016). However, only a fraction of those mutations are immunogenic. Further, the number of mutated neo-antigen candidates that can be targeted in parallel is limited due to restrictions by regulatory authorities as well as technical limitations of vaccine platforms. Currently, 10–20 mutations are typically addressed in clinical trials of individualized cancer vaccines (see Sect. 5). Selecting the mutated targets that are most likely immunogenic and therapeutically relevant is essential.

So far, there is no consensus on how to prioritize mutations in the most efficient way. Typically, MHC class I binding prediction is used which has been shown to enrich for immunogenic CD8$^+$ T cell recognized neo-antigens (Robbins et al. 2013; Van Rooij et al. 2013; Duan et al. 2014; Johanns et al. 2016; Matsushita et al. 2012; Yadav et al. 2014; Carreno et al. 2015; Gubin et al. 2014). Algorithms such as NetMHC (Hoof et al. 2009) and IEDB consensus (Vita et al. 2014) (available at www.iedb.org) are most frequently used to predict MHC binding affinity. For common MHC alleles, these algorithms show a very high specificity. This means that actual T cell epitopes usually have a very strong predicted MHC binding. However, as the false positive rate is high, the positive predictive value is rather poor. One reason for this may be that not every MHC ligand is recognized by T cells due to 'holes' in the repertoire. More recently, it has been proposed that the stability of the MHC–peptide complex is a better predictor for T cell immunogenicity as compared to MHC binding affinity. A weak binding stability could account for up to 30% of non-immunogenic ligands with good MHC class I binding affinity (Harndahl et al. 2012; Rasmussen et al. 2016; van der Burg et al. 1996). In silico prediction algorithms for MHC–peptide complex stability exist for only a few alleles (Jørgensen et al. 2014) and the underlying datasets are rather small and therefore are not broadly applicable.

MHC class II compared to MHC class I binding prediction is less accurate. One reason for this is that the algorithm is based on a much smaller dataset of binders. Further, rules for MHC class II binding are more promiscuous than for MHC class I. CD8 epitopes have a clear length restriction of about 8–11 amino acids with defined anchor positions. CD4 epitopes usually bind with a core region of nine amino acids. However, due to an open binding pocket, the core region can be extended by flanking residues of variable size ranging from a few amino acids to whole proteins (Arnold et al. 2002). Moreover, MHC class II ligands can bind in different registers complicating the exact epitope definition (Landais et al. 2009; Mohan et al. 2011). Since MHC class II-restricted neo-epitopes compared to MHC class I-restricted neo-epitopes are more abundant, MHC class II binding prediction was shown to be more efficient in enriching immunogenic neo-antigens (Kreiter et al. 2015).

The ability of a peptide to be presented on MHC class I furthermore depends on the expression levels of the MHC molecules, on transporter associated with antigen processing (TAP) (Peters et al. 2003) as well as C- and N-terminal cleavage (Kesmir et al. 2002; Saric et al. 2002). Algorithms that combine MHC binding prediction, proteasomal cleavage as well as TAP transport do exist (Tenzer et al. 2005), and their usefulness, however, is under debate.

Beyond MHC binding prediction, the expression level of the mutated gene is an important selection criterion. Expression levels are not directly involved in predicting immunogenic mutations but are factored in when selecting therapeutically relevant mutations. Only expressed mutated genes can give rise to processed and presented neo-epitopes on the surface of the tumor cell. It was shown that the expression level of a protein is correlated with the amount of MHC ligands generated from it (Bassani-Sternberg et al. 2015) which in turn influences T cell recognition and lysis (Christinck et al. 1991; Lethe et al. 1997; Kurts et al. 1998). The protein expression of a mutated allele is usually estimated via RNA sequencing and can be quantified by multiplying the mutation allele frequency by the transcript expression of the mutated gene. Although many factors such as the efficacy of RNA translation and protein stability influence the cellular protein amounts, RNA sequencing and protein levels, as determined via mass spectrometry, have been shown to significantly correlate (Schwanhäusser et al. 2011). Interestingly, there is evidence that a high RNA expression level which results in more MHC ligands can to some extent compensate for a weak predicted MHC class I binding and vice versa (Abelin et al. 2017). This suggests that MHC class I binding prediction and RNA expression levels of the mutated allele should be analyzed together to decide whether or not to select a mutation for vaccination.

Not many additional features beyond MHC binding prediction and RNA expression levels are currently in use for mutation selection. The fraction of tumor cells expressing a mutated epitope seems to be an important predictor of anti-tumoral activity (Mcgranahan et al. 2016). So-called clonal antigens are expressed on all tumor cells, whereas 'subclonal' antigens are found only on a fraction. Targeting clonal antigens is thought to be superior as this diminishes the likelihood of clonal escape after vaccination therapy. Other than that, factors such as the variant allele frequency (the proportion of sequencing reads covering the mutation), the function of the mutated gene, or the similarity of the epitope to a microbial peptide are hypothesized to influence the relevance of a neo-epitope. It is conceivable that the former two factors affect the chance of immune escape through epitope loss. Although a matter of debate, mutated genes crucial for proliferation, survival, or metastasis of tumor cells might be less easily lost upon T cell pressure. The resemblance of a neo-epitope to bacterial or viral antigens might influence the frequency, affinity, and hence the anti-tumoral activity of T cell responses. It has been proposed that the TCR repertoire is evolutionary biased for the recognition of pathogen-derived epitopes. Moreover, microbial antigens are completely foreign and respective T cell responses not affected by thymic negative selection. In this regard, several studies in mice demonstrated that the composition of the gut microbiome impacts the efficacy of cancer immunotherapy (Iida et al. 2013; Sivan et al. 2015; Vétizou et al. 2015; Routy et al. 2017). Whether this observation relies solely on pattern recognition receptor-mediated modulation of inflammation, or, as hypothesized, additionally on molecular mimicry between microbial and neo-antigens (Vétizou et al. 2015), is so far not clear. Initial supporting evidence for shared epitope patterns in patients treated with anti-CTLA-4 checkpoint blockade (Snyder et al. 2014) was not confirmed in two meta-analyses relying on larger patient cohorts (Van Allen et al. 2015; Nathanson et al. 2016). Two recent publications predicted neo-epitopes based on the resemblance to microbial epitopes as well as on the difference between the predicted binding of the mutated versus the wild-type epitope in pancreatic, lung tumor, and melanoma patients. These parameters were used to calculate a specific 'quality' value for each tumor clone. The 'quality' model in comparison with a model based on the quantity of predicted neo-epitopes was able to discriminate long- and short-term survivors (Balachandran et al. 2017; Łuksza et al. 2017).

5 Neo-Epitope Vaccines in Clinical Practice

Translation of neo-epitope vaccination into clinical practice requires a paradigm shift from a drug-centered to a patient-centered development. Instead of searching for patients that respond to certain medication (or express the targeted antigen in case of shared antigens), a neo-epitope vaccine is customized for every patient. This requires regulatory approvement not of a single compound but rather a whole process ranging from sample acquisition to vaccine production (Britten et al. 2013;

Türeci et al. 2016; Vormehr et al. 2015). As time is essential for tumor patients, a fast and reliable manufacturing process is a prerequisite for therapy success. Even though the safety of the vaccine platform can be tested, potential toxicities through T cells cross-reacting with the wild-type counterpart of the neo-antigen can vary from patient to patient. Although no such toxicities have been observed in any of the mouse studies (Castle et al. 2012; Kreiter et al. 2015) or the first published phase-I trials, conscientious personalized safety monitoring especially of organs that highly express the wild-type counterparts is advised. Additionally, safety aspects should already be considered in the selection process of the vaccine targets by omitting genes highly expressed in vital organs like the heart or the brain.

So far, three trials studying individualized neo-epitope vaccination in cancer have been published. A small study with three patients was published in 2015 by Carreno et al. out of Washington University in St. Louis (Carreno et al. 2015). They treated three melanoma patients with stage III resected cutaneous melanoma and prior ipilimumab treatment. Mutation identification and selection were done based on whole-exome sequencing (WES) from fresh frozen tumor samples and PBMC followed by RNA sequencing. The authors focused on the induction of $CD8^+$ T cells recognizing mutated neo-epitopes and on one common HLA allele and therefore filtered in silico for HLA-A*02:01 binding nonamers from the patients expressed mutations. The final validation step was done by wet-bench verification of HLA-A*02 binding. Autologous dendritic cells were used to deliver seven neo-epitopes plus two gp100-derived peptides per patient. The DC for vaccination were generated from PBMC by differentiation with GM-CSF and IL4 for 6 days followed by a maturation step for 16 h using CD40L-expressing K562, IFNγ, poly I:C and R848. Two hours prior to infusion, the DC were pulsed separately for each peptide and the patients received 5×10^6 DC i.v. per peptide. The patients received a total of three vaccinations (week 1, 7, and 13) with a single administration of cyclophosphamide (300 mg/m^2) 96 h prior to the first vaccination. To the first dose, a commercial seasonal influenza vaccine was added. In each patient, the authors identified one preexisting neo-epitope-specific T cell reactivity, which was amplified following the vaccinations. Moreover, each patient developed additionally two novel vaccine-induced T cell responses. Those T cell responses were not tested for recognition of autologous tumor cells; hence, their relevance remains uncertain. Importantly, two of the identified epitopes were afterward proven to be cryptic. The induction of T cells against two epitopes that are not processed naturally demonstrates the limitations of this peptide-based approach and bears the risk of toxicity. In the current study, no signs of autoimmune adverse events were observed. Concerning objective clinical responses, the authors shared no information.

In 2017, another clinical trial in patient with malignant melanoma (stage IIIB/C and IVM1a/b) was published again using peptide-based vaccination that was conducted by Catherine Wu and co-workers, who also play an active role in the establishment of Neon Therapeutics, a biotech company focusing on neo-antigen therapeutics (Ott et al. 2017). Also here, WES followed by RNA sequencing was employed to identify somatic mutations. Mutation prioritization was directed toward the enrichment of HLA-A and HLA-B binding epitopes. Patients received thirteen to twenty peptides with a length of fifteen to thirty amino acids. Peptides were split in four peptide pools (0.3 mg/peptide plus 0.5 mg poly-ICLC) and injected subcutaneously into the four extremities on days 1, 4, 8, 15, and 22, followed by two booster injections (week 12 and 20). Vaccine-induced immune responses were characterized by IFNγ ELISpot and techniques like intracellular cytokine staining (ICS) or MHC multimer technology. T cell responses against peptides incorporated into the vaccine were identified in all six treated patients (2–4 vaccine peptides were recognized per patient). In total, T cell responses for 73 of the 97 peptides used across all patients were detected after vaccination.

Of these, 19 responses were measurable ex vivo without prior in vitro expansion, and all of these were elicited by CD4$^+$ T cells and did not preexist prior vaccination. T cell responses were detected early after starting the vaccinations and persisted up to week 24. To identify also immune responses below the detection limit of the used assays, the group performed in vitro expansion cultures (10–21 days) followed by IFNγ ELISpot or ICS. With this approach, additional 39 CD4 responses and 15 CD8 responses were detected, and again no preexisting mutation-specific reactivities found. For 24 of 28 epitopes, it was shown that the expanded T cells only recognize the mutated epitope. Processing of the respective antigens was tested with B cells transfected with in vitro transcribed RNA encoding multiple minigenes. For 5 of 19 tested CD4 reactivities, antigen processing and presentation could not be verified, whereas all 15 CD8 reactivities tested recognized the transfected target cells. In four of six patients, the vaccine-primed T cells did not recognize autologous tumor cells. However, it has to be taken into account that only one of five investigated patients' tumor cells expressed HLA class II, and four patients' tumor cells expressed HLA class I. With respect to the anti-tumoral efficacy, the authors reported that no objective responses were observed. However, four patients who entered the study with stage IIIB/C disease remained without disease recurrence at a median follow-up of 25 months. The two patients with lung metastases (stage IV M1b) had disease recurrence at restaging following the last vaccination but achieved a complete response after subsequent anti-PD1 treatment. Under anti-PD1 therapy, vaccine-induced T cell responses persisted, and a couple of new mutation-specific T cell reactivities were induced.

Also in 2017, the largest clinical trial was published by Sahin et al. (2017). The biotech company BioNTech who acted as the sponsor of the study together with the independent research institute TRON (TRON—Translational Oncology at the University Medical Center of the Johannes Gutenberg University Mainz) reported the first RNA based fully individualized vaccine study in melanoma patients.

To identify non-synonymous mutations, WES and RNA sequencing were performed from routine tumor biopsies and healthy blood cells. To take into account their preclinical finding of dominant MHC class II neo-epitopes in murine model systems (Kreiter et al. 2015), the group combined two paths for mutation prioritization, one was directed toward enriching for mutated HLA class II ligands with predicted high-affinity binding and the other toward HLA class I ligands. Moreover, the mutations were selected for high expression. Patients received two synthetic RNAs (500 or 1000 µg dose levels per RNA) each encoding five linker-connected

27mer peptides with the mutated amino acid located centrally in position 14. In order to bridge the time required for vaccine manufacturing, patients with positive tumors were offered immunization with NY-ESO-1 and/or tyrosinase RNAs. After the release of their neo-epitope RNA vaccine, all patients had at least eight doses of neo-epitope vaccine which was injected percutaneously into the inguinal lymph node. At the time point of starting the neo-epitope vaccination, six patients were in stage III and seven in stage IV. Against 75 of the 125 (60%) predicted neo-epitopes used for vaccination a specific T cell response was detected, with 68% of the responses being de novo T cell reactivities. Again, the majority of these were CD4 responses (57%), a considerable amount of mixed CD4 and CD8 responses (26%), and a relevant percentage of CD8 T cell reactivities (17%). T cell responses against 20% of all immunogenic neo-epitopes were detectable without short-term in vitro stimulation directly from the patient's blood. Each patient mounted specific T cell responses against at least three predicted neo-epitopes. The eight patients entering neo-epitope vaccination without measurable disease remained disease-free for a prolonged period (12–23 months) demonstrating a significantly sustained progression-free survival. In the cohort of five patients, who had radiologically detectable and progressive lesions prior to starting the vaccination, the authors observed objective responses. Two of these patients developed vaccine-related objective responses; one was a partial response, the other a confirmed complete response sustained for 26 months. One patient had a mixed response. Another patient had a stable lymph node metastasis, which was dissected later. And finally, one patient reached a complete response under anti-PD-1 treatment which he received subsequent to the neo-epitope RNA vaccine.

In summary, these trials provide important data and answers to relevant questions concerning the therapeutic potential of neo-epitope vaccines. First of all, they show that de novo induction as well as the expansion of preexisting neo-epitope-specific T cell responses can be reproducibly and frequently achieved in melanoma patients. Moreover, they provide the first promising evidence for the clinical benefit of neo-epitope vaccination.

Future studies will need to examine single-agent activity and potential synergistic combination partners. One can only speculate in which setting and tumor types a cancer vaccine will be most successful. It is conceivable that, as a monotherapy, neo-epitope vaccines will be especially efficacious in highly mutated tumor types such as melanoma, smoking-induced lung cancer, bladder cancer, or hyper-mutated colorectal cancers (Vormehr et al. 2016). In such tumors, the chance to induce multiple high-affinity T cell responses and even a subsequent epitope spreading is assumed to be higher compared to cancers with the low mutational burden. Furthermore, tumors that exert no or little immunosuppressive activity such as in minimal residual disease or the adjuvant setting may be a promising area of application. Efficient targeting of larger tumors most probably will rely on combination treatments (Moynihan et al. 2016). One auspicious combination partner is PD-1/PD-L1 checkpoint blockade, as this treatment is known to depend on a preexisting immune response (Rizvi et al. 2015; Gubin et al. 2014). Vaccination has the potential to broaden the success rate of anti-PD-1/PD-L1 therapies to patients without an established T cell response (Woller et al. 2015). This might be especially valuable in tumors with a medium to low mutational burden lacking spontaneously immunogenic epitopes. In addition, as PD-1 re-invigorated T cells were shown to fail to develop robust memory (Pauken et al. 2016), vaccine-induced memory T cells might help to further extend the treatment durability. Currently, a phase-I clinical trial testing PD-L1 blockade in combination with RNA based neo-epitope vaccination is ongoing (NCT03289962). Similarly, inhibitors of LAG-3 (Matsuzaki et al. 2010; Grosso et al. 2007), TIM-3 (Sakuishi et al. 2010; Baghdadi et al. 2013), IDO (Holmgaard et al. 2015; Sharma et al. 2009) or TGF-β (Takaku et al. 2010) as well as stimulation of costimulatory molecules such as OX40 (Linch et al. 2016), GITR (Cohen et al. 2006), and CD137 (Bartkowiak et al. 2015) were shown to synergize with T cell vaccination. From the mechanistic standpoint, agents that promote an acute inflammation in the tumor ought to create a strong synergistic benefit for T cell vaccines. Tumor inflammation enhances T cell and APC infiltration, tumor antigen presentation and can modulate the suppressive microenvironment to support T cell function (Klug et al. 2013; Iwasaki and Medzhitov 2015; Wang et al. 2016; Lee et al. 2014). This can in principle be reached directly by pattern recognition receptor (PRR) agonists (Corrales et al. 2015; Manrique et al. 2016; Wang et al. 2016; Lee et al. 2014) or indirectly through promotion of immunogenic cell death (Galluzzi et al. 2016), for example, via tumor irradiation (Deng et al. 2014; Ganss et al. 2002; Klug et al. 2013) or immunogenic chemotherapy (Sistigu et al. 2014; Pfirschke et al. 2016; Manrique et al. 2016). Optimally, the induced inflammation should be restricted to the tumor site [e.g., by intratumoral injection (Wang et al. 2016; Corrales et al. 2015) or local irradiation (Klug et al. 2013)] to avoid systemic toxicity and to potentiate T cell attraction.

6 Conclusion and Outlook

Though the potential of vaccination with neo-antigens has been shown by various preclinical as well as early-phase clinical studies, there are challenges to be overcome in order to fully exploit its potency. Prediction algorithms used to identify MHC class I and class II binding neo-epitopes need to be further improved to increase the probability of detection for true neo-epitopes and to decrease false positive hits. Most of the current algorithms focus on the detection of single-nucleotide changes as well as insertions and deletions which should be expanded to other potentially neo-antigenic aberrations such as gene fusions and duplications. The power of such algorithms for assessing MHC binding strength, expression as well as immunogenicity of the candidate neo-epitopes can be further enhanced by machine learning based on the incoming data stream, e.g., from clinical studies. Moreover, NGS can be combined with mass spectrometry analysis of the tumor itself or cell lines derived from it in order to support genomic data with ligandome data. These cell lines can also be employed to evaluate the immunogenicity of the predicted epitopes—especially for the preexisting immune response against them—using in vitro assays with autologous T cells derived from the patient.

Tumor heterogeneity is yet another challenge for neo-antigen vaccines, which can occur within a given tumor lesion or between the primary tumor and different metastases (Mcgranahan et al. 2016). As a result, sampling from the primary tumor for identification of neo-antigens might be insufficient to target all tumor cells within the primary tumor or those in disseminated metastatic lesions. Therefore, a granular understanding of the neo-antigen landscape is of great importance. In addition to the natural heterogeneity of the tumor, dynamic changes in the neo-antigen repertoire can occur during tumor progression and upon treatment. Similar to other immunotherapeutic approaches, immune escape is an important mechanism responsible for these changes. It can manifest itself by downregulation of selected neo-epitopes (Matsushita et al. 2012; Marty et al. 2017; Verdegaal et al. 2016) as well as induced defects in the antigen processing and presentation machinery (e.g., HLA or B2M loss) due to the immune pressure generated upon vaccination (Sahin et al. 2017; Shukla et al. 2015; Zaretsky et al. 2016). A broad panel of neo-antigens can be utilized to address intratumoral heterogeneity. Sampling from metastases can further help to compare and select the neo-antigen repertoire shared by the primary tumor and metastases. Moreover, refreshment of these panels in the next rounds of vaccination based on information derived from the latest neo-antigen landscape can counteract against immune escape. To hinder immune escape, neo-antigen vaccination can also be combined with other immunotherapeutic interventions such as checkpoint blockade therapy or therapies against the inhibitory tumor microenvironment.

Two other key challenges for rolling out the use of personalized neo-antigen vaccines are the costs and time of production, which also conceptionally differ from manufacturing processes of conventional off-the-shelf pharmaceutical drugs. The continuous decrease in the cost of whole genome sequencing is expected to decrease the cost of neo-antigen vaccination. The improvements in prediction algorithms will further strengthen purely bioinformatical selection of neo-epitopes and shorten the time required for their selection. Moreover, automatized production processes and facilities can be designed and optimized specially for these novel drug products. Supported by the anticipated adaptation of regulatory policies, these will not only lead to a significant drop in cost but also decrease the time required from sample collection to the tailor-made vaccine enabling in-time preparation for many thousands of patients.

References

Abelin JG et al (2017) Mass spectrometry profiling of HLA-associated peptidomes in mono-allelic cells enables more accurate epitope prediction. Immunity 46(2):315–326

Alexandrov LB et al (2013) Signatures of mutational processes in human cancer. Nature 500 (7463):415–421

Arnold PY et al (2002) The majority of immunogenic epitopes generate CD4+ T cells that are dependent on MHC class II-bound peptide-flanking residues. J Immunol (Baltimore, Md.: 1950) 169(2):739–749

Baghdadi M et al (2013) Combined blockade of TIM-3 and TIM-4 augments cancer vaccine efficacy against established melanomas. Cancer Immunol Immunother: CII 62(4):629–637

Balachandran VP et al (2017) Identification of unique neoantigen qualities in long-term survivors of pancreatic cancer. Nature

Bartkowiak T et al (2015) Unique potential of 4-1BB agonist antibody to promote durable regression of HPV+ tumors when combined with an E6/E7 peptide vaccine. Proc Natl Acad Sci USA 112(38):E5290–E5299

Bassani-Sternberg M et al (2015) Mass spectrometry of human leukocyte antigen class I peptidomes reveals strong effects of protein abundance and turnover on antigen presentation. Mol Cell Proteomics: MCP 14(3):658–673

Bosch GJ et al (1996) Recognition of BCR-ABL positive leukemic blasts by human CD4+ T cells elicited by primary in vitro immunization with a BCR-ABL breakpoint peptide. Blood 88 (9):3522–3527

Britten CM et al (2013) The regulatory landscape for actively personalized cancer immunotherapies. Nat Biotechnol 31(10):880–882

Carreno BM et al (2015) A dendritic cell vaccine increases the breadth and diversity of melanoma neoantigen-specific T cells. Science (New York, N.Y.) 348(6236):803–808

Castle JC et al (2012) Exploiting the mutanome for tumor vaccination. Can Res 72(5):1081–1091

Christinck ER et al (1991) Peptide binding to class I MHC on living cells and quantitation of complexes required for CTL lysis. Nature 352(6330):67–70

Cohen AD et al (2006) Agonist anti-GITR antibody enhances vaccine-induced CD8(+) T-cell responses and tumor immunity. Can Res 66(9):4904–4912

Corrales L et al (2015) Direct activation of STING in the tumor microenvironment leads to potent and systemic tumor regression and immunity. Cell Rep 11(7):1018–1030

Coulie PG et al (1995) A mutated intron sequence codes for an antigenic peptide recognized by cytolytic T lymphocytes on a human melanoma. Proc Natl Acad Sci USA 92(17):7976–7980

Deng L et al (2014) STING-dependent cytosolic DNA sensing promotes radiation-induced type I interferon-dependent antitumor immunity in immunogenic tumors. Immunity 41(5):543–852

Duan F et al (2014) Genomic and bio-informatic profiling of mutational neo-epitopes reveals new rules to predict anti-cancer immunogenicity. J Exp Med 211(11):2231–2248

Foley EJ (1953) Antigenic properties of methylcholanthrene-induced tumors in mice of the strain of origin. Can Res 13(12):835–837

Galluzzi L et al (2016) Immunogenic cell death in cancer and infectious disease. Nat Rev Immunol, Oct 17, p.Epub ahead of print

Ganss R et al (2002) Combination of T-cell therapy and trigger of inflammation induces remodeling of the vasculature and tumor eradication. Can Res 62:1462–1470

Gjertsen M, Breivik J, Saeterdal I (1995) Vaccination with mutant ras peptides and induction of T-cell responsiveness in pancreatic carcinoma patients carrying the corresponding RAS mutation. Lancet 346(8987):1399–1400

Grosso JF et al (2007) LAG-3 regulates CD8+ T cell accumulation and effector function in murine self- and tumor-tolerance systems. J Clin Investig 117(11):3383–3392

Gubin MM et al (2014) Checkpoint blockade cancer immunotherapy targets tumour-specific mutant antigens. Nature 515(7528):577–581

Hanahan D, Weinberg RA (2011) Hallmarks of cancer: the next generation. Cell 144(5):646–674

Harndahl M et al (2012) Peptide-MHC class I stability is a better predictor than peptide affinity of CTL immunogenicity. Eur J Immunol 42(6):1405–1416

Herbst RS et al (2014) Predictive correlates of response to the anti-PD-L1 antibody MPDL3280A in cancer patients. Nature 515(7528):563–567

Hodi FS et al (2010) Improved survival with ipilimumab in patients with metastatic melanoma. New Engl J Med 363(8):711–723

Holmgaard RB et al (2015) Tumor-expressed IDO recruits and activates MDSCs in a Treg-dependent manner. Cell Rep 13(2):412–424

Hoof I et al (2009) NetMHCpan, a method for MHC class i binding prediction beyond humans. Immunogenetics 61(1):1–13

Houbiers JG et al (1993) In vitro induction of human cytotoxic T lymphocyte responses against peptides of mutant and wild-type p53. Eur J Immunol 23(9):2072–2077

Iida N et al (2013) Commensal bacteria control cancer response to therapy by modulating the tumor microenvironment. Science (New York, N.Y.) 342(6161):967–970

Iwasaki A, Medzhitov R (2015) Control of adaptive immunity by the innate immune system. Nat Immunol 16(4):343–353

Johanns TM et al (2016) Endogenous neoantigen-specific CD8 T cells identified in two glioblastoma models using a cancer immunogenomics approach. Cancer Immunol Res 4 (12):1007–1015

Jørgensen KW et al (2014) NetMHCstab—predicting stability of peptide-MHC-I complexes; impacts for cytotoxic T lymphocyte epitope discovery. Immunology 141(1):18–26

Kesmir C et al (2002) Prediction of proteasome cleavage motifs by neural networks. Protein Eng 15(4):287–296

Klein G et al (1960) Demonstration of resistance against methylcholanthrene-induced sarcomas in the primary autochthonous host. Can Res 20:1561–1572

Klug F et al (2013) Low-Dose Irradiation Programs Macrophage Differentiation to an iNOS(+)/M1 Phenotype that Orchestrates Effective T Cell Immunotherapy. Cancer Cell 24(5):589–602

Kreiter S et al (2015) Mutant MHC class II epitopes drive therapeutic immune responses to cancer. Nature 520(7549):692–696

Kurts C et al (1998) Major histocompatibility complex class I-restricted cross-presentation is biased towards high dose antigens and those released during cellular destruction. J Exp Med 188(2):409–414

Landais E et al (2009) New design of MHC class II tetramers to accommodate fundamental principles of antigen presentation. J Immunol 183(12):7949–7957

Lee M et al (2014) Resiquimod, a TLR7/8 agonist, promotes differentiation of myeloid-derived suppressor cells into macrophages and dendritic cells. Arch Pharmacal Res 37(9):1234–1240

Lennerz V et al (2005) The response of autologous T cells to a human melanoma is dominated by mutated neoantigens. Proc Natl Acad Sci USA 102(44):16013–16018

Lethe B et al (1997) MAGE-1 expression threshold for the lysis of melanoma cell lines by a specific cytotoxic T lymphocyte. Melanoma Res 7(Suppl 2):S83–S88

Linch SN et al (2016) Combination OX40 agonism/CTLA-4 blockade with HER2 vaccination reverses T-cell anergy and promotes survival in tumor-bearing mice. Proc Natl Acad Sci USA 113(3):E319–E327

Łuksza M et al (2017) A neoantigen fitness model predicts tumour response to checkpoint blockade immunotherapy. Nature

Lurquin C et al (1989) Structure of the gene of tum- transplantation antigen P91A: the mutated exon encodes a peptide recognized with Ld by cytolytic T cells. Cell 58(2):293–303

Manrique SZ et al (2016) Definitive activation of endogenous antitumor immunity by repetitive cycles of cyclophosphamide with interspersed Toll-like receptor agonists. Oncotarget 7 (28):42919–42942

Margulies M et al (2005) Genome sequencing in microfabricated high-density picolitre reactors. Nature 437(7057):376–380

Marty R et al (2017) MHC-I genotype restricts the oncogenic mutational landscape. Cell, 1–12

Matsushita H et al (2012) Cancer exome analysis reveals a T-cell-dependent mechanism of cancer immunoediting. Nature 482(7385):400–404

Matsuzaki J et al (2010) Tumor-infiltrating NY-ESO-1-specific CD8+ T cells are negatively regulated by LAG-3 and PD-1 in human ovarian cancer. Proc Natl Acad Sci USA 107 (17):7875–7880

Mcgranahan N et al (2016) Clonal neoantigens elicit T cell immunoreactivity and sensitivity to immune checkpoint blockade. Science (New York, N.Y.) 351(6280):1463–1469

Mohan JF, Petzold SJ, Unanue ER (2011) Register shifting of an insulin peptide-MHC complex allows diabetogenic T cells to escape thymic deletion. J Exp Med 208(12):2375–2383. Available at: http://www.pubmedcentral.nih.gov/articlerender.fcgi?artid=PMC3256971

Moynihan KD et al (2016) Eradication of large established tumors in mice by combination immunotherapy that engages innate and adaptive immune responses. Nat Med 22(12):1402–1410

Nathanson T et al (2016) Somatic mutations and neoepitope homology in melanomas treated with CTLA-4 blockade. Cancer Immunol Res, Dec 12, p.Epub ahead of print

Ott PA et al (2017) An immunogenic personal neoantigen vaccine for patients with melanoma. Nature

Pauken KE et al (2016) Epigenetic stability of exhausted T cells limits durability of reinvigoration by PD-1 blockade. Science (New York, N.Y.) 354(6316):1160–1165

Peters B et al (2003) Identifying MHC class I epitopes by predicting the TAP transport efficiency of epitope precursors. J Immunology (Baltimore, Md. : 1950) 171(4):1741–1749

Pfirschke C et al (2016) Immunogenic chemotherapy sensitizes tumors to checkpoint blockade therapy. Immunity 44(2):343–354

Popp MW-L, Maquat LE (2013) Organizing principles of mammalian nonsense-mediated mRNA decay. Annu Rev Genet 47:139–165

Prehn RT, Main JM (1957) Immunity to methylcholanthrene-induced sarcomas. J Natl Cancer Inst 18(6):769–778

Rasmussen M et al (2016) Pan-specific prediction of peptide-MHC class I complex stability, a correlate of T cell immunogenicity. Journal of immunology (Baltimore, Md. : 1950) 197 (4):1517–1524

Rizvi NA et al (2015) Mutational landscape determines sensitivity to PD-1 blockade in non-small cell lung cancer. Science (New York, N.Y.) 348(6230):124–128

Robbins PF et al (2013) Mining exomic sequencing data to identify mutated antigens recognized by adoptively transferred tumor-reactive T cells. Nat Med 19(6):747–752

Routy B et al (2017) Gut microbiome influences efficacy of PD-1–based immunotherapy against epithelial tumors. Science (New York, N.Y.) 3706(November), p.eaan3706

Sahin U et al (2017) Personalized RNA mutanome vaccines mobilize poly-specific therapeutic immunity against cancer. Nature 547(7662):222–226

Sakuishi K et al (2010) Targeting Tim-3 and PD-1 pathways to reverse T cell exhaustion and restore anti-tumor immunity. J Exp Med 207(10):2187–2194

Saric T et al (2002) An IFN-gamma-induced aminopeptidase in the ER, ERAP1, trims precursors to MHC class I-presented peptides. Nat Immunol 3(12):1169–1176

Schwanhäusser B et al (2011) Global quantification of mammalian gene expression control. Nature 473(7347):337–342

Sharma MD et al (2009) Indoleamine 2,3-dioxygenase controls conversion of Foxp3+ Tregs to TH17-like cells in tumor-draining lymph nodes. Blood 113(24):6102–6111

Shendure J et al (2005) Accurate multiplex polony sequencing of an evolved bacterial genome. Science (New York, N.Y.) 309(5741):1728–1732

Shukla SA et al (2015) Comprehensive analysis of cancer-associated somatic mutations in class I HLA genes. Nature Biotechnol 33(11):1152–1158

Sibille C et al (1990) Structure of the gene of tum- transplantation antigen P198: a point mutation generates a new antigenic peptide. J Exp Med 172(1):35–45

Sistigu A et al (2014) Cancer cell-autonomous contribution of type I interferon signaling to the efficacy of chemotherapy. Nat Med 20(11)

Sivan A et al (2015) Commensal Bifidobacterium promotes antitumor immunity and facilitates anti-PD-L1 efficacy. Science (New York, N.Y.) 350(6264):1084–1089

Snyder A et al (2014) Genetic basis for clinical response to CTLA-4 blockade in melanoma. N Engl J Med 371(23):2189–2199

Somasundaram R et al (2006) Human leukocyte antigen-A2-restricted CTL responses to mutated BRAF peptides in melanoma patients. Can Res 66:3287–3293

Takaku S et al (2010) Blockade of TGF-beta enhances tumor vaccine efficacy mediated by CD8(+) T cells. Int J Cancer 126(7):1666–1674

Tenzer S et al (2005) Modeling the MHC class I pathway by combining predictions of proteasomal cleavage, TAP transport and MHC class I binding. Cell Mol Life Sci 62(9):1025–1037

Tumeh PC et al (2014) PD-1 blockade induces responses by inhibiting adaptive immune resistance. Nature 515(7528):568–571

Türeci O et al (2016) Targeting the heterogeneity of cancer with individualized neoepitope vaccines. Clin Cancer Res 22(8):1885–1896

Van Allen EM et al (2015) Genomic correlates of response to CTLA-4 blockade in metastatic melanoma. Science (New York, N.Y.) 350(6257):207–211

van der Burg SH et al (1996) Immunogenicity of peptides bound to MHC class I molecules depends on the MHC-peptide complex stability. J Immunol 156(9):3308–3314

Van Rooij N et al (2013) Tumor exome analysis reveals neoantigen-specific T-cell reactivity in an ipilimumab-responsive melanoma. J Clin Oncol 31(32):e439–e442

Verdegaal EME et al (2016) Neoantigen landscape dynamics during human melanoma-T cell interactions. Nature 536(7614):91–95

Vétizou M et al (2015) Anticancer immunotherapy by CTLA-4 blockade relies on the gut microbiota. Science (New York, N.Y.) 350(6264):1079–1084

Vita R et al (2014) The immune epitope database (IEDB) 3.0. Nucleic Acids Res 43(D1):D405–D412

Vormehr M et al (2015) Mutanome engineered RNA immunotherapy : towards patient-centered tumor vaccination. J Immunol Res Article ID 595363:6

Vormehr M et al (2016) Mutanome directed cancer immunotherapy. Curr Opin Immunol 39:14–22

Wang RF et al (1999) Cloning genes encoding MHC class II-restricted antigens: mutated CDC27 as a tumor antigen. Science (New York, N.Y.) 284(5418):1351–1354

Wang S et al (2016) Intratumoral injection of a CpG oligonucleotide reverts resistance to PD-1 blockade by expanding multifunctional CD8+ T cells. Proc Natl Acad Sci USA 113(46): E7240–E7249

Wolchok JD et al (2013) Nivolumab plus ipilimumab in advanced melanoma. N Engl J Med 369 (2):122–133

Wölfel T et al (1995) A p 16INK4a-insensitive CDK4 mutant targeted by cytolytic T lymphocytes in a human melanoma. Science (New York, N.Y.) 269(5228):1281–1284

Woller N et al (2015) Viral infection of tumors overcomes resistance to PD-1-immunotherapy by broadening neoantigenome-directed T-cell responses. Mol Ther: The Journal of the American Society of Gene Therapy 10:1630–1640

Yadav M et al (2014) Predicting immunogenic tumour mutations by combining mass spectrometry and exome sequencing. Nature 515(7528):572–576

Zaretsky JM et al (2016) Mutations associated with acquired resistance to PD-1 blockade in melanoma. N Engl J Med 375(9):819–829

The Era of Checkpoint Inhibition: Lessons Learned from Melanoma

Annette Paschen and Dirk Schadendorf

1 Melanoma

Melanoma originates from the malignant transformation of pigment-producing melanocytes in different tissues. Depending on the tissue origin, different melanoma subtypes can be distinguished such as cutaneous, mucosal, and uveal melanoma. Since each of the subtypes is characterized by specific genetic alterations, melanoma has to be considered as a heterogeneous disease. Cutaneous melanoma dominates in the Western world (incidence of 15–25 per 100,000 individuals), with UV light being a major risk factor. Due to its early metastatic spread, melanoma is a highly aggressive disease that is responsible for 75% of skin cancer-related deaths (Schadendorf et al. 2015a).

Progress in sequencing technologies over the past decade allowed for mutation screening of large cohorts of melanoma samples, revealing genetic alterations involved in melanoma development and progression (Griewank et al. 2014). Mutations affecting components of the mitogen-activated protein kinase (MAPK) signaling pathway (NRAS-BRAF-MEK-ERK) have been identified as oncogenic drivers. Up to 30 and 50% of cutaneous melanomas show activating *NRAS* ($NRAS^{Q61}$, $NRAS^{Q61R}$) and *BRAF* ($BRAF^{V600E}$, $BRAF^{V600K}$) mutations, respectively. This leads to constitutive MAPK signaling, driving melanoma cell survival, and proliferation. Also, constitutive PI3K-AKT pathway activation contributes to melanoma development and progression, frequently achieved by genetic PTEN loss (Griewank et al. 2014).

A. Paschen (✉) · D. Schadendorf
Department of Dermatology, University Hospital Essen, University Duisburg-Essen, Hufelandstrasse 55, 45147 Essen, Germany
e-mail: annette.paschen@uk-essen.de

© Springer Nature Switzerland AG 2020
M. Theobald (ed.), *Current Immunotherapeutic Strategies in Cancer*,
Recent Results in Cancer Research 214,
https://doi.org/10.1007/978-3-030-23765-3_6

Of all human malignancies, melanomas show the highest somatic mutation rate (>10 mutations per megabase of DNA), with a typical UV-induced mutation signature (Lawrence et al. 2013; Alexandrov et al. 2013). This is in line with UV radiation as a risk factor for cutaneous melanoma, though the occurrence of tumors in non-sun-exposed skin or mucosa argues against an absolute UV dependency. The majority of mutations in melanoma are so-called passenger mutations of no relevance for tumor development and progression. But somatic mutations within expressed genomic regions can give rise to mutated tumor antigens (neoantigens) (Coulie et al. 2014; Lennerz et al. 2005; Gros et al. 2014, 2016), determining melanoma immunogenicity as described in the following.

2 Checkpoint Control of Cytotoxic Anti-tumor CD8⁺ T Cell Activity

Cytotoxic $CD8^+$ T cells of the adaptive immune system can recognize autologous melanoma cells as altered self. Recognition occurs via the T cell receptor (TCR) that engages specific tumor cell surface complexes consisting of antigen peptide epitopes bound to HLA class I molecules. Those peptides are produced in the course of endogenous protein (antigen) degradation by the proteasome, then loaded onto HLA class I molecules for transportation and presentation at the cell surface (Fig. 1). Upon recognition of specific antigen peptide–HLA class I complexes, $CD8^+$ T cells become activated and release cytolytic granules onto their target cells, leading to cell death (Martinez-Lostao et al. 2015). In addition, $CD8^+$ T cells secrete the pro-inflammatory cytokine interferon-γ (IFNγ) which can block proliferation or induce apoptosis of surrounding tumor cells (Sanderson et al. 2012) (Fig. 1). Recent studies in mouse melanoma models demonstrated that the immunotherapy can only be effective against tumor cells with intact IFNγ signaling (Manguso et al. 2017; Patel et al. 2017).

Melanoma cells present a unique repertoire of HLA class I–antigen peptide epitopes that are derived from mutant proteins not expressed in normal cells. T cells recognizing these so-called neoantigens are truly tumor-specific and do not attack normal cells (Coulie et al. 2014; Lennerz et al. 2005; Gros et al. 2014, 2016). Moreover, neoantigen-specific T cells express high-affinity T cell receptors that have not been subjected to negative selection in the thymus, making them highly potent anti-tumor effectors (Schumacher and Schreiber 2015). However, within the tumor microenvironment activity of those T cells is generally blocked. Different suppressive mechanisms have been described including the inhibition of T cell activity by regulatory immune cells like myeloid suppressor cells or regulatory T cells (Munn and Bronte 2016). In addition, inhibition of T cell activity by tumor cells plays a major role. Initially, T cells infiltrating the tumor microenvironment become activated upon recognition of cognate HLA class I–antigen peptide complexes, leading to cytolytic granule release and IFNγ secretion. On the one hand, IFNγ can act anti-tumorigenic by inducing death of surrounding tumor cells, and on the other hand, IFNγ can have pro-tumorigenic activity in that it elicits the

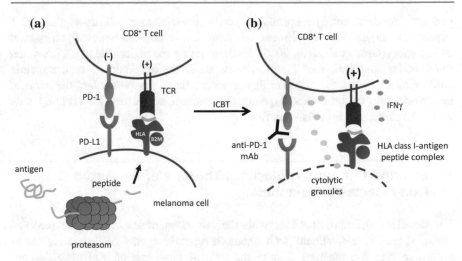

Fig. 1 Inhibition of CD8⁺ T cell activity by melanoma cells via the PD1-PD-L1 axis. a CD8⁺ T cells infiltrating melanoma lesions bind with the T cell receptor (TCR) to specific HLA class I–antigen peptide surface complexes on melanoma cells. The antigen peptides originate from the degradation of endogenous proteins by the proteasome. But TCR-dependent T cell activation is counteracted by inhibitory signals delivered via the co-receptor PD-1 upon engagement of its ligand PD-L1. Thus, the expression of PD-L1 enables tumor cells to put T cells on hold. **b** Blockade of the interaction between PD1 and its ligand PD-L1 by antibodies releases T cells from inhibitory checkpoint signaling and initiates T cell-dependent killing of tumor cells by cytolytic granule release and secretion of effector cytokines (e.g., IFNγ). ICBT, immune checkpoint blocking therapy; (−) inhibitory signaling, (+) activating signaling

expression of PD-L1 on neighboring melanoma cells (Fig. 1) (Spranger et al. 2013; Garcia-Diaz et al. 2017). PD-L1 functions as a ligand of PD-1, an inhibitory co-receptor on antigen-activated CD8⁺ T cells. Binding of PD-1 to its ligand on tumor cells dampens T cell proliferation and effector function. Under normal conditions, PD-1 act as a physiological brake (checkpoint) that limits T cell activity in order to maintain self-tolerance. But by the acquisition of PD-L1 surface expression, melanoma cells efficiently block CD8⁺ T cell activity.

Asides from PD-1, CTLA-4 acts as another checkpoint of T cell activation. Its ligands CD80 and CD86 are expressed on dendritic cells (DCs) but not on melanoma cells. DCs play a critical role in primary CD8⁺ T cell activation in tumor-draining lymph nodes, where they present tumor antigens, sampled in the periphery, to T cells (Merad et al. 2013). Upon primary TCR ligation, CTLA-4 is expressed on the surface of T cells and engages its ligands CD80/CD86 on DCs which in turn limits T cell activation (Krummel and Allison 1995). CTLA-4 similar to PD-1 is of importance for the maintenance of self-tolerance. Notably, while PD-1 knockout mice develop autoimmunity, animals which are deficient for CTLA-4 show massive lymphoproliferation associated with early lethality (Tivol et al. 1995). Expression of both checkpoints has been detected on tumor-reactive CD8⁺ T cells isolated from the peripheral blood and metastatic lesions of melanoma patients. Also, neoantigen-specific T cells show strong CTLA-4 and PD-1 expression suggesting impairment of their anti-tumor activities upon ligand engagement (Gros et al. 2014, 2016). Understanding the major role of CTLA-4 and PD-1 in the suppression of T cell activity led to the development of therapeutic antibodies blocking the receptor/ligand interactions. In particular, the clinical implementation of antibodies targeting the immune regulatory PD-1/PD-L1 axis was a breakthrough in melanoma therapy.

3 Immune Checkpoint Blocking Therapy of Advanced Non-resectable Melanoma

For decades, melanoma patients with the advanced metastatic disease received standard palliative treatment with chemotherapeutic agents (dacarbazine, temozolomide, and fotemustine), despite the lack of large randomized trials demonstrating an impact on overall survival for these drugs. This changed when the first checkpoint blocking antibody targeting CTLA-4 was approved by the US Food and Drug Administration (FDA) and European Medicines Agency (EMA) in 2011. Though anti-CTLA-4 antibody treatment can be considered an important step in melanoma therapy, more striking clinical responses are achieved with antibodies blocking PD-1 signaling. In the following, the clinical trials that led to therapy approval and available 3-year and 4-year follow-up data are shortly summarized.

3.1 Approved Anti-CTLA-4 Antibody

Approval of the first immune checkpoint blocking antibody ipilimumab, a fully human IgG1 antibody targeting CTLA-4, by the FDA and EMA was given for therapy of patients with advanced non-resectable melanoma based on two randomized trials. The NCT00094653 phase 3 trial compared ipilimumab to a gp100 peptide-based vaccine in HLA-A*0201 patients with previously treated unresectable melanoma (Hodi et al. 2010). The overall response rate (ORR) was 5.7% for ipilimumab plus gp100, 11.0% for ipilimumab alone, and 1.5% for the gp100 vaccine. The median overall survival (OS) for patients with ipilimumab plus gp100 and ipilimumab alone was 10.0 and 10.1 months, respectively, compared to 6.4 months for patients receiving gp100 alone (Table 1) (Hodi et al. 2010).

In the NCT00324155 phase 3 trial, patients were treated with ipilimumab plus dacarbazine or dacarbazine plus placebo (Robert et al. 2011). The ORR was 15.2 and 10.3% for patients being treated with ipilimumab plus dacarbazine and dacarbazine plus placebo, respectively. In the ipilimumab plus dacarbazine patient group, the median OS was significantly longer (11.2 months) compared in the group receiving dacarbazine plus placebo (9.1 months) (Robert et al. 2011).

Within the NCT00094653 trial (Table 1), severe adverse events (AEs), defined as grade 3–4, were noted in 10–15% of patients receiving ipilimumab compared to

Table 1 Phase 3 trials related to the approval of anti-CTLA-4 therapy

Agent	Trial	Patient cohort	Treatment arms	Outcome
Ipilimumab	ClinicalTrials.gov identifier: NCT00094653 Hodi et al. (2010)	Pretreated patients with unresectable stage III or stage IV melanoma Number of patients enrolled: n = 676	Ipilimumab + gp100 Versus Ipilimumab Versus gp100	Overall response rate: 5.7.0% versus 11.0% versus 1.5% Duration of response[a]: 11.5 versus not reached versus not reached Progression-free survival[a]: 2.76 versus 2.86 versus 2.76 Overall survival[a]: 10.0 versus 10.1 versus 6.4
	ClinicalTrials.gov identifier: NCT00324155 Robert et al. (2011) Maio et al. (2015)	Untreated patients with unresectable stage III or stage IV melanoma	Ipilimumab + dacarbazine Versus Placebo + dacarbazine	Overall response rate: 15.2.0% versus 10.3% Duration of response[a]: 19.3 versus 8.1 Progression-free survival[a]: similar in both groups Overall survival[a]: 11.2 versus 9.1

[a]Median, months

3% for patients treated with peptide alone, the most common being colitis, skin rash, and endocrinopathies. In the NCT00324155 study (Table 1), grade 3–4 AEs were observed in 56.3% of patients treated with ipilimumab plus dacarbazine, as compared to 27.5% for patients receiving dacarbazine and placebo.

Five-year follow-up data from the NCT00324155 trial (Table 1), as well as pooled follow-up data from 1861 patients with advanced metastatic disease receiving ipilimumab treatment within 12 clinical studies (including the NCT00094653 and NCT00324155 trials, Table 1), revealed a plateau in the survival curves after 3 years (Maio et al. 2015; Schadendorf et al. 2015b), demonstrating that approximately 20% of the anti-CTLA-4-treated patients who managed to survive till year 3 will show long-term benefit, compared to 10% historically expected for patients with stage IV melanoma.

In summary, immune checkpoint blockade with ipilimumab was the first therapy with a documented survival benefit in a subgroup of melanoma patients. In this regard, anti-CTLA-4 treatment can be considered a milestone in melanoma therapy, despite the fact that clinical benefit was still limited to only a small patient subset and that treatment was frequently associated with toxicities, in some cases life-threatening autoimmune pathologies.

3.2 Approved Anti-PD-1 Antibodies

Two antibodies, pembrolizumab and nivolumab, targeting the immune checkpoint PD-1 have been approved for the treatment of non-resectable metastatic melanoma. Treatment with both antibodies achieved higher durable response rates compared to ipilimumab and AEs occurred at a much lower frequency as described in the following.

3.2.1 Nivolumab-Based Clinical Trials

In December 2014, nivolumab was approved by the FDA for treatment of advanced melanoma, followed by EMA approval in June 2015. Approval was given based on the results of two clinical studies: CheckMate 066, a randomized, double-blind phase 3 study with 418 melanoma patients included (Robert et al. 2015a) and CheckMate 037, an open-label phase 3 study with 405 melanoma patients recruited (Weber et al. 2015) (Table 2). In both trials, patients received treatment with nivolumab (3 mg/kg body weight) every two weeks.

CheckMate 066: Melanoma patients without prior treatment received either nivolumab or dacarbazine. With nivolumab, the median ORR was 40.0 and 13.9% with dacarbazine (Robert et al. 2015a). An update on the clinical trial revealed a median OS of 37.5 months for the nivolumab arm and 11.2 months for dacarbazine treatment (Ascierto et al. 2018).

CheckMate 037: Patients enrolled in this study were refractory to ipilimumab or BRAF inhibitor (in case of BRAF-V600 mutant melanoma) and received treatment with either nivolumab or chemotherapy (dacarbazine or carboplatin and paclitaxel [investigators choice]) (Weber et al. 2015). The ORR was 27% for the nivolumab arm and 10% for the chemotherapy group. The clinical trial update revealed a median OS of 15.7 months for nivolumab and 14.4 months for chemotherapy treatment, but median duration of response was higher for nivolumab (32 months) compared to chemotherapy (13 months) (Larkin et al. 2018). Notably, this study demonstrated that patients pretreated with ipilimumab could still respond to nivolumab, which led to accelerated approval of nivolumab by the FDA.

Compared to ipilimumab, clinical response rates to nivolumab were much higher and ranged between 30 and 40%. Nivolumab was superior to ipilimumab also with regard to side effects that were less frequent and less severe, with most common being fatigue, pruritus, and nausea. Grade 3 or 4 drug-related AEs for nivolumab were approximately 15% in CheckMate 066 and CheckMate 037 (Table 2).

3.2.2 Pembrolizumab-Based Clinical Trials

In September 2014, pembrolizumab was approved by the FDA for treatment of patients with advanced unresectable melanoma who no longer responded to other

Table 2 Phase 3 trials related to the approval of anti-PD-1 therapy

Agent	Trial	Patient cohort	Treatment arms	Outcome and adverse events (AE) (based on latest updates)
Nivolumab	**CheckMate 066** ClinicalTrials.gov identifier: NCT01721772 Robert et al. (2015a) Ascierto et al. (2018)	Patients with unresectable stage III or IV melanoma and no prior systemic treatment, BRAF-V600 mutant melanoma excluded Number of patients enrolled: n = 418	Nivolumab Versus dacarbazine	Overall response rate: 40.0% versus 13.9% Duration of response[a]: not reached versus 6 Progression-free survival[a]: 5.1 versus 2.2 Overall survival[a]: 37.5 versus 11.2 AE grade 3 and 4: 15% versus 17.6%
	CheckMate 037 ClinicalTrials.gov identifier: NCT01721746 Weber et al. (2015) Larkin et al. (2018)	Patients with unresectable stage III or IV melanoma, after ipilimumab treatment or after therapy with ipilimumab and BRAF inhibitor for BRAF-V600 mutant melanoma Number of patients enrolled: n = 405	Nivolumab Versus Investigator's choice of chemotherapy: dacarbazine or paclitaxel + carboplatin	Overall response rate: 27% versus 10% Duration of response[a]: 31.9 versus 12.8 Progression-free survival[a]: 3.1 versus 3.7 Overall survival[a]:15.7 versus 14.4 AE grade 3 and 4: 14% versus 34%
Pembrolizumab	**KEYNOTE-006** ClinicalTrials.gov identifier: NCT01866319 Robert et al. (2015b) Schachter et al. (2017)	Patients with unresectable stage III or IV melanoma and no more than one prior systemic treatment Number of patients enrolled: n = 834	Pembrolizumab every 2 weeks Versus Pembrolizumab every 3 weeks Versus Ipilimumab	Overall response rate: 37% versus 36% versus 13% Duration of response[a]: not reached versus not reached versus not reached Progression-free survival[a]: 5.6 versus 4.1 versus 2.8 Overall survival[a]: not reached versus not reached versus 16 AE grade 3–5: 17% versus 17% versus 20%

[a]Median, months

drugs, followed by the EMA approval in July 2015. This decision was based on the outcome of phase 1 KEYNOTE-001 trial (Hamid et al. 2013; Robert et al. 2014), the phase 2 KEYNOTE-002 study (Ribas et al. 2015), and the phase 3 KEYNOTE-006 trial (Robert et al. 2015b).

In the KEYNOTE-006 randomized phase III trial, 834 patients with no more than one prior systemic therapy received treatment with either pembrolizumab or ipilimumab (Table 2). Pembrolizumab (10 mg/kg body weight) was administered either every two or every three weeks, whereas patients received ipilimumab (3 mg/kg body weight) in four doses every 3 weeks. For pembrolizumab administered every two and three weeks, the ORR for patients was 37 and 36%, respectively, compared to 13% for ipilimumab (Robert et al. 2015b; Schachter et al. 2017). The strikingly high response rate to pembrolizumab in ipilimumab-pretreated patients led to an accelerated FDA approval at a dose of 2 mg/kg body weight administered every three weeks since testing of different doses and schedules did not reveal significant difference.

Patients treated with pembrolizumab showed less frequent and severe AEs compared to patients receiving ipilimumab. Most common AEs were fatigue, diarrhea, endocrine disorders, rash, and pruritus. Drug-related AEs of grade 3 or 4 developed in 17% of the pembrolizumab-treated patients (independent of the administration interval) and in 20% of patients receiving ipilimumab.

3.3   Combined Anti-PD-1 and Anti-CTLA-4 Therapy

Since PD-1 and CTLA-4 receptors interact with its ligands in the tumor and the peripheral lymph nodes, respectively, it seemed reasonable to combine both antibodies for treatment. In a multicenter randomized phase 3 trial (CheckMate 067), a total of 945 melanoma patients without prior treatment received a combination of nivolumab and ipilimumab or monotherapy with either ipilimumab or nivolumab (randomization 1:1:1) (Table 3). The ORR for the combination therapy was 58%, compared to 44% with nivolumab or 19% with ipilimumab monotherapy (Larkin et al. 2015; Wolchok et al. 2017). This led to FDA and EMA approval of the nivolumab plus ipilimumab combination therapy for advanced-stage melanoma patients in 2015 and 2016, respectively.

Notably, the 4-year follow-up of the study showed that the median OS was still not reached in the nivolumab plus ipilimumab group, but was 36.9 months in the nivolumab and 19.9 months in the ipilimumab arm (Hodi et al. 2018). However, the improved clinical benefit of combined nivolumab plus ipilimumab treatment was associated with higher toxicity: Grade 3 and 4 AEs occurred in 59% of patients receiving the combination and in 22 and 28% of patients treated with nivolumab and ipilimumab, respectively.

Overall, anti-PD-1 antibodies have revolutionized the treatment of advanced metastatic melanoma, inducing clinical responses up to 40% of the treated patients. Response rates were increased up to 50% when anti-PD-1 antibodies were administered in combination with the anti-CTLA-4 antibody ipilimumab.

Table 3 Phase 3 trial related to the approval of anti-PD-1/anti-CTLA-4 combination therapy

Agents	Trial	Patient cohort	Treatment arms	Outcome and adverse events (AE) (based on latest updates)
Nivolumab + Ipilimumab	**CheckMate 067** ClinicalTrials.gov identifier: NCT01844505 Larkin et al. (2015) Wolchock et al. (2017) Hodi et al. (2018)	Patients with unresectable stage III or IV melanoma and no prior systemic therapies Number of patients enrolled: $n = 945$	Nivolumab + Ipilimumab Versus Nivolumab Versus Ipilimumab	Overall response rate: 58% versus 44% versus 19% Duration of response[a]: 50.1 versus not reached versus 14.4 Progression-free survival[a]: 11.5 versus 6.9 versus 2.9 Overall survival[a]: not reached versus 36.9 versus 19.9 AE grade 3 and 4: 59% versus 22% versus 28%

[a]Median, months

Follow-up data from different clinical trials suggest that a remarkable fraction of long-term responders might even be cured. But still, the majority of patients is primary resistant to ICBT or acquires resistance under treatment, indicating the medical need to understand therapy resistance, define biomarkers predicting therapy response, and screen for alternative combination therapies using PD-1 as a backbone.

4   Resistance to Immune Checkpoint Blocking Therapy

Intense studies aiming to understand primary and acquired resistance to ICBT are ongoing and led already to the identification of different genetic as well as non-genetic tumor cell-intrinsic resistance mechanisms.

CD8$^+$ T cells are critical mediators of clinical responses in ICBT, suggesting melanoma cells with genetic defects in the HLA class I antigen presentation machinery (APM) should be involved in therapy resistance. Indeed, genetic alterations affecting HLA class I APM components, including B2M and HLA heavy chains, have been detected in biopsies from patients with primary and acquired resistance to antibody treatment (Fig. 1) (Zaretsky et al. 2016; Sade-Feldman et al. 2017; Chowell et al. 2018). B2M is the constant component of all HLA class I–antigen peptide complexes and its mutational inactivation abrogates HLA class I surface expression, thereby establishing a CD8$^+$ T cell-resistant melanoma cell phenotype. Also, loss of an HLA haplotype (one set of parental *HLA-A, HLA-B,* and *HLA-C* genes) in tumor cells has been associated with impaired responsiveness to ICBT (Chowell et al. 2018). Conceivably, HLA haplotype loss could be a very efficient immune evasion strategy as long as it protects tumor cells from recognition by highly tumor-reactive neoantigen-specific T cells (Zhao et al. 2016; Schrors et al. 2017). While inactivating *B2M* mutations and loss of *HLA* genes enable melanoma cells to escape T cell recognition, recent studies suggest that evasion from T cell effector mechanisms is of equal importance in primary and acquired ICBT resistance. Inactivation of the IFNγ signaling pathway by genetic alterations in IFNGR1/2-JAK1/2-STAT1 pathway components protects tumor cells from the anti-proliferative and pro-apoptotic cytokine activity. Defective IFNγ signaling has been detected in biopsies from ICBT non-responders and resistant lesions developing after initial therapy response (Zaretsky et al. 2016; Gao et al. 2016; Sucker et al. 2017; Shin et al. 2017).

Generally, inactivation of IFNγ signaling and antigen presentation in tumor cells by JAK1/2 and B2M deficiency, respectively, is a 2-step evolutionary process: One of the two gene copies is lost relatively early in the course of disease due to chromosomal aberrations followed by the acquisition of an inactivating mutation in the remaining allele (Zhao et al. 2016; Sucker et al. 2014, 2017). In line with this observation, an abnormal number of chromosomes and chromosomal segments have been found associated with impaired ICBT efficacy (Roh et al. 2017; Davoli et al. 2017). Despite the importance of irreversible genetic alterations, the mechanisms of therapy resistance remain unknown in most cases. Though new genomic tumor alterations will most likely be defined, it is expected that also non-genetic mechanisms limit clinical benefit from therapy. Melanoma cells can switch their phenotypes to adapt and survive hostile conditions in the tumor microenvironment (Roesch et al. 2016), suggesting that melanomas can acquire a reversible state of resistance due to their phenotypic plasticity. In this regard, melanomas with activated WNT/beta-catenin signaling seem to be less infiltrated by T cells (Luke et al. 2019). Accordingly, a T cell exclusion program associated with ICBT resistance has recently been defined (Jiang et al. 2018). Ongoing studies will most likely identify additional mechanisms associated with resistance to anti-PD-1 treatment, including also tumor cell-extrinsic factors like different types of immune-suppressive cells (regulatory T cells and myeloid-derived suppressor cells) (O'Donnell et al. 2017; Pitt et al. 2016).

5 Predicting Response to Immune Checkpoint Blocking Therapy

To improve clinical outcomes, intense efforts of clinicians and researchers are ongoing also to identify biomarkers predicting ICBT response. A number of those markers have already been described. As such, a higher density of CD8$^+$ T cells at the tumor invasive margin and within the tumor parenchyma has been correlated with improved therapy response (Tumeh et al. 2014; Taube et al. 2014). Moreover, several studies demonstrated that clinical benefit from ICBT is linked to the number of mutations in the tumor (tumor mutational burden, TMB) (Van Allen et al. 2015). The higher the number of mutations within expressed coding regions, the higher the likelihood that neoantigens originate, which are considered the most potent tumor rejection antigens. These markers are in line with the critical role of $CD8^+$ T cells in ICBT, which is further corroborated by the finding of an IFNγ-related mRNA profile as a predictor of clinical response to PD-1 blockade (Ayers et al. 2017). Indeed, several studies identified, distinct but largely overlapping T cell-inflamed gene expression profiles, designate TIDE (Jiang et al. 2018) and IMPRES (Auslander et al. 2018) within metastatic melanoma lesions as a strong predictor of therapy response. Interestingly, the combination of a T cell-inflamed tumor microenvironment and a high TMB seems to be superior in predicting therapy response and has recently been proposed as a PAN-predictive combined biomarker of relevance not only for melanoma but also other tumor entities being treated with anti-PD-1 antibodies (Cristescu, 2018). Besides markers of the tumor microenvironment also systemic factors influencing response to ICBT have been identified. As such, an elevated frequency of classical $CD14^+CD16^-HLA-DR^{hi}$ monocytes in the peripheral blood seems to be a strong predictor of progression-free and overall survival in response to anti-PD-1 immunotherapy (Krieg et al. 2018). Comprehensive summaries of systemic, tumor cell-intrinsic and tumor cell extrinsic biomarkers in IBCT have been published recently (Havel et al. 2019; Keenan et al. 2019).

6 Current Developments and Perspective

The striking clinical responses in patients with advanced non-resectable melanoma led to ICBT trials also in the adjuvant setting, i.e., patients were treated after complete resection of all visible metastases (resection of regional lymph node metastasis in stage 3 disease or distant metastases in oligometastatic stage 4 disease). Adjuvant therapy of stage 3 patients with ipilimumab was associated with a modest but significant improvement of recurrence-free survival (RFS) and OS (Eggermont et al. 2016). Though long-term follow-up data are not yet available for adjuvant anti-PD1 therapy, first results on RFS from two clinical trials seem to be much more promising. In the CheckMate 238 phase 3 trial, 906 patients (stage IIIB, IIIC, IV) undergoing complete tumor resection were treated with nivolumab (3 mg per kilogram of body weight every 2 weeks; $n = 453$) or ipilimumab (10 mg per kilogram every 3 weeks for four doses and then every 12 weeks; $n = 453$). Patients were treated for a period of up to 1 year or until disease recurrence or occurrence of unacceptable side effects. At a minimum follow-up of 18 months, the 12-month RFS rate was 70.5% for the nivolumab and 60.8% for the ipilimumab arm. Treatment-related grade 3 or 4 adverse events were reported for 14.4 and 45.9% of the patients treated with nivolumab and ipilimumab, respectively (Weber et al. 2017). The results of this study led to the approval of nivolumab for adjuvant treatment of melanoma by the FDA in 2017 and EMA in 2018.

In the KEYNOTE-054 phase 3 trial, 1019 patients with completely resected stage III melanoma either received pembrolizumab (514 patients) or placebo (505 patients) every 3 weeks for a total of 18 doses (approximately 1 year) or until disease recurrence/occurrence of unacceptable side effects (Eggermont et al. 2018). At a median follow-up of 15 months, the 12-month RFS rate was 75.4% for pembrolizumab-treated patients and 61.0% for the placebo group. Adverse events of grades 3–5 occurred in 14.7% of the patients receiving pembrolizumab and 3.4% of placebo-treated patients (one treatment-related death in the pembrolizumab group). Based on this study, pembrolizumab was approved for adjuvant treatment of melanoma by EMA in 2018 and FDA in 2019.

Asides from adjuvant treatment, phase 1 clinical trials have been recently performed testing anti-PD-1/anti-CTLA-4 combination therapy in the neoadjuvant setting. First results seem to be encouraging, but therapy resistance and treatment-related toxicities still remain major challenges (Robert 2018).

Thus, experimental studies and clinical trials are ongoing testing combinations of anti-PD1 antibodies with alternative agents that might have improved safety profiles and induce clinical responses also in anti-PD-1 non-responders (Anderson et al. 2017; Smyth et al. 2016). In a significant number of clinical studies, anti-PD-1 antibodies are being tested in combination with antibodies targeting additional inhibitory immune checkpoints. This refers to the observation that T cells from melanoma metastasis are not only positive for PD-1 and CTLA-4 but frequently express additional inhibitory checkpoints such as LAG-3, TIM-3, and TIGIT which have non-redundant functions in the control of T cell activity (Anderson et al. 2016). These receptors bind to ligands expressed on melanoma cells. Intriguingly, the expression of those ligands on tumor cells is enhanced by IFNγ, similar to PD-L1 (Benci et al. 2016). A completely different approach is based on the combination of systemic nivolumab application with intratumoral administration of an oncolytic virus. Analyses of tumor biopsies revealed that the virus-induced local inflammation attracted $CD8^+$ T cells into metastatic lesions, with the result that clinical response to anti-PD1 therapy was no longer dependent on baseline $CD8^+$ T cell infiltration (Kohlhapp and Kaufman 2016; Ribas et al. 2017).

Another strategy follows the combination of BRAF/MEK inhibitors with anti-PD1 antibodies in patients with BRAF-V600 mutant melanoma (approximately 50%). Similar to anti-PD-1, treatment of patients with BRAF/MEK inhibitors induces striking clinical responses, but only in a subgroup of patients, and again, primary and acquired resistance are major challenges (Larkin et al. 2014; Long et al. 2015; Robert et al. 2015c). Interestingly, response to these inhibitors is associated with an infiltration of $CD8^+$ T cells into the lesion, providing a rational to combine inhibitor treatment with immune checkpoint blockade (Cooper et al. 2014; Wilmott et al. 2012). A comprehensive list of the different combination approaches tested in the clinics cannot be given here but is available at https://clinicaltrials.gov/.

In summary, the last few years demonstrated that ICBT can significantly prolong the survival of patients with advanced metastatic disease and a subgroup of patients might even be cured. Follow-up data from clinical trials in the adjuvant setting will demonstrate whether early treatment is advantageous. As therapy resistance still affects the majority of patients, there is a medical need for further improvement in predicting who will respond and in setting up new combination therapies building on the anti-PD-1 backbone. First results of some trials will be available soon but very likely, additional investigations might be needed to optimize schedules and dosing for combination therapies. Overall it can be expected that some of these trials will impact on melanoma therapy and provide improved treatment options for different patient's subgroups.

References

Alexandrov LB, Nik-Zainal S, Wedge DC, Aparicio SA, Behjati S, Biankin AV, Bignell GR, Bolli N, Borg A, Borresen-Dale AL, Boyault S, Burkhardt B, Butler AP, Caldas C, Davies HR, Desmedt C, Eils R, Eyfjord JE, Foekens JA, Greaves M, Hosoda F, Hutter B, Ilicic T, Imbeaud S, Imielinski M, Jager N, Jones DT, Jones D, Knappskog S, Kool M, Lakhani SR, Lopez-Otin C, Martin S, Munshi NC, Nakamura H, Northcott PA, Pajic M, Papaemmanuil E, Paradiso A, Pearson JV, Puente XS, Raine K, Ramakrishna M, Richardson AL, Richter J, Rosenstiel P, Schlesner M, Schumacher TN, Span PN, Teague JW, Totoki Y, Tutt AN, Valdes-Mas R, van Buuren MM, van 't Veer L, Vincent-Salomon A, Waddell N, Yates LR, Australian Pancreatic Cancer Genome I, Consortium IBC, Consortium IM-S, PedBrain I, Zucman-Rossi J, Futreal PA, McDermott U, Lichter P, Meyerson M, Grimmond SM, Siebert R, Campo E, Shibata T, Pfister SM, Campbell PJ, Stratton MR (2013) Signatures of mutational processes in human cancer. Nature 500:415–421
Anderson AC, Joller N, Kuchroo VK (2016) Lag-3, Tim-3, and TIGIT: co-inhibitory receptors with specialized functions in immune regulation. Immunity 44:989–1004
Anderson KG, Stromnes IM, Greenberg PD (2017) Obstacles posed by the tumor microenvironment to T cell activity: a case for synergistic therapies. Cancer Cell 31:311–325
Ascierto PA, Long GV, Robert C, Brady B, Dutriaux C, Di Giacomo AM, Mortier L, Hassel JC, Rutkowski P, McNeil C, Kalinka-Warzocha E, Savage KJ, Hernberg MM, Lebbe C, Charles J, Mihalcioiu C, Chiarion-Sileni V, Mauch C, Cognetti F, Ny L, Arance A, Svane IM, Schadendorf D, Gogas H, Saci A, Jiang J, Rizzo J, Atkinson V (2018) Survival outcomes in patients with previously untreated BRAF wild-type advanced melanoma treated with nivolumab therapy: three-year follow-up of a randomized phase 3 trial. JAMA Oncol
Auslander N, Zhang G, Lee JS, Frederick DT, Miao B, Moll T, Tian T, Wei Z, Madan S, Sullivan RJ, Boland G, Flaherty K, Herlyn M, Ruppin E (2018) Robust prediction of response to immune checkpoint blockade therapy in metastatic melanoma. Nat Med 24:1545–1549
Ayers M, Lunceford J, Nebozhyn M, Murphy E, Loboda A, Kaufman DR, Albright A, Cheng JD, Kang SP, Shankaran V, Piha-Paul SA, Yearley J, Seiwert TY, Ribas A, McClanahan TK (2017) IFN-gamma-related mRNA profile predicts clinical response to PD-1 blockade. J Clin Invest 127:2930–2940
Benci JL, Xu B, Qiu Y, Wu TJ, Dada H, Twyman-Saint Victor C, Cucolo L, Lee DS, Pauken KE, Huang AC, Gangadhar TC, Amaravadi RK, Schuchter LM, Feldman MD, Ishwaran H, Vonderheide RH, Maity A, Wherry EJ, Minn AJ (2016) Tumor interferon signaling regulates a multigenic resistance program to immune checkpoint blockade. Cell 167:1540–1554 e1512

Chowell D, Morris LGT, Grigg CM, Weber JK, Samstein RM, Makarov V, Kuo F, Kendall SM, Requena D, Riaz N, Greenbaum B, Carroll J, Garon E, Hyman DM, Zehir A, Solit D, Berger M, Zhou R, Rizvi NA, Chan TA (2018) Patient HLA class I genotype influences cancer response to checkpoint blockade immunotherapy. Science 359:582–587

Cooper ZA, Reuben A, Amaria RN, Wargo JA (2014) Evidence of synergy with combined BRAF-targeted therapy and immune checkpoint blockade for metastatic melanoma. Oncoimmunology 3:e954956

Coulie PG, Van den Eynde BJ, van der Bruggen P, Boon T (2014) Tumour antigens recognized by T lymphocytes: at the core of cancer immunotherapy. Nat Rev Cancer 14:135–146

Cristescu R, Mogg R, Ayers M, Albright A, Murphy E, Yearley J, Sher X, Liu XQ, Lu H, Nebozhyn M, Zhang C, Lunceford JK, Joe A, Cheng J, Webber AL, Ibrahim N, Plimack ER, Ott PA, Seiwert TY, Ribas A, McClanahan TK, Tomassini JE, Loboda A, Kaufman D (2018) Pan-tumor genomic biomarkers for PD-1 checkpoint blockade-based immunotherapy. Science 362(6411)

Davoli T, Uno H, Wooten EC, Elledge SJ (2017) Tumor aneuploidy correlates with markers of immune evasion and with reduced response to immunotherapy. Science 355

Eggermont AM, Chiarion-Sileni V, Grob JJ, Dummer R, Wolchok JD, Schmidt H, Hamid O, Robert C, Ascierto PA, Richards JM, Lebbe C, Ferraresi V, Smylie M, Weber JS, Maio M, Bastholt L, Mortier L, Thomas L, Tahir S, Hauschild A, Hassel JC, Hodi FS, Taitt C, de Pril V, de Schaetzen G, Suciu S, Testori A (2016) Prolonged survival in stage III melanoma with ipilimumab adjuvant therapy. New Engl J Med 375:1845–1855

Eggermont AMM, Blank CU, Mandala M, Long GV, Atkinson V, Dalle S, Haydon A, Lichinitser M, Khattak A, Carlino MS, Sandhu S, Larkin J, Puig S, Ascierto PA, Rutkowski P, Schadendorf D, Koornstra R, Hernandez-Aya L, Maio M, van den Eertwegh AJM, Grob JJ, Gutzmer R, Jamal R, Lorigan P, Ibrahim N, Marreaud S, van Akkooi ACJ, Suciu S, Robert C (2018) Adjuvant pembrolizumab versus placebo in resected stage III melanoma. New Engl J Med 378:1789–1801

Gao J, Shi LZ, Zhao H, Chen J, Xiong L, He Q, Chen T, Roszik J, Bernatchez C, Woodman SE, Chen PL, Hwu P, Allison JP, Futreal A, Wargo JA, Sharma P (2016) Loss of IFN-gamma pathway genes in tumor cells as a mechanism of resistance to anti-CTLA-4 therapy. Cell 167:397–404 e399

Garcia-Diaz A, Shin DS, Moreno BH, Saco J, Escuin-Ordinas H, Rodriguez GA, Zaretsky JM, Sun L, Hugo W, Wang X, Parisi G, Saus CP, Torrejon DY, Graeber TG, Comin-Anduix B, Hu-Lieskovan S, Damoiseaux R, Lo RS, Ribas A (2017) Interferon receptor signaling pathways regulating PD-L1 and PD-L2 expression. Cell Rep 19:1189–1201

Griewank KG, Scolyer RA, Thompson JF, Flaherty KT, Schadendorf D, Murali R (2014) Genetic alterations and personalized medicine in melanoma: progress and future prospects. J Natl Cancer Inst 106:djt435

Gros A, Robbins PF, Yao X, Li YF, Turcotte S, Tran E, Wunderlich JR, Mixon A, Farid S, Dudley ME, Hanada K, Almeida JR, Darko S, Douek DC, Yang JC, Rosenberg SA (2014) PD-1 identifies the patient-specific CD8(+) tumor-reactive repertoire infiltrating human tumors. J Clin Invest 124:2246–2259

Gros A, Parkhurst MR, Tran E, Pasetto A, Robbins PF, Ilyas S, Prickett TD, Gartner JJ, Crystal JS, Roberts IM, Trebska-McGowan K, Wunderlich JR, Yang JC, Rosenberg SA (2016) Prospective identification of neoantigen-specific lymphocytes in the peripheral blood of melanoma patients. Nat Med 22:433–438

Hamid O, Robert C, Daud A, Hodi FS, Hwu WJ, Kefford R, Wolchok JD, Hersey P, Joseph RW, Weber JS, Dronca R, Gangadhar TC, Patnaik A, Zarour H, Joshua AM, Gergich K, Elassaiss-Schaap J, Algazi A, Mateus C, Boasberg P, Tumeh PC, Chmielowski B, Ebbinghaus SW, Li XN, Kang SP, Ribas A (2013) Safety and tumor responses with lambrolizumab (anti-PD-1) in melanoma. N Engl J Med 369:134–144

Havel JJ, Chowell D, Chan TA (2019) The evolving landscape of biomarkers for checkpoint inhibitor immunotherapy. Nat Rev Cancer 19:133–150

Hodi FS, O'Day SJ, McDermott DF, Weber RW, Sosman JA, Haanen JB, Gonzalez R, Robert C, Schadendorf D, Hassel JC, Akerley W, van den Eertwegh AJ, Lutzky J, Lorigan P, Vaubel JM, Linette GP, Hogg D, Ottensmeier CH, Lebbe C, Peschel C, Quirt I, Clark JI, Wolchok JD, Weber JS, Tian J, Yellin MJ, Nichol GM, Hoos A, Urba WJ (2010) Improved survival with ipilimumab in patients with metastatic melanoma. N Engl J Med 363:711–723

Hodi FS, Chiarion-Sileni V, Gonzalez R, Grob JJ, Rutkowski P, Cowey CL, Lao CD, Schadendorf D, Wagstaff J, Dummer R, Ferrucci PF, Smylie M, Hill A, Hogg D, Marquez-Rodas I, Jiang J, Rizzo J, Larkin J, Wolchok JD (2018) Nivolumab plus ipilimumab or nivolumab alone versus ipilimumab alone in advanced melanoma (CheckMate 067): 4-year outcomes of a multicentre, randomised, phase 3 trial. Lancet Oncol

Jiang P, Gu S, Pan D, Fu J, Sahu A, Hu X, Li Z, Traugh N, Bu X, Li B, Liu J, Freeman GJ, Brown MA, Wucherpfennig KW, Liu XS (2018) Signatures of T cell dysfunction and exclusion predict cancer immunotherapy response. Nat Med 24:1550–1558

Keenan TE, Burke KP, Van Allen EM (2019) Genomic correlates of response to immune checkpoint blockade. Nat Med 25:389–402

Kohlhapp FJ, Kaufman HL (2016) Molecular pathways: mechanism of action for talimogene laherparepvec, a new oncolytic virus immunotherapy. Clin Cancer Res 22:1048–1054

Krieg C, Nowicka M, Guglietta S, Schindler S, Hartmann FJ, Weber LM, Dummer R, Robinson MD, Levesque MP, Becher B (2018) High-dimensional single-cell analysis predicts response to anti-PD-1 immunotherapy. Nat Med 24:144–153

Krummel MF, Allison JP (1995) CD28 and CTLA-4 have opposing effects on the response of T cells to stimulation. J Exp Med 182:459–465

Larkin J, Ascierto PA, Dreno B, Atkinson V, Liszkay G, Maio M, Mandala M, Demidov L, Stroyakovskiy D, Thomas L, de la Cruz-Merino L, Dutriaux C, Garbe C, Sovak MA, Chang I, Choong N, Hack SP, McArthur GA, Ribas A (2014) Combined vemurafenib and cobimetinib in BRAF-mutated melanoma. N Engl J Med 371:1867–1876

Larkin J, Chiarion-Sileni V, Gonzalez R, Grob JJ, Cowey CL, Lao CD, Schadendorf D, Dummer R, Smylie M, Rutkowski P, Ferrucci PF, Hill A, Wagstaff J, Carlino MS, Haanen JB, Maio M, Marquez-Rodas I, McArthur GA, Ascierto PA, Long GV, Callahan MK, Postow MA, Grossmann K, Sznol M, Dreno B, Bastholt L, Yang A, Rollin LM, Horak C, Hodi FS, Wolchok JD (2015) Combined nivolumab and ipilimumab or monotherapy in untreated melanoma. N Engl J Med 373:23–34

Larkin J, Minor D, D'Angelo S, Neyns B, Smylie M, Miller WH Jr, Gutzmer R, Linette G, Chmielowski B, Lao CD, Lorigan P, Grossmann K, Hassel JC, Sznol M, Daud A, Sosman J, Khushalani N, Schadendorf D, Hoeller C, Walker D, Kong G, Horak C, Weber J (2018) Overall survival in patients with advanced melanoma who received nivolumab versus investigator's choice chemotherapy in CheckMate 037: a randomized, controlled, open-label phase III trial. J Clin Oncol 36:383–390

Lawrence MS, Stojanov P, Polak P, Kryukov GV, Cibulskis K, Sivachenko A, Carter SL, Stewart C, Mermel CH, Roberts SA, Kiezun A, Hammerman PS, McKenna A, Drier Y, Zou L, Ramos AH, Pugh TJ, Stransky N, Helman E, Kim J, Sougnez C, Ambrogio L, Nickerson E, Shefler E, Cortes ML, Auclair D, Saksena G, Voet D, Noble M, DiCara D, Lin P, Lichtenstein L, Heiman DI, Fennell T, Imielinski M, Hernandez B, Hodis E, Baca S, Dulak AM, Lohr J, Landau DA, Wu CJ, Melendez-Zajgla J, Hidalgo-Miranda A, Koren A, McCarroll SA, Mora J, Lee RS, Crompton B, Onofrio R, Parkin M, Winckler W, Ardlie K, Gabriel SB, Roberts CW, Biegel JA, Stegmaier K, Bass AJ, Garraway LA, Meyerson M, Golub TR, Gordenin DA, Sunyaev S, Lander ES, Getz G (2013) Mutational heterogeneity in cancer and the search for new cancer-associated genes. Nature 499:214–218

Lennerz V, Fatho M, Gentilini C, Frye RA, Lifke A, Ferel D, Wolfel C, Huber C, Wolfel T (2005) The response of autologous T cells to a human melanoma is dominated by mutated neoantigens. Proc Natl Acad Sci U S A 102:16013–16018

Long GV, Stroyakovskiy D, Gogas H, Levchenko E, de Braud F, Larkin J, Garbe C, Jouary T, Hauschild A, Grob JJ, Chiarion-Sileni V, Lebbe C, Mandala M, Millward M, Arance A, Bondarenko I, Haanen JB, Hansson J, Utikal J, Ferraresi V, Kovalenko N, Mohr P, Probachai V, Schadendorf D, Nathan P, Robert C, Ribas A, DeMarini DJ, Irani JG, Swann S, Legos JJ, Jin F, Mookerjee B, Flaherty K (2015) Dabrafenib and trametinib versus dabrafenib and placebo for Val600 BRAF-mutant melanoma: a multicentre, double-blind, phase 3 randomised controlled trial. Lancet 386:444–451

Luke JJ, Bao R, Sweis RF, Spranger S, Gajewski TF (2019) WNT/beta-catenin pathway activation correlates with immune exclusion across human cancers. Clin Cancer Res

Maio M, Grob JJ, Aamdal S, Bondarenko I, Robert C, Thomas L, Garbe C, Chiarion-Sileni V, Testori A, Chen TT, Tschaika M, Wolchok JD (2015) Five-year survival rates for treatment-naive patients with advanced melanoma who received ipilimumab plus dacarbazine in a phase III trial. J Clin Oncol 33:1191–1196

Manguso RT, Pope HW, Zimmer MD, Brown FD, Yates KB, Miller BC, Collins NB, Bi K, LaFleur MW, Juneja VR, Weiss SA, Lo J, Fisher DE, Miao D, Van Allen E, Root DE, Sharpe AH, Doench JG, Haining WN (2017) In vivo CRISPR screening identifies Ptpn2 as a cancer immunotherapy target. Nature 547:413–418

Martinez-Lostao L, Anel A, Pardo J (2015) How do cytotoxic lymphocytes kill cancer cells? Clin Cancer Res: An official Journal of the American Association for Cancer Research 21:5047–5056

Merad M, Sathe P, Helft J, Miller J, Mortha A (2013) The dendritic cell lineage: ontogeny and function of dendritic cells and their subsets in the steady state and the inflamed setting. Annu Rev Immunol 31:563–604

Munn DH, Bronte V (2016) Immune suppressive mechanisms in the tumor microenvironment. Curr Opin Immunol 39:1–6

O'Donnell JS, Long GV, Scolyer RA, Teng MW, Smyth MJ (2017) Resistance to PD1/PDL1 checkpoint inhibition. Cancer Treat Rev 52:71–81

Patel SJ, Sanjana NE, Kishton RJ, Eidizadeh A, Vodnala SK, Cam M, Gartner JJ, Jia L, Steinberg SM, Yamamoto TN, Merchant AS, Mehta GU, Chichura A, Shalem O, Tran E, Eil R, Sukumar M, Guijarro EP, Day CP, Robbins P, Feldman S, Merlino G, Zhang F, Restifo NP (2017) Identification of essential genes for cancer immunotherapy. Nature 548:537–542

Pitt JM, Vetizou M, Daillere R, Roberti MP, Yamazaki T, Routy B, Lepage P, Boneca IG, Chamaillard M, Kroemer G, Zitvogel L (2016) Resistance mechanisms to immune-checkpoint blockade in cancer: tumor-intrinsic and -extrinsic factors. Immunity 44:1255–1269

Ribas A, Puzanov I, Dummer R, Schadendorf D, Hamid O, Robert C, Hodi FS, Schachter J, Pavlick AC, Lewis KD, Cranmer LD, Blank CU, O'Day SJ, Ascierto PA, Salama AK, Margolin KA, Loquai C, Eigentler TK, Gangadhar TC, Carlino MS, Agarwala SS, Moschos SJ, Sosman JA, Goldinger SM, Shapira-Frommer R, Gonzalez R, Kirkwood JM, Wolchok JD, Eggermont A, Li XN, Zhou W, Zernhelt AM, Lis J, Ebbinghaus S, Kang SP, Daud A (2015) Pembrolizumab versus investigator-choice chemotherapy for ipilimumab-refractory melanoma (KEYNOTE-002): a randomised, controlled, phase 2 trial. Lancet Oncol 16:908–918

Ribas A, Dummer R, Puzanov I, VanderWalde A, Andtbacka RHI, Michielin O, Olszanski AJ, Malvehy J, Cebon J, Fernandez E, Kirkwood JM, Gajewski TF, Chen L, Gorski KS, Anderson AA, Diede SJ, Lassman ME, Gansert J, Hodi FS, Long GV (2017) Oncolytic virotherapy promotes intratumoral T cell infiltration and improves anti-PD-1 immunotherapy. Cell 170:1109–1119 e1110

Robert C (2018) Is earlier better for melanoma checkpoint blockade? Nat Med 24:1645–1648

Robert C, Thomas L, Bondarenko I, O'Day S, Weber J, Garbe C, Lebbe C, Baurain JF, Testori A, Grob JJ, Davidson N, Richards J, Maio M, Hauschild A, Miller WH Jr, Gascon P, Lotem M, Harmankaya K, Ibrahim R, Francis S, Chen TT, Humphrey R, Hoos A, Wolchok JD (2011) Ipilimumab plus dacarbazine for previously untreated metastatic melanoma. N Engl J Med 364:2517–2526

Robert C, Ribas A, Wolchok JD, Hodi FS, Hamid O, Kefford R, Weber JS, Joshua AM, Hwu WJ, Gangadhar TC, Patnaik A, Dronca R, Zarour H, Joseph RW, Boasberg P, Chmielowski B, Mateus C, Postow MA, Gergich K, Elassaiss-Schaap J, Li XN, Iannone R, Ebbinghaus SW, Kang SP, Daud A (2014) Anti-programmed-death-receptor-1 treatment with pembrolizumab in ipilimumab-refractory advanced melanoma: a randomised dose-comparison cohort of a phase 1 trial. Lancet 384:1109–1117

Robert C, Long GV, Brady B, Dutriaux C, Maio M, Mortier L, Hassel JC, Rutkowski P, McNeil C, Kalinka-Warzocha E, Savage KJ, Hernberg MM, Lebbe C, Charles J, Mihalcioiu C, Chiarion-Sileni V, Mauch C, Cognetti F, Arance A, Schmidt H, Schadendorf D, Gogas H, Lundgren-Eriksson L, Horak C, Sharkey B, Waxman IM, Atkinson V, Ascierto PA (2015a) Nivolumab in previously untreated melanoma without BRAF mutation. N Engl J Med 372:320–330

Robert C, Schachter J, Long GV, Arance A, Grob JJ, Mortier L, Daud A, Carlino MS, McNeil C, Lotem M, Larkin J, Lorigan P, Neyns B, Blank CU, Hamid O, Mateus C, Shapira-Frommer R, Kosh M, Zhou H, Ibrahim N, Ebbinghaus S, Ribas A, Investigators K (2015b) Pembrolizumab versus ipilimumab in advanced melanoma. N Engl J Med 372:2521–2532

Robert C, Karaszewska B, Schachter J, Rutkowski P, Mackiewicz A, Stroiakovski D, Lichinitser M, Dummer R, Grange F, Mortier L, Chiarion-Sileni V, Drucis K, Krajsova I, Hauschild A, Lorigan P, Wolter P, Long GV, Flaherty K, Nathan P, Ribas A, Martin AM, Sun P, Crist W, Legos J, Rubin SD, Little SM, Schadendorf D (2015c) Improved overall survival in melanoma with combined dabrafenib and trametinib. N Engl J Med 372:30–39

Roesch A, Paschen A, Landsberg J, Helfrich I, Becker JC, Schadendorf D (2016) Phenotypic tumour cell plasticity as a resistance mechanism and therapeutic target in melanoma. Eur J Cancer 59:109–112

Roh W, Chen PL, Reuben A, Spencer CN, Prieto PA, Miller JP, Gopalakrishnan V, Wang F, Cooper ZA, Reddy SM, Gumbs C, Little L, Chang Q, Chen WS, Wani K, De Macedo MP, Chen E, Austin-Breneman JL, Jiang H, Roszik J, Tetzlaff MT, Davies MA, Gershenwald JE, Tawbi H, Lazar AJ, Hwu P, Hwu WJ, Diab A, Glitza IC, Patel SP, Woodman SE, Amaria RN, Prieto VG, Hu J, Sharma P, Allison JP, Chin L, Zhang J, Wargo JA, Futreal PA (2017) Integrated molecular analysis of tumor biopsies on sequential CTLA-4 and PD-1 blockade reveals markers of response and resistance. Sci Transl Med 9

Sade-Feldman M, Jiao YJ, Chen JH, Rooney MS, Barzily-Rokni M, Eliane JP, Bjorgaard SL, Hammond MR, Vitzthum H, Blackmon SM, Frederick DT, Hazar-Rethinam M, Nadres BA, Van Seventer EE, Shukla SA, Yizhak K, Ray JP, Rosebrock D, Livitz D, Adalsteinsson V, Getz G, Duncan LM, Li B, Corcoran RB, Lawrence DP, Stemmer-Rachamimov A, Boland GM, Landau DA, Flaherty KT, Sullivan RJ, Hacohen N (2017) Resistance to checkpoint blockade therapy through inactivation of antigen presentation. Nat Commun 8:1136

Sanderson NS, Puntel M, Kroeger KM, Bondale NS, Swerdlow M, Iranmanesh N, Yagita H, Ibrahim A, Castro MG, Lowenstein PR (2012) Cytotoxic immunological synapses do not restrict the action of interferon-gamma to antigenic target cells. Proc Natl Acad Sci U S A 109:7835–7840

Schachter J, Ribas A, Long GV, Arance A, Grob JJ, Mortier L, Daud A, Carlino MS, McNeil C, Lotem M, Larkin J, Lorigan P, Neyns B, Blank C, Petrella TM, Hamid O, Zhou H, Ebbinghaus S, Ibrahim N, Robert C (2017) Pembrolizumab versus ipilimumab for advanced melanoma: final overall survival results of a multicentre, randomised, open-label phase 3 study (KEYNOTE-006). Lancet 390:1853–1862

Schadendorf D, Fisher DE, Garbe C, Gershenwald JE, Grob JJ, Halpern A, Herlyn M, Marchetti MA, McArthur G, Ribas A, Roesch A, Hauschild A (2015a) Melanoma. Nat Rev Dis Primers 1:15003

Schadendorf D, Hodi FS, Robert C, Weber JS, Margolin K, Hamid O, Patt D, Chen TT, Berman DM, Wolchok JD (2015b) Pooled analysis of long-term survival data from phase II and phase III trials of ipilimumab in unresectable or metastatic melanoma. J Clin Oncol 33:1889–1894

Schrors B, Lubcke S, Lennerz V, Fatho M, Bicker A, Wolfel C, Derigs P, Hankeln T, Schadendorf D, Paschen A, Wolfel T (2017) HLA class I loss in metachronous metastases prevents continuous T cell recognition of mutated neoantigens in a human melanoma model. Oncotarget 8:28312–28327

Schumacher TN, Schreiber RD (2015) Neoantigens in cancer immunotherapy. Science 348:69–74

Shin DS, Zaretsky JM, Escuin-Ordinas H, Garcia-Diaz A, Hu-Lieskovan S, Kalbasi A, Grasso CS, Hugo W, Sandoval S, Torrejon DY, Palaskas N, Rodriguez GA, Parisi G, Azhdam A, Chmielowski B, Cherry G, Seja E, Berent-Maoz B, Shintaku IP, Le DT, Pardoll DM, Diaz LA Jr, Tumeh PC, Graeber TG, Lo RS, Comin-Anduix B, Ribas A (2017) Primary resistance to PD-1 blockade mediated by JAK1/2 mutations. Cancer Discov 7:188–201

Smyth MJ, Ngiow SF, Ribas A, Teng MW (2016) Combination cancer immunotherapies tailored to the tumour microenvironment. Nat Rev Clin Oncol 13:143–158

Spranger S, Spaapen RM, Zha Y, Williams J, Meng Y, Ha TT, Gajewski TF (2013) Up-regulation of PD-L1, IDO, and T(regs) in the melanoma tumor microenvironment is driven by CD8(+) T cells. Sci Transl Med 5:200ra116

Sucker A, Zhao F, Real B, Heeke C, Bielefeld N, Mabetaen S, Horn S, Moll I, Maltaner R, Horn PA, Schilling B, Sabbatino F, Lennerz V, Kloor M, Ferrone S, Schadendorf D, Falk CS, Griewank K, Paschen A (2014) Genetic evolution of T-cell resistance in the course of melanoma progression. Clin Cancer Res: An Official Journal of the American Association for Cancer Research 20:6593–6604

Sucker A, Zhao F, Pieper N, Heeke C, Maltaner R, Stadtler N, Real B, Bielefeld N, Howe S, Weide B, Gutzmer R, Utikal J, Loquai C, Gogas H, Klein-Hitpass L, Zeschnigk M, Westendorf AM, Trilling M, Horn S, Schilling B, Schadendorf D, Griewank KG, Paschen A (2017) Acquired IFNgamma resistance impairs anti-tumor immunity and gives rise to T-cell-resistant melanoma lesions. Nature Commun 8:15440

Taube JM, Klein A, Brahmer JR, Xu H, Pan X, Kim JH, Chen L, Pardoll DM, Topalian SL, Anders RA (2014) Association of PD-1, PD-1 ligands, and other features of the tumor immune microenvironment with response to anti-PD-1 therapy. Clin Cancer Res 20:5064–5074

Tivol EA, Borriello F, Schweitzer AN, Lynch WP, Bluestone JA, Sharpe AH (1995) Loss of CTLA-4 leads to massive lymphoproliferation and fatal multiorgan tissue destruction, revealing a critical negative regulatory role of CTLA-4. Immunity 3:541–547

Tumeh PC, Harview CL, Yearley JH, Shintaku IP, Taylor EJ, Robert L, Chmielowski B, Spasic M, Henry G, Ciobanu V, West AN, Carmona M, Kivork C, Seja E, Cherry G, Gutierrez AJ, Grogan TR, Mateus C, Tomasic G, Glaspy JA, Emerson RO, Robins H, Pierce RH, Elashoff DA, Robert C, Ribas A (2014) PD-1 blockade induces responses by inhibiting adaptive immune resistance. Nature 515:568–571

Van Allen EM, Miao D, Schilling B, Shukla SA, Blank C, Zimmer L, Sucker A, Hillen U, Geukes Foppen MH, Goldinger SM, Utikal J, Hassel JC, Weide B, Kaehler KC, Loquai C, Mohr P, Gutzmer R, Dummer R, Gabriel S, Wu CJ, Schadendorf D, Garraway LA (2015) Genomic correlates of response to CTLA-4 blockade in metastatic melanoma. Science 350:207–211

Weber JS, D'Angelo SP, Minor D, Hodi FS, Gutzmer R, Neyns B, Hoeller C, Khushalani NI, Miller WH Jr, Lao CD, Linette GP, Thomas L, Lorigan P, Grossmann KF, Hassel JC, Maio M, Sznol M, Ascierto PA, Mohr P, Chmielowski B, Bryce A, Svane IM, Grob JJ, Krackhardt AM, Horak C, Lambert A, Yang AS, Larkin J (2015) Nivolumab versus chemotherapy in patients with advanced melanoma who progressed after anti-CTLA-4 treatment (CheckMate 037): a randomised, controlled, open-label, phase 3 trial. Lancet Oncol 16:375–384

Weber J, Mandala M, Del Vecchio M, Gogas HJ, Arance AM, Cowey CL, Dalle S, Schenker M, Chiarion-Sileni V, Marquez-Rodas I, Grob JJ, Butler MO, Middleton MR, Maio M, Atkinson V, Queirolo P, Gonzalez R, Kudchadkar RR, Smylie M, Meyer N, Mortier L, Atkins MB, Long GV, Bhatia S, Lebbe C, Rutkowski P, Yokota K, Yamazaki N, Kim TM, de Pril V, Sabater J, Qureshi A, Larkin J, Ascierto PA, CheckMate C (2017) Adjuvant nivolumab versus ipilimumab in resected stage III or IV melanoma. New Engl J Med 377:1824–1835

Wilmott JS, Long GV, Howle JR, Haydu LE, Sharma RN, Thompson JF, Kefford RF, Hersey P, Scolyer RA (2012) Selective BRAF inhibitors induce marked T-cell infiltration into human metastatic melanoma. Clin Cancer Res 18:1386–1394

Wolchok JD, Chiarion-Sileni V, Gonzalez R, Rutkowski P, Grob JJ, Cowey CL, Lao CD, Wagstaff J, Schadendorf D, Ferrucci PF, Smylie M, Dummer R, Hill A, Hogg D, Haanen J, Carlino MS, Bechter O, Maio M, Marquez-Rodas I, Guidoboni M, McArthur G, Lebbe C, Ascierto PA, Long GV, Cebon J, Sosman J, Postow MA, Callahan MK, Walker D, Rollin L, Bhore R, Hodi FS, Larkin J (2017) Overall survival with combined nivolumab and ipilimumab in advanced melanoma. N Engl J Med 377:1345–1356

Zaretsky JM, Garcia-Diaz A, Shin DS, Escuin-Ordinas H, Hugo W, Hu-Lieskovan S, Torrejon DY, Abril-Rodriguez G, Sandoval S, Barthly L, Saco J, Homet Moreno B, Mezzadra R, Chmielowski B, Ruchalski K, Shintaku IP, Sanchez PJ, Puig-Saus C, Cherry G, Seja E, Kong X, Pang J, Berent-Maoz B, Comin-Anduix B, Graeber TG, Tumeh PC, Schumacher TN, Lo RS, Ribas A (2016) Mutations associated with acquired resistance to PD-1 blockade in melanoma. N Engl J Med 375:819–829

Zhao F, Sucker A, Horn S, Heeke C, Bielefeld N, Schrors B, Bicker A, Lindemann M, Roesch A, Gaudernack G, Stiller M, Becker JC, Lennerz V, Wolfel T, Schadendorf D, Griewank K, Paschen A (2016) Melanoma lesions independently acquire T-cell resistance during metastatic latency. Can Res 76:4347–4358